"take as diRected"

OUR MODERN MEDICINES

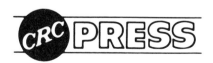

a division of

THE **CHEMICAL RUBBER** CO.

18901 CRANWOOD PARKWAY   CLEVELAND, OHIO 44128

USE OF PROPRIETARY NAMES

iv

PUBLISHER'S PREFACE

While virtually a stranger to the general public, The Chemical Rubber Co., is widely known to the scientific world as one of the foremost publishers of scientific reference works. In 1913, it began the publication of the Handbook of Chemistry and Physics, which is currently in its 48th Edition. Often referred to as the "scientist's bible", at least one edition can be found on the book shelf of almost every scientist in the world.

In addition to the Handbook of Chemistry and Physics, the company publishes basic reference works in other scientific fields such as the biosciences, medicine and mathematics. Each publication is revised frequently to include the latest information available.

The underlying principle of its publishing program is to provide the scientist with convenient access to the huge and rapidly expanding body of scientific data. The accuracy and authenticity of these data are assured by a system of Scientific Advisory Boards consisting of world-recognized authorities in each field.

"Take as Directed" is the first effort by The Chemical Rubber Co. to publish for the general public. The company believes, however, that its fifty-three years of experience in the collection and dissemination of authentic scientific information uniquely qualifies it to undertake the task of this particular book.

Within the past few years, the public has become acutely aware of the fantastic pace at which scientific laboratories are developing a multiplicity of drugs for every conceivable purpose. Overwhelmed by the confusion of claims and counter-claims, politics and partisanship, half-truths and misinformation, the intelligent citizen is deeply concerned—and rightly so. Obviously, an urgent and compelling need exists to provide the public with authentic information about the entire field of our modern medicines—what they are and how they work; their promise and potential, as well as hazards and limitations—in short, to differentiate as clearly as possible between the miracle and the myth.

To accomplish this noteworthy objective, the publisher enlisted a group of outstanding authorities to constitute a Scientific Advisory Board under the extremely capable editorship of Dr. Frederick Shideman, Chairman of the Pharmacology Department, University of Minnesota. These eminent scientists devoted their expertise to the creation of this book, and to assure the accuracy of its information. To present the material in a style both interesting and understandable has been the work of John Paul Russo, a Teaching Fellow in the Department of English at Harvard University.

In publishing a book on this subject, the role of the publisher is seen as a form of trusteeship: to make available to the general public an invaluable legacy of information contributed by highly qualified representatives of the scientific community. To discharge the responsibility of this trust—and with a great sense of satisfaction—the publisher presents "Take as Directed".

B. J. Starkoff, President
THE CHEMICAL RUBBER CO.

WRITER'S ACKNOWLEDGMENTS

I appreciate the aid of a small and invaluable group of friends who formed a staff and who brought their own special interests and talents to the work. In doing research and writing in certain chapters, I am grateful to Mr. Michael LeR. Donnelly, Mr. Robert Ferguson, Mr. Robert H. Anschuetz, Mr. Francis H. Martin, Miss Heather Dubrow, Mr. Richard Savage and Mr. O. Calvin Puckett. In an enterprise that attempts to cover so many areas of a vastly complicated field, they were extraordinarily observant, but I take upon myself the responsibility for any lapses.

Mr. Grant Ujifusa examined the manuscript with patience and applied his skillful editorial hand to many chapters. Without him the book would certainly have been longer, and, I believe, less concise.

Drs. Anthony J. Minichiello, Morton J. Olin and Earle H. Rosenberg were helpful in clearing up points in the section on dentistry and oral medicine.

I was fortunate that the Francis A. Countway Library of Medicine of the Harvard Medical School was just opened when I began work in earnest. To the Library of the Boston Athenaeum, and in particular to Miss Margaret Hackett, Reference Librarian, I owe a never-ending debt of gratitude.

There is considerable advantage in having a critical audience upon which to test thorny passages prior to publication, and I am thankful to my parents and to Mrs. F. E. Shideman who were always willing to read and more often to reread a chapter.

J. P. R.

Boston

May, 1967

TABLE OF CONTENTS

INTRODUCTION

by F. E. SHIDEMAN, M.D., Ph.D.
Editor

"Every scientist should, after all,
regard it as his duty to tell the public,
in a generally intelligible way,
about what he is doing."

Konrad G. Lorenz
King Solomon's Ring

EDITOR'S INTRODUCTION

Twenty-five hundred years ago, the Assyrians observed a growth, now called the ergot fungus, affecting their grain crops. The Assyrians did not know that when this grain was eaten it produced disease. In the Middle Ages, the disease was called Holy Fire or Saint Anthony's Fire by theologians who believed that afflicted unfortunates were merely doing penance for their sins.

The malady was given a secular name, ergotism, by the end of the seventeenth century. A relationship was established between the illness and ingestion of the tainted grain. Later, scientists isolated the substances responsible for ergotism. Now these chemicals and their derivatives provide drugs used in the treatment of migraine, high blood pressure, and the control of bleeding after child birth. Scientific research and the judicious application of its findings have turned blight into something more noble. But the chemicals derived from ergot, if used unwisely, can still be harmful. Consider the indiscriminate use by the uninformed of LSD-25, the hallucinogenic drug, closely related to the substances found in ergot.

Today, to call ergotism Holy Fire seems preposterous. Yet much of modern medicine has its origins in folk remedies, and in a few instances such remedies have not been replaced with better drugs. A certain kind of unknowing, and yet intelligent, empiricism still attends their use. The advice of the first physician who employed them is still valid—a testimony to his astute powers of observation. An example is William Withering's recommendation on the use of digitalis, or foxglove. This substance he used to treat dropsy and heart disease. Properly administered it can prolong life for years; improperly taken, it can cause quick death. Such is the nature of drugs. Fortunately most have a greater margin of safety than digitalis. No drug, however, is without potential harm.

The scientific literature is full of information on drugs, old and new. Since World War II, the rate at which such information has been published is astonishing. The pharamacologist's task—to be familiar with what these chemical substances do in the living organism—has become almost impossible. No wonder he has been remiss, neglecting to transmit important advances in his field to an interested but scientifically unprepared public. In a small measure, the book hopes to do this. No attempt will be made to be comprehensive. The book will emphasize recent advances in drug therapy, but will also discuss many drugs that have been used for centuries.

In preparing this book, reader interest and accurate communication of scientific fact are both prime concerns. Few people do not have some occasion to take a drug. My experience has been that they are interested in what the drugs they take do, how they work. Information of such a nature is presented here—hopefully in an understandable and clear manner.

Sometimes the effects of a drug are unpleasant. Why? It must be understood that a hazard is always associated with taking a drug, greater in some cases than in others. Moreover, no two individuals react in precisely the same way to a drug. The reactions may be so dissimilar that while one person is helped the other is poisoned. Finally, some people abuse drugs. Possible reasons for their abuse and resulting hazards will be explored.

Chapter 1

Contraception and "The Pill"

When primitive tribes wished to control their numbers, they generally resorted to abortion and infanticide. Contraception began when early man observed the relationship between intercourse and pregnancy. One of the oldest methods of birth control is withdrawal. Many authorities interpret Genesis 38:9–10, which states that Onan spilled his seed on the ground, as a reference to this method. But even primitive societies attempted contraception through drugs—we might as well call them drugs—often combining various potions and magic rituals. A tribe in Oceania practices the *egoro* rite.

> Bark is scraped with a *rikerike* from the two nut-trees called *ngari* and *vino* and from the *petepete* tree. The bark is mixed with scrapings from a special reddish stone procured from the island of Gizo, and the mixture put inside a betel leaf and given to the woman to be eaten with a nut of anggavapiru and lime, to the accompaniment of the following formula:
>
> "Ngge va pialia nu reknoreko pini: mi patu to pa na soloso; mi ke pondu komburu; mi egoro tu."
>
> ("I make this woman here eat betel: let her be as the stone on the mountain; let her not make child; let her be barren.")

It is rare for a small tribe to practice contraception, usually a procedure for more "civilized" cultures trying to stem their unwanted growth.

By comparison the contraceptive pill represents a very sophisticated use of drugs to prevent pregnancy. The pill results from careful medical research in a highly technical culture, but it might also be regarded as the product of more or less continuous search since ancient times for an ideal contraceptive method.

3

Contraception in History

The Petrie papyrus, an Egyptian medical document dating back to about 1850 B.C., contains the oldest prescriptions for contraception. Yet another document written around 1550 B.C., is scientifically more interesting:

> Beginning of the recipes made for women in order to cause that a woman should cease to conceive for one year, two years, or three years.

The recipe calls for the "tips of acacia." A thorny shrub-like tree, the acacia used to grow up and down the Nile valley; the locust is its American cousin. The directions say to "triturate (the acacia) with a measure of honey, moisten therewith, and place in her vulva."

The tips of acacia contain gum arabic. Fermentation of this substance liberates lactic acid anhydride, which, when dissolved in water, forms lactic acid. Today, the active agent in some contraceptive jellies is nothing else but lactic acid. So while most drugs used in primitive contraceptives were wholly ineffective, some of the ancients had stumbled on "prescriptions" with real contraceptive value.

Although early Jewish law stressed that every man has a religious obligation to father at least two children, Talmudic-Rabbinic law did not forbid birth control. In fact, Jewish documents contain extensive references to methods of contraception. These range from violent movements after coitus to complicated and sometimes effective "drugs."

Many well-known Greek and Roman writers discussed birth control. Aristotle, for example, notes that one can "anoint that part of the womb on which the seed falls with oil of cedar or with ointment of lead or with frankincense, commingled with olive oil." Although Aristotle probably did not understand the reason for its efficacy, his advice is not bad: oil both lowers the motility of sperm and prevents them from entering the uterus.

The *Gynaecology* of Soranos of Ephesus (98–138 A.D.) is an amazing document written by an amazing man. Soranos studied in Alexandria and then practiced medicine in Rome. During his career, he probably turned out nearly forty treatises. Those which dealt with contraception are particularly brilliant. He warned his readers against superstitious practices like the "delusive" use of an amulet made of the uterus of a mule. Instead he advocated measures like introducing wool soaked in various substances into the vagina before intercourse. Some of these substances, as it turns out, have genuine contraceptive value. For instance, Soranos recommended several fruit acids, including those from the pomegranate and gallnut. We know today that if the vagina is strongly acidic or strongly alkaline, spermatozoa cannot flourish. Moreover, Soranos also recognized that pregnancy is more likely at some points in a woman's cycle than at others.

During the Middle Ages, contraceptive knowledge went into decline. The Europeans of that period probably knew less about the subject than the Greeks a thousand years before. However, in addition to many magical potions—some of which survive in the folk medicine of modern Europe—the drinking of drugs was a common method of contraception. One such simple prescription reads: "drink sabina from the *Juniperus sabine,*" (and we are getting fairly close to gin).

The nineteenth century saw a revolutionary change in attitudes toward birth control, plus many technological advances in contraception. Until the last century, contraceptives were generally used for protection in illicit affairs rather than for "family planning." Then the English parson Thomas Robert Malthus emphasized the social dangers of overpopulation. While some heeded his warning, few approved his recommendation—sexual abstinence. Instead, the neo-Malthusians crusaded for widespread distribution of birth control information, especially to poor families. Meanwhile, the population of England and other industrializing nations skyrocketed.

One neo-Malthusian was the British social reformer Francis Place. In 1822 he published *Illustrations and Proofs of the Principles of Population,* a book which pointed out the need for contraception. Many pamphlets that detailed methods of contraception soon followed. (Place himself probably wrote and distributed many of these anonymous works.) And a few years later a volume with the innocuous title *What is Love?* was published in London. It proved to be a woman's handbook of birth control.

Another bland title, *The Fruits of Philosophy,* introduced a pamphlet published in the United States in 1832. Although it appeared with the anonymous byline "A Physician," people soon discovered that the author was one Charles Knowlton, a Massachusetts physician. Doctors now consider this thoughtful treatise the most important work in the field since Soronos. It advocates postcoital douching and also includes prescriptions of solutions of alum and "astringent vegetables." Knowlton was arrested, tried, fined, and sentenced to three months in prison.

As the opposition to Knowlton's work suggests, many people bitterly—and not ineffectively—fought the popularization of contraception during the nineteenth, and even the twentieth, centuries. A crusader against "immorality and indecency," one Anthony Comstock was sure that the practice of contraception involved both. As Head of the Society for the Suppression of Vice, Comstock lobbied successfully for a federal law against contraception. Passed in 1873—after less than ten minutes of debate—the law made it a criminal offense to import, mail, or transport in interstate commerce "obscene literature and articles of immoral use"—including "any article for the prevention of conception or for causing abortion." Encouraged by the congressional action, many states passed their own "Comstock laws."

It was not until 1930 that a federal court ruled that the national Comstock law should not be interpreted to prevent "the proper medical use of contraceptives." Three years later the courts decided that pharmacists should not be included in the ban against the distribution of contraceptives.

Contraceptive Devices

In 1936, Dr. Hannah Stone, like Margaret Sanger a leader in the birth control movement, imported a package of diaphragms from Japan. The customs authorities confiscated the package, and Dr. Stone immediately appealed to the courts where the case became known as "The United States vs. 'One Package.'" When a lower court decided in favor of Dr. Stone, the government appealed; finally, under the late Learned Hand, the Court of Appeals upheld Dr. Stone. Around this time, most states were repealing their bans on birth control, but it was not until the 1960's that Connecticut and Massachusetts relaxed their restrictions, and under court pressure at that.

At the same time that significant changes in public attitudes and in the legal status of contraception were taking place, several new methods of contraception appeared. These include vaginal creams, jellies, and foams, all recent inventions. Intrauterine devices have also joined the ranks of modern contraceptive methods during the twentieth century, although primitive versions of intrauterine contraceptives have existed for nearly two thousand years. The first modern reports on these devices appeared in 1928–30. Dr. Grafenburg examined at length the use of rings made of silkworm gut and silver or gold wire. Fearing pelvic infection, most gynecologists in the United States violently repudiated Grafenburg's work. In 1959, however, both Dr. Ishihama, a Japanese physician, and Dr. Oppenheimer, an Israeli doctor, published the results of their separate research about modified versions of the Grafenburg ring. Both reported a very low pregnancy rate and minimal problems with pelvic infection and other side effects. Because of their work, American physicians reconsidered the merits of intrauterine devices; today both Planned Parenthood clinics and many private physicians distribute them.

The Condom

The invention of the condom marked a major advance in contraception. The exact date of this event, however, remains unknown. Fallopius, an Italian anatomist, mentions the device in a work published in 1564, claiming that he invented it. (The Fallopian tubes, the female organs which transport eggs from the ovaries to the uterus, are, of course, named after Fallopius.) His account emphasizes the use of the condom to prevent syphilis. Other sources believe that the condom was invented by a Dr. Conton or Condom. He is believed to have been either a physician attached to the court of Charles II (1660–1685), or a physician living at that time but not connected with the court, or simply a courtier of the monarch. But no one has discovered any authoritative evidence of the existence of Dr. Conton.

Many seventeenth and eighteenth century works mention the condom, referring to it as a device used by libertines rather than by married couples. In 1671, Madame de Sévigné, a famous French woman of letters, referred to a condom as "armor against enjoyment and a spider web against danger." Casanova called this method of birth control, among other things, "the English riding coat," "the English vestment which puts one's mind at rest," "the preservation sheath," and "the assurance cap."

The condom described by Fallopius was made of skin; later models used the intestines of animals. When rubber was vulcanized in 1843–4, condoms became much cheaper—and more widely used. In the 1930's, manufacturers began to make condoms of latex, lowering the price even further.

Despite its comparative safety, the condom suffers from several aesthetic and psychological disadvantages. Many couples dislike interrupting sex play to put on the condom. Some men and women feel that the sheaths dull sensation. And, because they associate the condom with their premarital experiences, certain married men dislike using one.

The pregnancy rate for the condom, or sheath, is six to sixteen, (see Table 1). The chance of pregnancy can be lessened by lubricating the condom with a spermicidal cream or jelly or by introducing a spermicide into the vagina before intercourse. Moreover, if a man withdraws immediately after ejaculation and holds onto the condom, he can decrease the chances of leakage or spillage.

The Diaphragm

A German, Friedrich Wilde, invented the diaphragm in 1838, but it was not used extensively for several decades. Manufacturers started to use vulcanized rubber in diaphragms around 1880.

Until the pill became popular, many considered the diaphragm the most effective means of birth control. Placed in the vagina so that sperm cannot enter the uterus, this dome-shaped device provides the mechanical barrier to conception. Since a contraceptive cream or jelly is spread on the diaphragm before insertion, it also offers chemical protection against pregnancy.

The principal advantage of the diaphragm is its low failure rate; figures range from around six to twenty-nine. If a patient is intelligent, highly-motivated, and has a sub-pubic angle well-suited to fitting a diaphragm, this may be a good method of contraception for her.

But the cumbersome ritual of inserting the device is its major disadvantage. After a tiring day, a patient may neglect to use any contraceptives, let alone a diaphragm. Moreover, some women, such as those whose organs have been excessively relaxed by childbirth, are anatomically unsuited for this means of contraception. Some patients in lower socioeconomic groups lack the privacy needed to put in the diaphragm. There is another serious problem. The doctor must fit a woman with the correct size and shape diaphragm, and she must learn to insert it correctly. This is troublesome, particularly at a time of some emotional involvement.

More commonly used in Europe than in the United States, is the cervical cap, a dome-shaped instrument which fits snugly over the cervix, or opening of the uterus. Whereas a diaphragm cannot be left in place for more than sixteen hours, the cervical cap can remain within a patient for days. This is an obvious advantage. Furthermore, the efficacy of this method is quite high. Some sources report a pregnancy rate of eight.

Unfortunately, only a limited number of women can use the cervical cap. Fitting it correctly can be difficult. Moreover, a woman must be able to insert and remove the cap herself, and many find that they cannot do so. Women who have not had children can seldom wear one.

Intrauterine Devices

Intrauterine contraceptive devices (IUD) are instruments that a doctor places within a woman's uterus. The device remains there unless removed by the doctor, or unless the woman inadvertently passes it. Those currently in wide use are plastic rings or spirals. Some have long string-like attachments which hang down from the uterus into the vagina. By checking for the string, a patient can find out whether the device is still in place.

Where these IUD's are used, the pregnancy rate seems to be around five, although more research must be done before an accurate rate can be established. Their main advantage is that, once they are securely in place, the patient is not required to make any effort to insert or remove them. Therefore, the device becomes particularly useful for patients whose motivation toward contraception may not be continuing or strong. The devices seem to be an excellent means of birth control in many underdeveloped countries.

But a woman may pass the device without realizing it; in fact, the expulsion rate is as high as twenty percent. This is less of a problem when one uses the IUD's which have strings that permit regular checks. Moreover, the devices sometimes cause side effects such as bleeding and pelvic pain, although these reactions usually disappear promptly. While insertion in a woman who has had children is usually a fairly simple procedure, insertion of the device in a patient who has not given birth can be much more difficult and may cause some pain.

Jellies and Foams

Vaginal jellies, creams and foams all contain a spermicidal agent. Although they are not as successful as other methods (the pregnancy rate for the creams and jellies is eighteen to twenty-five, while the pregnancy rate for the foams is fifteen to twenty), these methods do offer some advantages. They are very simple to use. In fact, these means of birth control are of some value for a few women who cannot employ more complex means of birth control, and in whom the intrauterine devices have not been satisfactory.

Vaginal Suppositories

Vaginal suppositories, made with cocoa-butter or from a glycero-gelatin base, have a failure rate of about eight to twenty-seven. One of the easiest methods to use, they are simply inserted ten to fifteen minutes before intercourse. In addition to the comparatively high failure rate, they suffer from several drawbacks. Because they melt at body temperatures, suppositories will also melt if stored at temperatures above 90°F; in some climates the patient must store them in the refrigerator.

The Rhythm Method

The rhythm method is based on an attempt to pinpoint the time when a woman ovulates and becomes fertile. Couples using this method avoid intercourse at these times. To determine the exact time of ovulation is difficult even with technical knowledge and equipment. We do know that ovulation usually occurs around fourteen days before the next period begins and that the egg is susceptible to fertilization for only about twelve hours. To calculate the time when a particular woman will ovulate, authorities recommend that she measure her cycles over the space of at least eight months and preferably one year. However, one cannot rely completely on such calculations because even women with the most regular menstrual cycles do not always ovulate at a predictable time. Moreover, a patient may occasionally ovulate on two separate occasions during one cycle.

To increase the efficacy of the rhythm method, doctors have formulated various methods of determining the time of ovulation. One depends on recording the basal body temperature which usually rises slightly at the time of ovulation. The woman determines her basal body temperature by taking it as soon as she wakes up in the morning and before any activity at all, keeping a daily graph of her findings. When the thermometer shows a rise, she knows that ovulation has occurred. Three days later, the egg can no longer be fertilized, and she is almost completely safe. This permits her to recognize the "safe days" after ovulation, but it does not help to identify those "safe days" which precede ovulation. Most failures with this method are probably due to intercourse a few hours before an unusually early ovulation.

Artificial means of contraception are not currently approved by the Roman Catholic Church, though the Church has been studying the question. Thus, many Catholic couples choose to space their children by using the rhythm method.

One problem with the method is, of course, that even the most elaborate calculations sometimes do not accurately predict the time of ovulation. In fact, the failure rate ranges from fourteen (in a group of women selected for this method because of the regularity of their menstrual cycle) to thirty-eight. Another disadvantage is that the couple must remain continent for prolonged periods of time, often around ten days.

Withdrawal

Withdrawal before ejaculation is one of the most time-honored methods of contraception. The method is presumably simple and always available, but its pregnancy rate ranges from twelve to as high as thirty-eight. Men may emit some sperm before ejaculation, which means that a woman can be impregnated before the man withdraws. Other drawbacks include many emotional factors. The woman may be unable to reach climax if the man withdraws before ejaculating, and concern about the need to withdraw may injure the couple's sexual relationship.

Douches

Few doctors would recommend *douching* as a reliable means of contraception. After all, sperm travel one-fourth of an inch in two minutes on a glass slide and may move even more quickly in the favorable environment of the vagina. Therefore, even if a woman douches immediately after intercourse, she cannot be sure of removing the spermatozoa. It is not surprising that the pregnancy failure rate ranges from twenty-one to forty-one. Douching can, however, be useful in an occasional emergency, as in the breakage of the condom or indiscretion when no prior precaution has been taken.

Determination of Pregnancy Rate

To evaluate the efficacy of contraceptive methods, one must weigh such tangible factors as the number of pregnancies which occur because of—or, rather, in spite of—the method, as well as such intangibles as psychological appeal. To measure the failure rate of each method, scientists employ "Pearl's formula," introduced by Raymond Pearl in the 1930's:

$$R = \frac{(\text{Number of pregnancies} \times 12)}{\text{Total months of use}} \times 100$$

This formula applies to a large group over an extended period of "total months." The "number of pregnancies" is the total for the entire group divided by the number of women in the group.

The formula shows the failure rate per one hundred woman-years or the average percentage of women who will become pregnant within one year. A high failure rate, R, indicates a low level of effectiveness for a contraceptive, while a low rate signifies a high level of effectiveness.

Using this formula, researchers have discovered that the pregnancy rate for fertile women not using any means of contraception is about eighty. In other words, if one hundred women of proven fertility have sexual relations, eighty will conceive within a year. The figure of eighty shows us that even the comparatively ineffective methods of birth control are valuable. Some of the less effective methods have pregnancy rates of forty—which, after all, cuts in half the number of pregnancies which would otherwise result.

TABLE 1

EXAMPLES OF PREGNANCY RATES WITH USE OF VARIOUS CONTRACEPTIVE PROCEDURES

Procedure	Number of patients	Number of cycles	Years of exposure	Number of pregnancies	Pregnancy rate per 100 woman-years*
Cervical cap (diaphragm)	143	4,784	368	28	8
Condom (sheath)	387	8,437	649	72	11
Safe period (rhythm)	409	7,878	606	87	14
Jelly (only)	3,139	40,391	3,107	727	11–38
Jelly and diaphragm	99,815	147,459	11,343	943	6–29
Suppositories	516	5,639	433	74	8–27
Foam tablets	2,313	14,105	1,085	195	13–49

From: *Drill's Pharmacology in Medicine* 3rd Edition, McGraw, 1965
* This is equivalent to the average percentage becoming pregnant in one year. When no contraceptive is used, this percentage is about eighty.

When listing pregnancy rates (Table 1), we may indicate the range of rates reported by reliable authorities. For example, one survey yields the figure of eight for the diaphragm, while another reports a rate of fourteen for women using the same device. Since researchers use varying groups of the population in their surveys, rates can vary widely. Thus, some studies include people who are very eager to avoid conception, while others involve patients who, because they plan to have a child soon anyway, may use a method inconsistently. Thus, rates vary for many different reasons.

Physicians prefer to analyze the failure of a given type of contraceptive more closely. A pregnancy may result either from a deficiency in the method or from a deficiency in the manner the patient uses the method. If a woman conceives after taking the pills according to directions, the pregnancy must be blamed on the method of contraception. If, on the other hand, the patient forgets to take some of her pills, the method itself is not at fault. Therefore, doctors attempt to differentiate between "method failures" and "patient failures."

To judge a type of contraception, one may try to measure the factors which will affect the patient's willingness and ability to use it consistently; such factors include the temperament, religion and socioeconomic background of the patient and her mate. The diaphragm may yield a low failure rate among patients suited to this means of birth control—and a high failure rate among people who dislike the trouble of inserting the device or who, because of their living conditions, lack the privacy to insert it. Aesthetic and psychological considerations may also become relevant. A couple may dislike interrupting sexual play to put on a condom. In short, a method which is ideal for one couple may not be for another.

Planned Parenthood suggests three axioms to consider when judging types of contraceptives:

1. Any method of birth control is better than no method.
2. The most effective method is the one the couple will use with the greatest consistency.
3. Acceptability by both members of the team is the most critical factor in the effectiveness of any contraceptive method.

"The Pill"—How It Works

Many effective contraceptive drugs, such as those described by Aristotle, were discovered by accident. The contraceptive pill, however, resulted from logical developments based on existing scientific knowledge. Birth control pills are effective because they inhibit ovulation. A normal woman, not taking the pills, ovulates (produces an egg) every lunar month. Pregnancy occurs upon fertilization by sperm. Since taking birth control pills prevents a patient from ovulating, she cannot become pregnant.

To understand "the pill" it is necessary first to be familiar with the events that take place during a normal menstrual cycle. At the beginning of each month a small gland at the base of the brain, called the pituitary gland (see the chapter "Hormones as Drugs"), begins to secrete what is called the follicle-stimulating hormone (FSH). This FSH travels in the blood to the ovary and causes the development of an egg. At about the middle of the month, the pituitary gland then secretes another hormone which causes the egg to be liberated from the ovary; and this is the process of ovulation. As these hormones from the pituitary gland stimulate the development and release of the egg, they also cause the ovary to liberate two hormones. During approximately the first 14 days of the cycle the secretion of one hormone, estrogen, from the ovary slowly increases reaching a peak at about the time of ovulation. After ovulation the ovary secretes a second hormone, progesterone.

The secretion of estrogen and progesterone from the ovary does two things. First, these two hormones stimulate the growth of the endometrium, which is the inner lining of the uterus. In this way the uterus is prepared for the implantation of a fertilized egg. At the same time the increasing concentrations of estrogen and progesterone that are secreted from the ovary begin to exert a depressing effect on the pituitary gland. As the pituitary gland is depressed, it secretes less of its stimulating factors. Therefore, its effect on the ovary begins to diminish and the ovary secretes lesser amounts of estrogen and progesterone. The level of estrogen and progesterone then drops below a critical level and menstruation occurs. At this point the pituitary gland is no longer depressed by estrogen and progesterone and it begins a new cycle.

It should be obvious from the above account that estrogen and progesterone can exert an inhibiting effect on the pituitary gland and it is logical to suppose that if these hormones were administered as drugs, the depression of the pituitary gland would prevent the occurrence of ovulation. Such is indeed the case, and during the 1940's estrogens alone were employed to inhibit ovulation in patients with dysmenorrhea (painful menstruation). Unfortunately, however, such estrogens are not effective cycle after cycle in inhibiting ovulation. Moreover, the administration of estrogens by themselves tends to cause in some patients an overstimulation of the lining of the uterus, possibly leading to bleeding problems. The other hormone, progesterone, will also inhibit ovulation but it is not completely effective when given by mouth and therefore has to be given by injection. The injections of progesterone are, at times, quite painful and it is, of course, impractical to give multiple injections of this type during the month in order to inhibit ovulation. Thus, for practical purposes estrogens and progesterone could not be employed successfully as oral contraceptives.

Because of these complications, scientists attempted to develop new chemical substances that would have the properties of progesterone but that would be active in tablet form for oral use. In 1952, the laboratories of two pharmaceutical companies began to study this problem with the objective of developing more potent progesterone-like chemicals. It was thought that such compounds might be useful in their own right for the treatment of menstrual disorders (where progesterone was—and still is—frequently employed), and possibly as oral contraceptives. These compounds, first synthesized in 1952, eventually led to the development of oral contraceptives.

These new steroids which have the properties of progesterone were called progestins. They were first shown to inhibit ovulation and to be devoid of any undesirable or toxic effects in animals, even when administered in high doses. Following such studies, the first of the compounds were then shown to be active in inhibiting ovulation in women. The initial studies were soon expanded to cover a large number of patients in the United States and other countries.

Although these new progestins were active in inhibiting ovulation, a fairly high percentage of patients experienced spotting or bleeding while the tablets were being taken. It was thus found necessary to add a small amount of estrogen to the progestin in order to stabilize the lining of the uterus. Thus the oral contraceptives are now a combination of a progestin with an estrogen. In 1957, the first of these oral contraceptives was used by physicians for the treatment of various menstrual disorders. The study of these compounds, conducted during the years at various clinics in the United States and abroad, established, with more and more data, that the compounds were effective and safe for the purpose of controlling ovulation. In 1960 the first of these compounds, Enovid, was approved for use as an oral contraceptive on prescription of a physician.

To insure that oral contraceptives will work in the ways described, the patient must follow a precise schedule. Counting the first day of bleeding as Day 1, she begins to take pills on Day 5. She then usually takes one at the same time each day for a total of twenty days. About one to three days after she has stopped taking the pills, bleeding starts. Now this is not a true menstrual period as it has not been preceded by ovulation, and, therefore, doctors sometimes refer to the period of a woman who is taking oral contraceptives as "withdrawal bleeding." In fact, the bleeding of a patient using this form of contraception tends to be lighter than normal for many women. Also, sufferers from dysmenorrhea, or painful periods, find that their "withdrawal bleeding" is usually painless. The pills create a cycle very similar to the twenty-eight day cycle of a woman not taking them.

Although all of the oral contraceptives on the market operate in the same manner, the various preparations differ in two ways. The first kind of tablet to be developed is known as the "combination" tablet and contains both a progestin and an estrogen. The progestin and estrogen are taken in a fixed dosage for 20 or 21 days each month, as described above. The contraceptives first appeared on the market in a 10-milligram dose combination of progestin and estrogen. Shortly afterwards, the normal dose was reduced to 5 milligrams; subsequently, many companies brought out 2- or 2.5-milligram doses and recently a 1-milligram pill has appeared on the market. The low-dose tablets are as effective as are the high-dose tablets in controlling ovulation. These combination tablets, when taken correctly, are practically 100 percent effective in preventing ovulation and pregnancy.

The second kind of pill available has been called the sequential tablet. The sequential brands include 15 tablets of estrogen to be taken on the first 15 days and 5 tablets containing a combination of progestin and estrogen for the remaining 5 days. The sequential tablets are slightly less effective than the combination tablets in controlling ovulation but they are still much more effective than jellies, creams, or mechanical methods of contraception.

During the normal cycle, women may spot or bleed before

the menstrual period and occasionally a patient taking the pills will experience bleeding or spotting before the last tablet has been taken; physicians refer to this phenomenon as "breakthrough bleeding." It occurs because the dosage of hormone is insufficient. In patients taking the combination pill, the spotting can usually be stopped if the patient takes two pills per day for a few days. The problem of spotting or bleeding with the sequential pills is such that in the summer of 1966 Planned Parenthood chapters would no longer supply them. Moreover, because these pills are designed to be taken on designated days, taking an extra pill to control the bleeding can become very confusing.

Most women, even illiterate patients, can be relied upon to take a daily tablet for 20 or 21 days a month. To achieve best effectiveness it is necessary that the tablets be taken correctly; even missing one or two tablets may allow ovulation to occur with the subsequent risk of pregnancy. The incidence of pregnancy increases quite dramatically if five or six pills are missed during a cycle, particularly if this occurs at the beginning of the cycle. When taken correctly, the combination tablets are practically 100 percent effective.

Side Effects and Long-Term Usage of "The Pill"

The side effects of the pill are minimal. A few women may experience mild nausea as the first few tablets are taken. A rare patient may have severe nausea and even vomiting and may not be able to tolerate the pill. This situation has been minimized by the lower dosage pills now available. The pills do not have a significant effect on body weight as the number of women taking the pills and gaining weight is similar to the number losing weight. During a normal cycle certain women may complain of breast tenderness or some water retention during the menstrual cycle and those conditions may also appear with women taking oral contraceptives. In some cases the oral contraceptives may increase the size of the patient's breasts, but many women do not consider this a problem.

There have been tabulations on the frequency of coitus during the use of the pill. Increased frequency was reported by 50 percent, decreased frequency by 40 percent, and no change by 10 percent.

It seems likely that any reported increase in frequency of coitus is an indirect effect of the oral contraceptives. It is probably related to freedom from fear of pregnancy—once the woman's confidence in oral contraceptives has been established.

Many questions have arisen regarding the pill, particularly as regards thrombophlebitis. Thrombophlebitis, which is a blood clot- (thrombus) and inflammation of the veins (phlebitis), is a naturally-occurring disease found in both the male and female. No one has proven a cause-and-effect relationship between attacks of this disease and the administration of oral contraceptives, although a great number of researchers have made studies on this subject. In a study of over 14,000 women made at a Planned Parenthood Clinic the conclusion was reached that "the percentage of thrombophlebitis in this series is lower than the 'expected rate' when compared to women not receiving oral contraceptives."

The physician will usually not administer oral contraceptives to patients with cysts of the breast. Other patients may have fibroids (a non-cancerous growth) of the uterus and in some patients the fibroid may increase in size when oral contraceptives are taken; it will usually regress when the oral contraceptives are discontinued.

Some women may hesitate to take oral contraceptives because they fear possible ill effects of taking the pill over a prolonged period of time. Of course, no one can be certain whether women taking the pill will suffer ill effects 20 years later. Thus far, all of the detailed studies indicate that there are no such risks. The fact that such pills have been taken for many years leads reputable physicians across the country to believe that this fear is unfounded.

None of the studies conducted to date show any increase in the incidence of cancer or abnormal "Pap" smears when oral contraceptives are taken. The incidence seems to be somewhat lower. In fact, estrogens are at times used in the treatment of certain types of breast cancer, and studies are now in progress to assess the roll of the pill in the incidence of cancer of the breast or uterus.

Further Use of Oral Contraceptives

Physicians prescribe "birth control pills" for other reasons than birth control. First of all, administering these hormone preparations will alleviate dysmenorrhea (a condition in which periods are highly painful) and menorrhagia (excessive bleeding) and metrorrhagia (irregular periods). If a patient has endometriosis, a disease of the lining of the uterus which causes highly painful menstrual periods, the pills will not only relieve her discomfort but will also prevent the disease from worsening.

The oral contraceptives also serve functions even further removed from their original purpose. Many medical conditions improve if the female hormone estrogen is administered, and doctors now prescribe this hormone in the convenient form of birth control pills. If the patient is also concerned about birth control, she can accomplish two things at once. Physicians have also attempted to give estrogens to men suffering from conditions which respond to female hormones. But the side effects which the physician might expect from administering a female sex hormone—enlargement of the breasts is one—have proved so distressing to men that such therapy has generally been discontinued.

Estrogens can also alleviate dryness of the skin and of the mucous membranes. This characteristic of these hormones has created a controversial problem: whether or not to administer the pill that contains estrogen and a progestin to middle-aged women to keep them looking and feeling younger. The pill certainly can make a woman appear younger, as it alleviates dryness. And oral contraceptives seem to prevent the appearance of symptoms of menopause, or "change of life," the time when the production of estrogen by the ovaries slows down and the menses eventually ceases. A woman taking the tablets experiences withdrawal bleeding each month. Certain doctors, eager to avoid the negative emotional reaction which women may have to the cessation of menstruation, feel that postponing "change of life" is an excellent idea. Moreover, the menopause often involves physiological reactions, such as "hot flashes," which probably result from the progesterone level remaining fairly constant while the estrogen level decreases. Prescribing estrogen in the form of the birth control pills can delay these problems, presumably indefinitely.

In some cases giving estrogen to middle-aged women can be dangerous as well as useless. One signal that cancer of the female organs may be present is vaginal bleeding or spotting in a post-menopausal woman. Thus when doctors do feel it necessary to administer the pills to menopausal women, they emphasize strongly that any irregular bleeding must be reported promptly.

Some physicians believe that estrogens help to prevent heart disease. This could be one of the reasons women suffer from heart attacks far less frequently than do men. If a female patient has a heart condition, she is often given birth control pills. Osteoarthritis is an inflammation of the finger joints and the weightbearing joints of the body; estrogen administered in the form of oral contraceptives, will frequently relieve this condition.

The Future

Although the pill is certainly the most effective contraceptive developed to date, researchers are continuing to investigate ways of improving it. They are eager, for instance, to find a pill which would inhibit ovulation by affecting the woman's sexual organs directly, rather than by affecting the pituitary gland. Such a discovery would eliminate some of the side effects which are occasionally present, but a new tablet may have side effects of its own.

Scientists are also searching for a pill which could be taken just once a month. This would help the many patients who lack the motivation or intelligence to take the oral contraceptives regularly for twenty days. Similarly, researchers hope to discover a substance which, when administered by a doctor once a month, could eliminate ovulation. This would, of course, eliminate "patient failures."

Current studies are examining the feasibility of a "morning-after pill." Taken after coitus, it may prevent pregnancy by interfering with the transport of the egg down the tubes, by inhibiting development of the fertilized egg, or by changing the endometrium (the lining of the uterus) so that a fertilized egg could not implant there. But both religious groups and private individuals might disapprove of tampering with the normal growth of a fertilized egg, and might consider the effect of a "morning-after pill" very much like an abortion. Practical as well as ethical problems complicate the research. These tablets at present produce side-effects. Also, it may be necessary to take the tablets not only *the* morning after but for several mornings after.

Another type of research is attempting to prevent pregnancy by limiting the fertility of the male. The male contraceptive pill currently under investigation decreases the production of the sperm. A few effective drugs have been produced, but they may cause some side effects. For example, a man taking one type of such tablets will become ill after drinking a cocktail or highball. And some of the experimental pills have an even more undesirable side effect. They decrease sexual desire—a drastically effective mode of contraception, to be sure, but one which most patients probably would not accept.

Perhaps both the biological and psychological aspects of the pill will reverse the old theory of "the biological tragedy of women." With this theory some anthropologists have described how women came to take second place in the battle between the sexes. It was not because of less keen minds, or weaker strength or less endurance, but rather for purely biological reasons. Women were effectively removed from the arenas of action every month, and sometimes for nine-month periods. Handicapped by this condition, women in both early and more civilized societies were not given any positions of importance. Consequently, their contribution in many areas of learning and their political power have lagged far behind men's, until recently. The increased freedom that women may now enjoy should have many beneficial social consequences, besides the obvious one of saving the world from overcrowding. Even the "sexual revolution" which has been in progress since the beginning of the century may, for better or worse, receive strong reinforcement from the pill.

SUPPLEMENTAL READING

Drill, V. A., Oral Contraceptives, McGraw-Hill, New York, 1966.
Goldzicher, J. W. and Rice-Wray, E., Oral Contraception, Charles C Thomas, Springfield, Illinois, 1966.
Pincus, G., The Control of Fertility, Academic Press, New York, 1965.

Chapter 2

Drugs and the Unborn Child

R ecently in Boston a pregnant mother was given sedatives to quiet the child in her womb. The woman's blood was Rh-positive, her husband's Rh-negative. About one of twenty offspring suffers severe consequence from this circumstance. Doctors found that the Rh-factor was stifling the child's life, and the baby had to be given several intrauterine (within-the-womb) transfusions only days before birth. This technique had been mastered by Dr. A. W. Liley in New Zealand in 1963.

The sedative drugs in the mother here had a beneficial effect. The chemicals coursed through her blood stream across the placenta, and into the fetus to reduce its activity and thus possibly to save its life. But the fetus is not so favorably affected by all drugs given to the mother. One example is the thalidomide disaster in which thousands of unborn children suffered drastic anatomical consequences. Thalidomide is now banned; but it nonetheless remains an embarrassing enigma. We actually know very little more about the mechanism of its disruptive action than when it was first implicated in the world-wide tragedy a few years ago. It is a sober reminder that heroic measures are needed to avoid a similar occurrence in the future.

A New Science: Teratology

The study of the types, frequency, and mechanisms of abnormal embryonic development is called teratology; the chemical agent that causes the abnormality is a teratogen. Man has long been aware of and curious about his abnormal offspring. Considerable scientific writing has been devoted to documentation of the types and the degrees of human variations. But characterization of congenital disease is not enough. Today, previously unsuspected biochemical disorders are being analyzed to determine whether they are the result

of the inheritance of faulty genes or of drugs that might have inter-
fered with the normal development of the fetus. Recent controlled
surveys reveal that a surprisingly high percentage of human deliveries
yield individuals that have demonstrable structural or functional defects, not all of which are traceable to genetic factors. Studies are
being planned and carried out, not only to obtain a more accurate
figure on occurrence, but also in the hope that suitable statistical
analyses of large numbers of cases will reveal correlations with unsuspected causative factors.

It is becoming increasingly apparent that no single agent,
perhaps no one class of agents, is responsible for a large portion
of human abnormal development. Genetic factors, once regarded as
a major cause of congenital abnormalities, are now estimated to account for no more than 20 percent of the total. A considered guess
is that infectious agents, endocrine diseases, radiations, antigrowth
substances and such drugs as thalidomide—all known to be capable
of producing malformations in man—are probably not responsible
for more than 5 percent of congenital disease.

Abnormalities in the genes (linked together they make up
the chromosomes) have been shown to be regularly connected with
certain aggregates of defects. Yet genes seem not to be the cause
of most *specific* birth defects, and present indications are that only a
very limited number of congenital "syndromes" involve deviations
in the number or form of the chromosomes. Thus it appears at
present that most human malformations have no recognizable cause.

Since scientists have been unable to uncover any widely applicable single cause or causes, they have had to consider the highly
complicated phenomena of interacting causes. Conceivably, these
multiple causes could be combinations of two or more genetic factors,
two or more environmental factors, or a mixture of two or more
of each variety. Multifactorial genetic systems have been understood
for some time and new ones with special relevance to malformations
will doubtless continue to be revealed. Interaction between genetic
and environmental agents (such as a drug) has several times been
demonstrated in laboratory animals. For example, one researcher
found that a strain of rats with a low incidence of hereditary dia-
phragmatic defect could be made to show a remarkable increase

in its occurrence if the pregnant females were fed a vitamin A deficient diet.

Drugs and Pregnancy

The following table enumerates possible effects of drugs on pregnancy or its outcome. With the probable exception of the first item in the table, which refers in part to the popularly known "pill," our knowledge of most of them is very limited:

TABLE 1
POSSIBLE EFFECTS OF DRUG ACTION ON PREGNANCY OR ITS OUTCOME

1. Failure of ovulation—secondary to endocrine or metabolic imbalance.
2. Prevention of fertilization—by destroying or intefering with fertilizability of germ cells.
3. Interference with migration of the ovum or early embryo.
4. Abnormal or no implantation—owing to damaged blastocyst or inappropriate uterine conditions.
5. Indirect damage to embryo, as a result of:
   a. altered placental function,
   b. altered maternal metabolism.
6. Direct damage to embryo or fetus.

The action of several drugs has been charted at least as far as their effects on lower forms of life is concerned. Actinomycin D, a powerful antibiotic crystallized from a *Streptomyces* in 1940, acts by binding with DNA in a way which prevents the synthesis of "messenger" RNA (see Chapter 18). Ultimately the genetic information encoded in the genes cannot be expressed. It is therefore not surprising that even minute quantities of actinomycin have a devastating effect on the early embryo. At this stage the organism presumably would be especially dependent upon a steady flow of information from the genes if differentiation and growth are to proceed on schedule.

Actinomycin D will not lead to malformation unless it is given in a sufficient dosage. And yet, when minute doses were combined with such drugs as cyclophosphamide or 5-fluorouracil, unexpected numbers of malformations began to occur in rats. This result strongly supports the possibility that at least a part of the unexplained birth defects can be attributed to the interaction of agents neither of which would be recognized by ordinary survey methods. Drugs that are ordinarily considered safe could conceivably be teratogenic if they interacted with other drugs, or perhaps with some other unfavorable condition such as a borderline dietary deficiency. No such interaction has yet been demonstrated in human beings, but the animal experiments have shown that the possibility exists.

Occasionally in embryonic development there is a delay in the alteration of the fetus' cells, a phenomenon which is impossible to observe except in abortions. In a mother who has been on narcotics or barbiturates, for example, an unborn child may develop a tolerance for barbituric drugs. Some fundamental cellular change occurs in the child. As a result, the child may be far more susceptible to drug addiction in later life. Some physicians now feel that some of the inexplicable diseases that develop as a patient grows older may be explained by altered cellular metabolism induced during intrauterine life by some drug taken by the mother. Some of the diseases remain unsolved: multiple sclerosis and myasthenia gravis may yet be traced to some noxious agent innocently taken by the pregnant woman.

Animal Experimentation

It is probable that even the intensified animal tests to which new drugs are now subjected would have failed to identify thalidomide as the devastating teratogen it has proved to be. Of the various laboratory animals in which new drugs are tried, only certain strains of rabbits, mice, and rats have since been shown to be susceptible to the teratogenic influences of thalidomide. Moreover, in these instances dosages considerably *above* the human equivalent were required. It is also likely that some drugs in use today, such as Adrenalin, salicylates, meclizine, certain antibiotics, insulin, and several others would have difficulty passing, had they been initially tested according to the more stringent standards for teratogenicity used today. These substances are all known to be capable of causing malformation in laboratory animals in relatively modest doses, but none of them has been shown to be teratogenic in man. The only known human teratogens to have been first identified as teratogenic in animals were folic acid antagonists, sex hormones, and possibly X-radiations. This knowledge, however, did not prevent their use with unfortunate consequences in several instances during human pregnancy. Thus, in the face of wide-species, subspecies, and even individual variation in reaction to teratogenic agents, it appears that little reliance can be placed in information obtained from one animal when applied to another—or to man.

When a new drug is found to cause malformation in an animal, scientists are obliged to proceed with greater caution in making the first clinical tests. However, the greatest benefits derived from animal experimentation with teratogenic or potentially teratogenic agents lie more in the basic science than in the clinical realm. Animal studies designed to reveal mechanisms of teratogenic action would, like all well-conducted basic science efforts, have potential value far beyond any immediate application. A knowledge of mechanism could permit preventive measures to be taken. Such knowledge might also lead to therapeutic measures: possibly the supplying of a deficient chemical or the bypassing of a missing enzyme. Relatively few teratogenic mechanisms are positively known at the present time. This emphasizes the need for the subject to be intensively studied in experimental animals.

Agents of Destruction

Strictly speaking, there are two primary embryonic considerations in teratogenesis, the genetic make-up of the embryo and the developmental stage at which it is confronted with a damaging influence from the environment. In simplest terms, genetic make-up is important because it determines the inherent susceptibility of an embryo to a given agent at a given time of development. Physical environment of the embryo is, of course, the maternal organism. This provides the immediate source of materials needed for growth and maintenance; the physiologic state of the mother, therefore, is of great importance to the embryo. Factors such as maternal weight and age under the right conditions are correlated positively with the occurrence of maldevelopment in the embryo. But the mechanisms by which this comes about are obscure.

The mother is often able to protect her child from poten-tially-damaging chemical substances. This is done primarily by two means, either by rapid excretion or by detoxification. In fact, it is now well established that special detoxification mechanisms can be developed in response to noxious substances which are repeatedly or chronically administered. For instance, pretreatment of mice with mitomycin C before pregnancy tends to reduce the expected terato-genicity of this substance when given during pregnancy.

Malfunction of the placenta may be responsible for faulty development of the child. This organ provides for the communica-tion, as it were, between the mother and her baby. The placenta could possibly affect the embryo adversely in three ways: excluding materials essential for growth; admitting substances not ordinarily admitted; or failing to perform its usual excretory or endocrine func-tions. None of these functional disorders of the placenta is actually known to have resulted in malformation of an embryo, although some suggestive evidence has been advanced. On the whole, however, it seems unlikely that the placenta is responsible for appreciable teratogenesis.

In general, the embryonic stage at the time an agent acts determines which tissues are susceptible to teratogenesis. Susceptibil-ity has been shown to vary greatly during the course of embryonic development (see Figure 1).

The precise mechanism by which the great majority of very early embryos resist teratogenic damage is unknown. In any case the onset of teratogenic susceptibility occurs at about the time the germ layers are formed. In mammals this is several days after con-ception, about five days in the hamster and mouse, eight days in a rat, nine in a rabbit, assumed to be ten days in a monkey, and as early as twelve or thirteen in man. The onset of susceptibility is sudden and many teratogenic substances produce their highest numbers of malformation shortly thereafter. This occurs when the embryo consists of two or three simple layers of cells arranged as an embryonic disc, with little if any indication of future organs and tissues. Nevertheless, at the early stages it is possible to demonstrate by transplantation or by chemical means that localized areas of the disc have acquired specific organ-forming potential; in other words, chemical differentiation has set in. Thus, chemically differentiated cells may be subject to teratogenesis several hours or possibly days before their ultimate role in development is indicated by structural differentiation. Kidney anomalies, for example, can be induced by irradiating rat embryos on the ninth day, but the kidney does not

Usually Not Susceptible to Teratogenesis

Pre differentiation Period

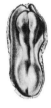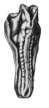

Highly Susceptible to Teratogenesis

Period of Early Differentiation

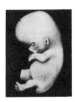

Increasingly Resistant to Teratogenesis With Increasing Age

Period of Advanced Organogenesis

FIGURE 1. *Schematic representation of the changing susceptibility of the mammalian embryo to teratogens. The stages depicted are drawn from or are retouched photographs of actual human specimens that have appeared in several papers in the Contributions to Embryology of the Carnegie Institution. (Annals New York Academy of Sciences)*

appear till the twelfth day and only somewhat later does specific malformation of the kidney appear.

There is also the matter of dosage, not as simple as might be assumed. All dosage levels of a known teratogen are not teratogenic. Typically there is a lower range that permits normal development and a higher range that kills all of the embryos and perhaps also the mothers, if extended far enough. Between these there may be a narrow teratogenic zone, in which dosage is just sufficient to interfere with specific developmental events without destroying the whole embryo. And, of course, to complicate matters, teratogenic dosage is dependent on the age of the embryo.

Thus far, a number of drugs have been implicated as causing teratological or other undesirable effects in the newborn infant. Progestins, for example, have masculinized female monkeys as embryos and have produced permanent alterations in their sexual behavior. Androgens and estrogens may be also responsible for accelerated bone age. Chloroquine, the antimalarial drug, may lead to retinal damage. Reserpine given during pregnancy causes nasal congestion and drowsiness in the newborn infant. Antihistamines have an uncertain effect. Potassium iodide and methimazole cause goiter. Nitrofurantoin (Furadantin) break up the red blood cells in the fetus. Smoking by the mother can precipitate premature births. Heavy smoking leads to a universal incidence of low birth weight among infants.

It is probably unavoidable that children yet unborn will also be damaged by teratogenic drugs because only widespread usage in human beings can reveal the unusual and infrequent reactions. Animal experiments and analytic studies will continue at an increasing pace, but they can never be conclusive as far as human hazard is concerned. Probably, the most critical method of final testing would be administering the drug to a woman who is scheduled to have a therapeutic abortion. At least some effects might be apparent in the fetus, effects not apparent in animal tests. Despite its scientific limitations and probable reluctant acceptance by the public, this method could be justified on the grounds that it might protect the lives of many by prudently using the unhappy loss of a few.

SUPPLEMENTAL READING

Apgar, V., Drugs in pregnancy. JAMA, *190*, 840–841, 1964.

Cohlan, S. O., Fetal and neonatal hazards from drugs administered during pregnancy. N.Y. Med. J., *64*, 493–499, 1964.

Karnofsky, D. A., Drugs as teratogens in animals and man. Ann. Rev. Pharm., *5*, 447–472, 1965.

Lenz, W., Chemicals and Malformations in Man. Congenital Malformations, Papers and discussions presented at the Second International Conference, International Medical Congress Ltd., New York, 1964.

Lucey, J. F., Drugs and the intrauterine patient. Proceedings: Symposium on the Placenta, Its Form and Function, Birth Defects Original Article Series, *1*, 46–61. National Foundation.

Robson, J. M., Sullivan, F. M., and Smith, R. L., Embryopathic Activity of Drugs. Little, Brown and Co., Boston, 1965.

Villee, C. A., Placental transfer of drugs. Ann. N.Y. Acad. Sci., *123*, 237–244, 1965.

Wilson, J. G., Experimental teratology. Am. J. Obst. Gynec. *90*, 1181–1192, 1964.

Chapter 3

Vitamins

Being betwixt three or four degrees
of the Equinoctial line, my Company
within a few days began to fall sick, of
a disease which Sea-men are wont to call
the Scurvy; and seemeth to be a kind of
dropsy, and reigneth most in this climate
of any that I have heard or read of in
the World; though in all Seas it is wont
to help and increase the misery of
man . . .
The cause of this sickness, some
attribute to sloth; some to conceit,
and divers men speak diversely . . .
That which I have seen most fruitful
for this sickness is sour Oranges and
Lemons . . .

Sir Richard Hawkins
Observations in his Voyage
to the South Sea (1593)

S hould we take one a day, or is that so much nonsense? Since people in wealthier nations have been relatively free from vitamin deficiencies, they may not have understood their importance. Most people do know that a deficiency of vitamin C brought scurvy and death to many seamen in old vessels sent out on long ocean voyages. These seamen spent prolonged periods of time away from fresh fruits and vegetables that contain one vitamin or another essential to life. Unawareness of the importance of vitamins is still widespread. In the Near East, Africa, and the Orient, millions suffer from malnutrition. For many nations, disease, including vitamin deficiency, poses a larger problem than a stable economy.

As early as 1601 the mariners of the East India Company were regularly eating oranges and lemons to prevent scurvy. In 1720, fruits and juices were shown both to prevent and cure the disease, and to cure it in a dramatically short time. Captain Cook, for example, lost few men to scurvy. His ships carried crates of fruit, brought aboard regularly from the fruit-laden islands of the southern Pacific. In 1804, the Royal Navy of Great Britain made daily consumption of lemon juice compulsory: the number of cases of scurvy in the Haslar Naval Hospital dropped from 1,457 in 1780 to 1 in 1806. (British sailors required to drink lemon and lime juices were thus nicknamed "limeys.") But why fruits and vegetables prevented various diseases could not be answered at that time. The practical application of dietary supplements was far ahead of the understanding of their physiological functions—or even of the existence of such a thing as a "vitamin." As with scurvy, so with beriberi and rickets, the other two diseases of this powerful triumvirate. In 1882 the Japanese naval doctor, Kanehiro Takaki, found that beriberi could be cured by a proper diet. He won great fame for ridding the Japanese Navy of the disease. Takaki did not, however, interpret beriberi as vitamin deficiency (the term was still unborn) but rather

37

as a lack of protein. The fact remains that he accurately attributed the problem to a poor diet.

The next contribution was made by the Dutch physiologist Christiaan Eijkman; he induced experimental beriberi in chickens. But it was his astute colleague, Grijns, who first suggested that the disease was caused by a deficiency of some substance or substances essential to the metabolism of the central nervous system. This substance was found in rice hulls that were polished away when rice was prepared for storage and use. In 1906 Grijns and Eijkman began trying to isolate these unknown substances and met with some success. The discovery that rickets was caused by a food deficiency followed similar lines.

Funk's "Vitamines"

Most of our knowledge about vitamins, their existence and functions, has been gained in this century. The crucial contribution came in 1912 with the "vitamine hypothesis" of Casimir Funk, then only twenty-six years old. Based upon the work that had been done by other scientists, along with his own research, Funk provided the necessary theory in the field of deficiency disease. He postulated that there were four *vitamines* (amines he considered *vital* to life), each of which protected the body from a corresponding deficiency— beriberi, scurvy, rickets and pellagra. His thinking soon superseded the nutritional theory that held the only components of value in foodstuffs to be proteins, carbohydrates, fats, minerals and water.

Funk's theory led to the discovery of more vitamins and to their eventual synthesis in the laboratory. Today the little vitamin pills, synthetic dietary supplements, have the same chemical properties and physiological effect as "natural" vitamins in food. And it is clearly easier to take a pill than to peel an orange.

Scientific research on a given problem proceeds from many approaches. Work on the chemical analysis of the diet supplemented research on the deficiency diseases. In 1888 Dr. Lunin showed that rats could not survive on an artificial diet consisting of only five principal components present in foodstuffs (i.e. fats, proteins, sugars, minerals, and water). This meant that other things had to be present in food. But what are they? Clearly they could only exist in minute amounts, for quantitative analysis showed that the vast bulk of food is made of the five elements already known. A few milligrams of these "X" substances were enough to determine life or death.

In the same year that Funk's "vitamine" theory appeared, the British biologist Sir Frederick Hopkins published a crucial study on "synthetic diets." He proved beyond doubt that previous ideas positing the existence of some unknown substances in foodstuffs were correct. By 1912 it was clear that there were such substances as vitamins, and since the fundamental question of their existence was settled, the scientists proceeded with confidence.

Then in 1915 it was shown that rats needed two factors to keep alive. One was found in fats and was called "fat-soluble A"—later to be renamed vitamin A; the other was found in watery food extracts and was called "water-soluble B." This discovery made it clear that at least two, and probably many more, vitamins existed, all of which were essential to life. The discovery of vitamins D, C, and K followed. Then, in 1926, vitamin B was found to be a complex rather than a single vitamin. We now have vitamins B_1 (thiamine), B_2 (riboflavin), B_6 (pyridoxine), nicotinic acid (niacin), and so on. Knowledge advanced rapidly in the field once the work of Funk and Hopkins became known.

There are now nearly 30 vitamins that have been isolated. At least 8 of these are absolutely essential in the diet of man. In what follows, some of the more important vitamins will be discussed in detail.

The Nature of Vitamin C

While they were working on beriberi, two Norwegian scientists, A. Holst and T. Frohlich, induced scurvy experimentally. They went on to show that the scurvy-preventing (antiscorbutic) factor was distinct from the factor that prevented beriberi. At first the antiscorbutic factor was called "water-soluble C," but later it was changed to vitamin C. It was understood at that time, 1920, that vitamins would be labeled in alphabetical order. Subsequent discoveries of vitamin complexes have foiled the scheme.

Considerable time was required to establish the identity of vitamin C. Eventually it was found to be the same hexuronic acid which had earlier been isolated from pepper, and studied by A. Szent-Gyorgyi in Hungary. In the laboratory many foods were analyzed chemically to find the amount of hexuronic acid in each; in every case the anti-scurvy potency of the food was in exact proportion to the amount of hexuronic acid the food was known to contain. The acid was put through many tests. These proved other particles were not clinging to the acid, which alone possesses the actual vitamin value. The name of the acid was soon changed to ascorbic acid to remind people of its antiscorbutic action.

Finally, in 1933, vitamin C was synthesized almost simultaneously in England and Switzerland. Dr. E. L. Hirst and four collaborators in Birmingham, England, were among the first to postulate its theoretical structure. They began with d-galactose (a sugar) and after nine steps arrived at 1-ascorbic acid, the vitamin.

This chapter began with a few words about scurvy. Its cure—fruit juices—was popularized in James Lind's *A Treatise on the Scurvy,* published in 1757, though the author was not the first to know of such a cure (Kramer, 1720). Not remiss about his experimental methods, Lind took twelve scurvy patients on a cruise and treated all but two of them with various traditional remedies. To the remaining two he gave lemons and oranges. The results were, of course, as one would expect. "The consequence was that the most sudden and visible effects were perceived from the use of the oranges and lemons . . . Some persons cannot be brought to believe that a disease so fatal and dreadful can be prevented or cured by such easy means."

And indeed the disease was dreadful. Scurvy is usually discovered through excessive bleeding, which is seen in the gums, under the surface of the skin, and in the joints. The skin may become horribly spotted and soft; the joints may swell to the point where it becomes unbearable for the victim to be touched. Because of their heavy milk diet, babies have been especially prone to the disease in this century. Parents must see that the baby gets adequate vitamin C through strained fruits and fruit juices. Baby cannot live on milk alone.

Scurvy: Pathology and Treatment

A dog can synthesize vitamin C. The human body cannot. Hence we depend entirely on an intake of vitamin C for survival.

As babies we may receive the vitamin through our mother's milk, *if* her intake of it is adequate. Human milk is normally richer in the vitamin than cow's milk. Later we must either eat properly or supplement our diets with vitamin pills. Food-processing often destroys some of the vitamin C content; but a great many foods contain this vitamin, and even if processed, still retain substantial amounts of it.

Vitamin C is rapidly and completely absorbed in the intestine. The amount of vitamin C in any given organ seems to be determined by the metabolic needs of the organ. High concentrations are found, for example, in the adrenal gland, in the pituitary gland, and in the tissues of the intestinal wall. The vitamin leaves the body through ordinary internal breakdown, perspiration, through tears, and urine.

Vitamin C is necessary for the maintenance of the normal structure and proper function of the intercellular ground substance (substance between cells) of mesothelial tissue such as connective tissue, bone, teeth, and capillaries. This intercellular ground substance contains tiny reserves of protein, known as collagen bundles. Collagen is a major supportive protein in the formation of skin, tendons, bones, and cartilage. Vitamin C seems to control the making of collagen. In the absence of the vitamin new intercellular substance is not laid down and the pathologic changes appear. For example, in the absence of the vitamin the teeth can no longer produce adequate quantities of dentine and enamel.

The pathological lesion of scurvy results from the body's inability to make the intracellular ground substance of mesothelial tissue. Distribution of lesions becomes wide-spread, making the disease easily recognizable. The capillaries, bones, teeth and gums are the areas usually affected. Capillary walls become defective, and bleeding occurs. This of course happens all over the body—even in the muscles. Bleeding in the eye and in the gastrointestinal tract is also common.

Skeletal changes seem particularly common in infantile scurvy. Bone growth slackens and stops. Irregularities develop in the cartilage, and fibrous tissue replaces the normal calcified cartilage. Bones become brittle and fractures occur easily. Sometimes bones get so thin that they are no stronger than the cartilage itself. Fortunately, recovery is rapid and normal bone growth will begin almost at once when the individual is treated with vitamin C. The same is true with the lesions and infections of the gums.

The milder deficiency, hypovitaminosis C, is in many ways more dangerous today than scurvy, primarily because it is harder to diagnose. Slight deficiencies may interfere with the healing of a wound, with the development of strong connective tissue, and with the body's capacity to defend itself against infections.

Diagnosis of hypovitaminosis C must be done in the laboratory. In the United States the deficiency is fairly common among the lower economic classes, though the presence of the disease often goes undetected. There are now five generally-accepted methods that may be used to detect the disease:

1. Urine Test
2. Blood Test
3. Load Test
4. Capillary Resistance Test
5. X-Ray

In the urine and blood tests a simple check exists to determine the amount of the vitamin in the sample. The load test consists of giving a large dose of the vitamin to the patient. If the body is deficient in ascorbic acid most of the dosage will remain in the tissues. If, on the other hand, there is an adequate supply in the body, the bulk of the dosage will be excreted. When this happens the doctor can assume that the problem is something other than vitamin C deficiency. To be accurate, however, these three tests must be given several times over a period of days because the amounts of the vitamin in the body will vary from day to day under *any* conditions. For the other two tests this is not a problem. The capillary resistance test consists simply of increasing the pressure in the capillaries by means of a tourniquet or by increasing the blood pressure, and then seeing if the walls of the capillaries will hold. In a condition of severe deficiency, the weakened walls will not be able to withstand the increased pressure. Finally, the X-ray is used to check for rather typical defects in bone and cartilage.

Treatment for ascorbic acid deficiency is relatively simple. An otherwise healthy person is given an increased amount of vitamin

C through dietary regulation. People sick with such ailments as fever or infection need larger doses, which sometimes have to be given intravenously or intramuscularly. The exact vitamin requirements vary with bodily weight and the rate of metabolism, but generally an extra 10 milligrams a day (over the 50–100 normally required) is enough to cure mild or latent scurvy. Since vitamin C has no toxic effect in large doses, an overdose need not be feared. Broken bones that often result from severe scurvy are treated like any other broken bones.

One well-known professional athlete was struggling through two seasons with one cartilage tear after another. A large number of clinical tests were made before one doctor noticed that his problem was due to a deficiency of vitamin C. The mild shortage of the vitamin was enough to weaken the cartilage and to slow down the healing process when the cartilage was torn. Treatment returned him to the lineup quickly. A native of the South, the player had inadvertently reduced his C intake on moving to the North. His legs had needed the extra fortification to stand the stress of his profession, and the reduction of vitamin C intake was too much for his legs to take.

Beriberi and Vitamin B_1—Thiamine

Before the discoveries of Kanehiro Takaki, beriberi affected 40 percent of the men of the Japanese navy. As late as 1947, the Philippines were plagued by the disease. Since a majority of all those afflicted eventually died, the widespread existence of the deficiency was made even more frightening; the annual death rate was at one time nearly 132 per 100,000 population.

Since Japanese sailors were as hygienic as any others, Takaki reasoned that the cause of the disease lay in a faulty diet. He found that wherever polished rice was the staple in the diet, beriberi existed. We know now that the outer husky part of the rice grain is the portion that contains vitamin B_1. If this part is left on the rice, no deficiency arises. If it is "polished" off, beriberi may occur.

Results obtained when the new diet was introduced into the Japanese navy were startling. From 1,789 reported cases in 1879, the number had fallen to 3 by 1886. Takaki thought that the results were due to an increased protein intake, but it was actually vitamin B_1. Later, Eijkman's work put the labors of the Japanese on sound scientific footing.

The isolation and synthesis of B_1 were both difficult. W. Murk Jansen and Julius Donath finally isolated the vitamin in 1926. Nine years later a group of American scientists synthesized B_1. The synthesis was very important, for nature is stingy with vitamin B_1, lending few foods very much of it. Hence if no supplement is taken, an extremely well-balanced diet is necessary for adequate supplies of the vitamin. A synthetic substitute, of course, may provide a plentiful and effective supply of B_1. Of the foods in the home, egg yolk, peas, liver, and cereal germ possess B_1. White bread, unless enriched, has virtually none. But the vitamin may be easily destroyed by heat, and the housewife must remember this when preparing foods containing vitamin B_1.

A shortage of thiamine in the body produces an excess of pyruvic and lactic acids in the tissues. Normally these acids, as products of carbohydrate metabolism, are oxidized as fast as they are formed. The vitamin promotes the oxidation of these acids. When their utilization is decreased, the cell is deprived of normal nutrition. In man, B_1 seems necessary for the maintenance of nerve tissue, appetite, normal intestinal and cardiovascular functions, and the normal growth and development of the young.

The body disposes of thiamine through the urine in amounts that reflect intake and storage. Thus the "load test", mentioned earlier, can be effectively used to test for thiamine deficiency as well as for ascorbic acid deficiency.

In the early stages of deficiency, or in cases of hypovitaminosis B_1 (subclinical deficiency), the symptoms lack specificity. In other words, the symptoms could be those of many diseases and must often be checked through laboratory tests rather than by simple observation. From autopsies we know that in the late stages of the disease noticeable changes occur in the structure of the heart and that lesions of the peripheral nerves appear. The muscles that are controlled by these nerves are affected by loss of striation or fatty degeneration. But these changes are also nonspecific, being found in other forms of neuritis as well. In general, the lesions at the early stages of deficiency must be found in the area of function.

Severe beriberi comes in two forms, the so-called wet and dry. The wet form affects the cardiovascular functions and is far more likely to produce early death. Dry beriberi affects the nervous system. (So may wet beriberi in some instances.) With the onset of beriberi, edema—swelling due to fluid in the tissues—occurs along with congestion and shortness of breath.

Neuritic symptoms and signs of the dry form are muscular tenderness, neuritis, burning and tingling sensations, numbness and loss of coordination. Limbs can actually waste away. Often, in the later stages of deterioration, mental confusion occurs. Fortunately, however, these severe forms are not common, and recovery is normally very rapid, except in cases where excessive neural damage has occurred. In such cases complete recovery is improbable.

The sufferer of a subclinical deficiency may often experience shortness of breath, have mild indigestion, muscular aches and pains and a general rundown feeling. Since symptoms are vague, the disease must be diagnosed through specific tests as suggested earlier. Unfortunately those most likely to have a mild deficiency are also least likely to receive regular and thorough medical attention. These are the indigent, the aged, the infirm, and the institutionalized. It is also important to remember that the requirements for vitamin B_1 are increased by pregnancy, growth, fever, increased metabolism and heavy work. The minimum requirement for a given person is hard to determine.

Often, if the doctor is informed of the patient's dietary history, diagnosis is greatly simplified. Electrocardiograms will sometimes expose the deficiency if it is the type that affects the heart. Laboratory and therapeutic tests are used as well. In the latter physicians simply prescribe the vitamin and then wait to see its effect on the patient. If the illness is indeed a deficiency, improvement will result. The laboratory tests are made on blood and urine. In the laboratory tests, if a patient has thiamine deficiency after exercise, the concentration of pyruvic acid in the blood returns to normal only slowly.

The treatment for B_1 deficiency falls into three different areas. They are preventive, protective, and curative. Preventive treatment is, of course, dietary. If one suspects that the diet is not supplying enough B_1, one should take vitamin pills as a supplement. Fortunately our white bread is generally enriched with thiamine so that we are assured of a significant amount of B_1—if we eat the enriched bread. People who have a high carbohydrate diet need more B_1 to metabolize carbohydrates; in a simple formula, the more carbohydrates in the diet, the more B_1 required.

Protective treatment is given to pregnant and nursing women, to chronic alcoholics, to those with gastrointestinal problems that affect digestion, to people with modified diets, to psychoneurotics and psychiatric patients, and to patients with chronic infections. Infants who have digestive problems are usually given extra thiamine. Sometimes a mild deficiency will cause a child to lose appetite, thus increasing the need for protective doses. Chronic alcoholics pose a particularly difficult problem, because their diet is very high in carbohydrates. At the same time it is invariably lacking in other nutrients.

In curative treatment pure crystalline thiamine is given in dosages ranging from 10 to 20 milligrams daily. Generally this is given orally, except with patients who have severe digestive problems. Here it may be given intramuscularly or intravenously. Such injections assure prompt action, adequate dosage, and certain absorption. Infants are often treated through their mother's milk.

In addition to thiamine, the patient is kept on a high-calorie diet and is given other supplementary vitamins after the major symptoms have disappeared. Commercial multiple vitamin pills may be helpful in balancing the diet, but the quantity of each ingredient is too small for therapeutic use. Massage and controlled exercises can be used to speed recovery in neuritic cases.

Pellagra and Niacin

Pellagra (from the Italian *pelle agra,* "rough skin") was first recognized as a distinct disease in 1735. It was not known in this country until the latter part of the nineteenth century. Yet in America pellagra has been a much greater problem than scurvy and beriberi. In 1927 there were over 120,000 cases reported in the United States, most in the South; in 1930 at least 7,000 people died from pellagra. Impoverished people in the deep South ate maize, bacon, and molasses almost exclusively; and the staple, maize, is inadequate in niacin, just as polished rice is deficient in thiamine.

As early as 1914 pellagra was recognized as a deficiency disease. Joseph Goldberger found that he could induce the disease in human subjects by a simple dietary change. Furthermore, all attempts to transmit the disease by inoculation failed, ruling out the possibility that the disease was caused by infection. However, the deficiency was first thought to be a protein deficiency (Takaki thought as much of beriberi), but Carl Voegtlin proved this incorrect in 1920. He was able to cure pellagra patients with extracts containing no trace of protein. In essence, then, the anti-pellagra factor seemed to be something in vitamin B, but it was not the part that was to be known as B_1. By 1926 Goldberger and his colleagues had proved that this new factor was more stable to heat than the anti-beriberi factor. They called it the P-P (pellagra-preventing) factor. The following year the two factors were classified as vitamin B_1 and B_2. Then B_2 itself proved to be a complex consisting of riboflavin, sometimes referred to as B_2 (1933), pyridoxine (1934), and finally nicotinic acid (1937). The name of the latter was quickly changed to niacin because of possible confusion with nicotine found in tobacco. Thus ten years after its discovery, the P-P factor was resolved to niacin.

Inside the body, niacin combines with phosphoric acid, adenine, and ribose to form two coenzymes, which are necessary for the oxidation of certain metabolites in cells, specifically for the transfer of hydrogen. When the supply of niacin is inadequate, certain enzyme systems are disturbed, there is an inflammation of the outer layers of skin (epithelial tissue) and changes in the nervous system. But the more intimate details regarding the means by which these pathologic changes are produced are unknown. This is just one of innumerable areas in the field of vitamin research where much more needs to be done.

Niacin is readily absorbed from the gastrointestinal tract. Soon after absorption the nicotinic acid becomes an amide, in which form the vitamin becomes a part of a coenzyme, a factor (nonprotein) necessary for an enzyme to function. The vitamin is stored in the tissues longer than vitamin C; much of it is found in the liver, kidney, and muscle, where the metabolism is high. Niacin appears in the urine in several forms and for this reason it is difficult to test for deficiency by urinalysis. Niacin also has a mildly toxic action if given in an overdose to people not grossly deficient. Resultant flushing and itching disappears when administration is stopped.

The symptoms, signs, and pathology of the deficiency may be discussed together. Dermatitis (skin lesions) and gastrointestinal symptoms are most frequent. The skin breaks out with symmetrical rashes on the hands, feet, neck, and across the nose and cheeks. Reddening, swelling slightly, the skin stings and itches—the characteristics of mild sunburn. In chronic cases, there may be ulceration and infection. The skin may become either brown, dry and thickened, or thin and atrophied.

The alimentary canal may be affected at any point. A sore tongue is one of the symptoms of the disease. Or the pharynx and the esophagus may be inflamed. With stomach irritation, salivation can occur. Diarrhea is common, with mucus and blood often accompanying the loose stools. The manifestations vary little according to sex and age, except that the female might well have vaginitis along with the other symptoms and signs, and the male, scrotal dermatitis. In both sexes there may be lesions of the colon in the latter stages, as well as lesions of the kidneys and degeneration of the liver. Usually the early symptoms are the same: weakness, lassitude, loss of appetite, indigestion, mental depression, irritability, and a tendency toward diarrhea. The skin will be easily subject to irritation, especially when exposed to the sun. It should be noted that some of these symptoms and signs might well be due to a coexisting riboflavin deficiency and that other symtoms are nonspecific in nature. A person whose diet is lacking in niacin is probably suffering from more than one B-vitamin deficiency. For example, many of the mental symptoms of a pellagrin are due to thiamine deficiency. Thus it is difficult to diagnose pellagra in its milder forms. The fact that there is no convenient laboratory test to uncover deficiency of niacin further complicates matters.

Diagnosis must depend upon obvious signs, a knowledge of the patient's prior diet, and a therapeutic test. A thorough examination is necessary, for obvious symptoms like dermatitis are not always present to aid the inexperienced or hasty examiner. The tongue, vagina, and rectum often will give clues to the presence or absence of the deficiency. Except in severe cases, the symptoms are elusive.

Fortunately, once diagnosed, the disease is easily cured. Nicotinic acid given orally or by injection produces a steady—often rapid—improvement. Somewhere between 250 and 350 milligrams a day is the average dose given to an adult sufferer. This greatly exceeds the 10–15 milligrams per day which is the minimum adult requirement. If the patient has obstructions along the alimentary canal that interfere with digestion, these are either removed or treated in some other way. Problems of absorption may have to be circumvented. This is sometimes done by injecting the vitamin rather than giving it orally.

Of course, a well-balanced diet will prevent pellagra in the first place. The diet should consist of a variety of vegetables, both fresh and properly canned, milk, eggs, and yeast. No cure of a deficiency disease is final. If the patient returns to a poor diet, trouble returns. Thus, the patient must understand clearly the nature of his problem. If he maintains a diet sufficient in niacin, thiamine, and riboflavin, he has little to fear. Since one symptom of the deficiency is loss of appetite, the patient will often have to force himself to eat enough. To make things worse, the mouth may be very sore and the digestion poor; but cure still requires eating.

Vitamin D and Rickets

Daniel Whistler published his classic thesis on rickets in 1645. Whistler's ideas began the intriguing story leading to discovery of vitamin D, the lack of which causes rickets, the all-too-common crippler of children and adults. Rickets is a bone disease, caused by the failure of the body to utilize calcium and phosphates. It was very common in America and Northern Europe until relatively recently and it is still common in the Near and Middle East. In 1928, 87 percent of all London school children examined were found to have rickets of varying degrees of severity. In New London, Connecticut, during the mid-twenties, M. M. Eliot showed that almost 5 percent of all infants examined were rachitic. As late as 1944, over 24,000 children in Great Britain were afflicted with the disease annually.

It had been known for a long time that people living in warmer climates were relatively free from rickets. In 1890 an Englishman, with the appropriate name T. A. Palm, explained why the Riviera was safer than the Oder. He attributed the disparity to exposure to sunlight. Wherever the sun shone abundantly, rickets was rare. Of course, there were exceptions to the rule. In some warm climates the women were kept inside, as in Kashmir, and such sheltering did little for their health. But in general Dr. Palm's observation was valid, and he was the first to advocate sunlight as a therapeutic measure. Later, in 1912, J. Raczynski showed in experiments with dogs that sunlight could promote an increase of the mineral substance of the bones. But it was many years later before this phenomenon was completely understood.

The realization that sunlight was not the only cure deepened the mystery of the disease. Traditionally, cod-liver oil had been used with success to treat rickets. In 1776 it was used as a remedy in the Manchester Infirmary, and in the 1820's the cure was introduced on the European Continent. Yet cod-liver oil was never an accepted means of treating the disease until this century, even though the noted French scientist Armand Trousseau endorsed it as early as 1865, and not without good evidence. Jules Guerin in 1838 produced experimental rickets in puppies, showing that the disease was caused by a faulty diet. Here, as in other cases we have examined, the problem was not understood as a vitamin deficiency. Working from the theories of Funk and Hopkins, Sir Edward Mellanby, in 1918, proved conclusively that there was an anti-rickets vitamin.

Sir Edward Mellanby found that cod-liver oil and other animal fats protected puppies against rickets. At first it was thought that the vitamin was fat-soluble A, discovered by E. V. McCollum and M. Davis in 1915. After further experimentation, it was shown that the anti-rickets vitamin was not vitamin A. Certain foods known to be rich in vitamin A failed to prevent rickets, and processes known to destroy vitamin A failed to reduce the anti-rickets potential of cod-liver oil. Finally an American chemist, T. F. Zucker, separated the two factors, and in 1923 the antirachitic vitamin was named vitamin D.

The vitamin was isolated, but its nature was still not understood. And the question remained, how could sunlight produce an anti-rickets factor? Furthermore, were the two antirachitic factors the same? These questions were not answered until World War I had long since ended, while rickets went unchecked in a devastated Europe. It was discovered that ultraviolet rays would cure rickets; scientists prevented rickets by irradiating the food that subjects ate. It seemed that the vitamin was manufactured in the presence of sunlight or ultraviolet rays, as shown by the Wisconsin scientists Harry Steenbock and E. B. Hart. But upon what substance did the light act? Soon it was ascertained that the sterols, waxy materials associated with fats, were those substances. Further research pin-pointed ergosterol as the sterol that was the parent of "sunshine vitamin D." Finally, in 1932, pure crystalline vitamin D was isolated from irradiated ergosterol. Many scientists were involved in the pro-cess of discovery, and no attempt is made here to list them all.

Vitamin D is a term used to describe a group of similar compounds. However, only D_2 (irradiated ergosterol) and D_3 (found in cod-liver oil) are of significant value in fighting rickets. Other sterols besides ergosterol, when irradiated, can have antirachitic properties. But it is D_2 (called calciferol after irradiation) that is primarily used in cases of rickets. When cows are fed irradiated yeast, calciferol is the form of vitamin D excreted in the milk. Milk can also be activated by direct exposure to the ultraviolet rays. Still, we are dependent on sunlight, acting on the sterols of the skin, for our basic supply of vitamin D. The amount in natural foodstuffs is small, and the normal, unenriched diet alone is inadequate, even though the amazingly small amount of one ounce of the pure vitamin is enough to treat one million children for one day.

When there is a deficiency of vitamin D, the net absorption of calcium and phosphates into the blood stream is reduced. And much more of these two substances is excreted in the feces. The bones, deprived of an adequate supply of calcium and phosphates, will not continue their normal growth. A deficient calcification of the bones follows, with inadequate mineralization. The junctures of the long bones swell; the soft osteoid tissue (uncalcified bone) grows irregularly. Soon the bones start bending. In addition, a loss of mus-cle tone and the protruding belly become noticeable features. In one case, a six-year-old child, from impoverished parentage in the northwestern part of this country, was brought to a clinic by state health authorities. His legs were so bent by severe rickets that he could not stand; he moved by crawling. The length of the child's body from head to toe was about six inches less than if his legs had been normal. In other cases, less severe, the legs will look knock-kneed.

Early signs and symptoms of this deficiency include night sweats, flabbiness, obesity, lack of color, and spasms. Rickets usually appears first between the ages of eight and fifteen months, though there is also an adult form of rickets, termed osteomalacia. Where overall nutrition is poor, symptoms are less apparent. Large and fast-growing children are most likely to show symptoms quickly, but there is seldom any evidence of the deficiency before the age of three months. The principal evidence of the disease is the obvious alteration in the skeleton; cranial deformities will appear, along with the many other defects.

For proper formation and maintenance, bones require both calcium and phosphorus. A lack of these elements in the diet is as detrimental to health as vitamin-D deficiency. Sometimes, a diet rich in both calcium and phosphorus might not be available, or the body might have difficulty utilizing these elements because of the chemical forms in which they are ingested. Phosphorus, for instance, cannot be used by the body in its organic form. Moreover, the need for the elements may be increased, as during rapid growth, while the supply stays constant. Even an excess of one mineral can make absorption of the other more difficult. There is, furthermore, a relationship between the parathyroid gland and the calcium content of the blood and bones. A low level of the parathyroid hormone causes a drop in the calcium level of the blood; this resembles the effects of vitamin-D deficiency. Thus it was believed that by giving the parathyroid hormone to a D-deficient patient one could gain a cure. The blood-calcium level would return to normal. This has proven both incorrect and dangerous. While an increase in vitamin D causes a greater amount of calcium to pass through the intestine into the blood stream, an increase of the hormone does not. It raises the calcium content of the blood, by removing it from the bone. This downright theft compounded the problem, and it is fortunate that the error was discovered quite early.

Besides skeletal changes, the deficiency is diagnosed by X-ray examination, by the determination of phosphate levels in the blood, or by therapeutic trial. Analysis of the diet in this case really offers little help. The early symptoms have been mentioned previously, but unfortunately most of the signs of the disease come relatively late. X-rays are not helpful in mild cases, but in moderate and severe cases they can be used both for diagnosis and for observation of the reaction to treatment. The blood serum enzyme, alkaline phosphatase, usually is increased in rickets and this may happen well before blood phosphorus and X-ray changes occur. Its measurement is consequently a valuable tool in early diagnosis. The therapeutic test is probably most valuable, though it is a method of trial and error. In adults mild vitamin-D deficiency is difficult to diagnose by any means.

Preventive treatment may be complicated by environmental factors. Industrialized areas with smog and high buildings cut down the amount of effective sunlight one receives. Long nights and short days in the winter add to the problem. It is essential to supplement the diet of infants with vitamin D even though many infant foods are already vitamin-enriched. In the United Kingdom during the Second World War, the government had to reinforce margarine with vitamin D_2. Such supplemented foods are especially important to the pregnant and nursing mother, as the mother loses calcium and phosphorus to the fetus and she must at the same time keep her own supply at an adequate level. Since vitamins A and D are companions in nature, if one is deficient the other is likely to be also. Hence it would be wiser to take vitamin A and D capsules than simply A alone.

For the treatment of rickets, as much as 5 to 10,000 units of vitamin D per day, even 50,000, may be required in some cases, though three teaspoons of good cod-liver oil should suffice in the average case. Generally all doses are given by mouth. After convalescence is established the cod-liver oil should be adequate in any case. Ultraviolet radiation may be used, though this was far more common twenty-five years ago than now. Signs of healing, which can be detected by X-ray, will appear two to three weeks after treatment is begun, if, of course, the dosage is adequate. Since their cases are usually milder, adults usually respond faster than do children.

Hypervitaminoses

Some vitamins become poisonous if used to excess. Niacin administered in sufficient doses produces a characteristic train of symptoms. A sensation of heat in the upper body and head begins, soon merging into stinging and tingling. The use of niacin in extremely high doses—to lower excessive blood cholesterol—has produced toxic effects such as peptic ulcer and impaired liver function. Vitamin A is stored in the liver; taken in large quantities it is toxic to that organ. Eskimos used to get deathly ill from eating polar bear liver which contains 18,000 units of vitamin A per gram. Though for many years a toxic reaction has been noted in animals, only recently has awareness of toxic effects in man been common. The symptoms and signs in adults may be a greasy, odorous skin, bone and joint pain, weakness and loss of weight and appetite, as well as others.

Vitamin D also may be toxic when taken in large amounts. Poisoning has occurred when massive doses were given for arthritis. Even relatively small doses have been fatal to children. Following several overdoses, there is a deposition of calcium in the various tissues, the danger to the kidneys being particularly great. In less severe cases, there is nausea, vomiting, diarrhea and loss of appetite, as well as weakness and headache. This is not to imply that any danger exists if vitamins are administered therapeutically. It simply is to point out that carelessness or overuse can bring about serious toxic results.

The Vitamin Profile

Many vitamins have been omitted. We have neglected vitamin A, the lack of which causes blindness; nothing has been said of vitamin K, essential for the synthesis of prothrombin in the liver. The K substance assures the proper clotting of the blood. Vitamin B_{12}, essential to growth, normal development of red blood cells and proper peripheral nerve function, has also been omitted. The same for biotin, riboflavin and pantothenic acid, inositol and other members of the B complex.

Besides omission of these vitamins, each of which has its own interesting history and function, we have not discussed the role of vitamins in such things as pregnancy, gastrointestinal diseases, liver diseases, hematology, surgery, and allergic conditions, among others. But hopefully the reader has become aware of two things. First, vitamins do play a vital role in our lives. Secondly, much more remains to be discovered about the function of vitamins. The field of clinical nutrition has yielded much valuable information, but there is much left to be done.

Do vitamins serve as a "tonic" to promote physical fitness? There is no doubt that much exercise creates a greater demand for certain vitamins. If one does not get these additional supplies, the individual will become fatigued. There is no evidence, however, that vitamins can be used to increase one's output in work and/or exercise. Simply by taking vitamins a discus thrower will not add two or three feet to his distance. Vitamins can help keep him fit, but they will not make him a superman.

There *is* a definite relationship between vitamin deficiency and infection. A deficiency of vitamin A makes the epithelial tissues more susceptible to infection. But administration of the vitamin does not cure the infection by acting directly upon it. The susceptibility alone is reduced. In general, infections tend to reduce the amount of vitamin A in the body and supplements may be needed. Likewise, infection increases the demand for vitamin C. The amount of vitamin C in human beings is inadequate to have bactericidal properties, though it no doubt must be present in sufficient amounts to aid the body in fighting infection. An individual with a disease like tuberculosis or malaria requires more vitamin C, but there is no evidence to show any beneficial effects of the supplement upon healing lesions. It is simply fulfilling a general body need. In some instances, when the invading organism needs more of a vitamin than the host, a deficiency might contribute to resistance.

Perhaps the wisest view on vitamins is that of Roger Williams. In his thinking, each of us is as highly individualistic in his chemical make-up as in his own unique facial features. Consequently the need for particular vitamins varies greatly from person to person. One thing is certain: vitamins have a value, though it is sometimes overestimated and at other times underestimated. Certainly they are not miracle drugs or panaceas; but they are essential, and we cannot live without them.

SUPPLEMENTAL READING

Kreig, M. B., Green Medicine: The Search for Plants That Heal, Bantam Books, New York, N.Y., 1966.

Harris, L. J., Vitamins and Vitamin Deficiencies, Churchill, London, 1938.

McCollum, E. V., The Newer Knowledge of Vitamins, Macmillan, New York, N.Y.

Chapter 4

Hardening of the Arteries

The heart in itself is not the beginning
of life; it is a vessel made of dense muscle,
vivified and nourished by the artery
and vein, as are the other muscles.

Leonardo da Vinci
The Notebooks

The heart rests, between beats. Otherwise, its incessant beatings drive the blood, nearly 2,000 gallons of it a day, through 60,000 miles of arteries and veins; drive the blood everywhere and back again in a minute of time. Some think this sturdy organ is as close as nature can come to an unmoved mover. Actually it is not.

The heart, too, has to be fed, and like the rest of our organs, it is fed by arteries and veins which course through this strongest of muscles, and prime it with oxygen and energy. Even the major arteries and veins are traversed by blood vessels, for the feeders must be self-fed. The outer layers of an artery are bathed and nourished by a fine network of vessels; inner layers of blood vessels are fed by nutrients flowing in the onrush of the blood stream. The extensive system of blood vessels, called the vascular system, ramifies like the branches of a bush.

Major diseases of the heart and the vascular system involve:

1. The heart muscle itself. The term "myocarditis" refers to injury, inflammation, or other disease which impairs the strength of the muscle. A damaged heart may not be able to contract as effectively as a normal one. The myocardium is the muscular layer of the heart wall.

2. The rhythm of the heartbeat. For example, tachycardia ("rapid heart") is a condition in which the heart beats very quickly, exceeding one hundred times per minute (adult average is seventy-two). The chambers of the heart fill during *diastole*, the rest period in the beating cycle. If this period is too brief, the chambers cannot fill adequately and the efficiency of the pump declines.

59

3. The valves. The efficiency of a valve may be impaired by (a) incomplete opening, (b) defective closing, and (c) a combination of both. Due most commonly to inborn defects or to the chronic valvulitis or inflammation of the valves in the heart associated with rheumatic fever, the efficiency of the heart's contraction may be reduced through improper fit of the valves, although the strength of contraction may be normal.

4. Diseases of the arteries. The major disease of the arteries is arteriosclerosis, of which atherosclerosis is, by far, the most important kind. Some arteriosclerosis is prevalent among older people and, as such, may be more a natural condition than a disease. Commonly called "hardening of the arteries," arteriosclerosis can, with the onset of age, affect every artery in the body, particularly the larger arteries—the aorta, the coronary arteries that nourish the heart, and the arteries that feed the brain and kidneys. Hardening of the arteries is often accompanied by fat deposits which accumulate in the walls of the arteries' inner lining; this disease is called *atherosclerosis*. These fat deposits or plaques may form in an abnormally rapid manner, so that the arterial walls thicken as well as harden. The blood cannot flow at a sufficient rate through the arteries, thus cutting off the food and oxygen needed by the organs of the body.

Atherosclerosis

The disease does not make a sudden or violent appearance. It takes years for the fatty deposits to accumulate in the arterial walls, to harden, and thus to impede the coursing blood. The name derives from the Greek *athere* meaning "porridge," and *scleros,* "hard." The disease begins with soft, porridge-like deposits in the wall; soon these deposits cement themselves in the blood vessel. Gradually the supply of blood to a given area will be reduced. At this point atherosclerosis begins to have serious consequences. When the narrowed vessel restricts the blood to any extremity, gan-

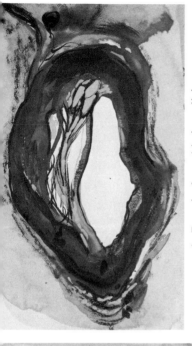

b. Deposits formed in inner lining

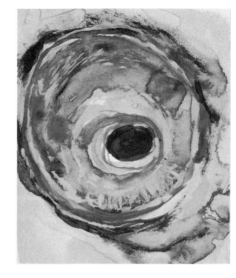

d. The narrowed channel is blocked by a blood clot

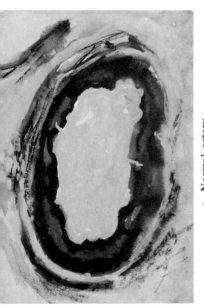

a. Normal artery

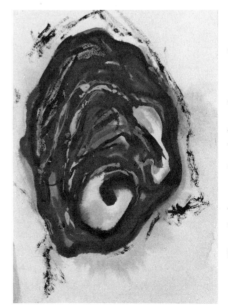

c. Deposits increased and channel narrowed

FIGURE 1. *Gradual development of atherosclerosis in a coronary artery leading to a heart attack. Deposits slowly narrow the artery opening*

grene may set in. When a diseased artery fails to feed the brain properly, a massive or a partial "stroke" may result (Fig. 1).

Quite commonly, atherosclerosis may involve one or more of the arteries in the heart itself: these are called the coronary arteries. The chief diseases of the heart from atherosclerotic vessels are angina pectoris and myocardial infarction. Coronary thrombosis is a synonym for infarction, implying that the damaged artery has been finally closed by the development of a small clot or "thrombus."

Nearly everyone in the United States over the age of 12 has some degree of atherosclerosis. Responsible for 95 percent of all heart attacks, the disease is now the major cause of disability and death and it is clearly on the rise. In a twenty-year study, David M. Spain and his associates showed that in Westchester County, New York, groups of people in similar age range (from 20 to 60) had "a significantly greater amount of atherosclerosis" in the 1950's than in the 1930's. A comparatively similar study by Swedish scientists confirmed this finding in their country (Fig. 2).

Atherosclerosis is not a new disease. Exhumed Egyptian mummies have been autopsied and their arteries have been found to be atherosclerotic. In 1850, Richard Quain published an astonishing treatise, *The Fatty Degeneration of the Heart*; in his study of eighty-three cases, he noted that the arteries in the heart were rough and hardened, some obstructed and nearly ossified. Only in the twentieth century, however, has the disease reached epidemic proportions. Before searching for the cause of the disease, we shall first consider its more serious manifestations.

Angina Pectoris

Atherosclerosis has its chief effect in the arteries of the heart. Even if these arteries are partly clogged, the heart may still be nourished sufficiently—under normal conditions. But the partially diseased arteries may not be able to supply the heart with extra blood when a person has exerted himself. Shoveling snow from a sidewalk, hurrying to catch a bus, walking uphill, any exertion might tip the scales. Walking after meals, even sexual intercourse may possibly be too much effort or excitement for the heart muscle. As

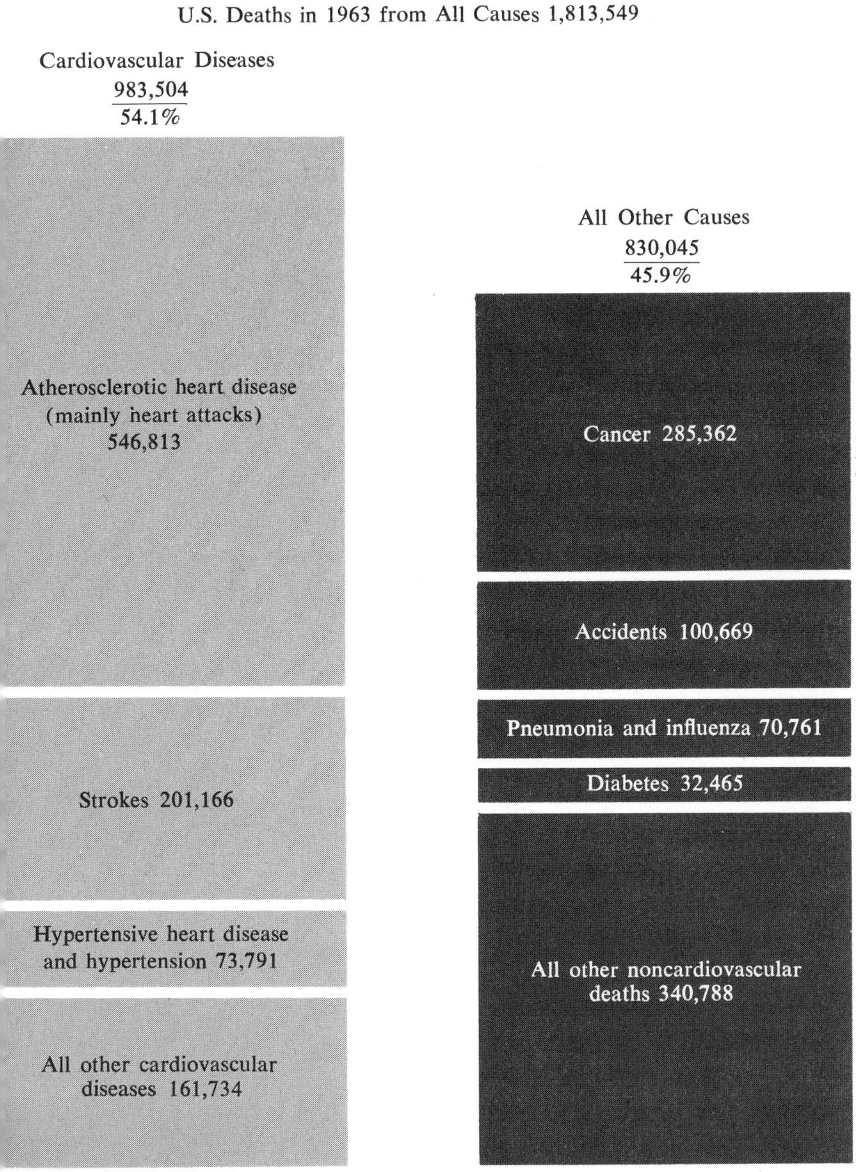

U.S. Deaths in 1963 from All Causes 1,813,549

Cardiovascular Diseases
983,504
54.1%

All Other Causes
830,045
45.9%

Atherosclerotic heart disease
(mainly heart attacks)
546,813

Cancer 285,362

Accidents 100,669

Pneumonia and influenza 70,761

Strokes 201,166

Diabetes 32,465

Hypertensive heart disease
and hypertension 73,791

All other noncardiovascular
deaths 340,788

All other cardiovascular
diseases 161,734

FIGURE 2. *Comparison of deaths from cardiovascular diseases with all other causes. Source: Public health service of the U.S. Dept. of Health, Education and Welfare*

a result, the heart does not stop beating, but a sharp pain, as drastic as a knife-wound, may shoot through the chest.

No one has improved upon William Heberden's first clinical description of the disorder, which he himself named angina pectoris, "a pain of the chest":

> But there is a disorder of the breast marked with strong and peculiar symptoms, considerable for the kind of danger belonging to it, and not extremely rare, which deserves to be mentioned more at length. The seat of it, and sense of strangling, and anxiety with which it is attended, may make it not improperly to be called angina pectoris. Those who are afflicted with it, are seized while they are walking (more especially if it be uphill and soon after eating) with a painful and most disagreeable sensation in the breast, which seems as if it would extinguish life, if it were to increase or to continue; but the moment they stand still, all this uneasiness vanishes.
>
> In all other respects, the patients are, at the beginning of this disorder, perfectly well, and in particular have no shortness of breath from which it is totally different. The pain is sometimes situated in the upper part, sometimes in the middle, sometimes at the bottom of the *os sterni,* and often more inclined to the left than to the right side. It likewise very frequently extends from the breast to the middle of the left arm. The pulse is, at least sometimes, not disturbed by this pain, as I have had opportunities of observing by feeling the pulse during the paroxysm. Males are most liable to this disease, especially such as have passed their fiftieth year. The termination of angina pectoris is remarkable. For, if no accident intervenes, but the disease goes on to its height, the patients all suddenly fall down and perish almost immediately.

So William Heberden wrote from London in 1768. Samuel Johnson called him *ultimus Romanorum,* for he thought of Heberden as the last and the best of the great doctors.

Heberden, of course, did not recognize the relation between the coronary arteries and the pain in the chest. In fact, however, there may be little direct correlation between the amount of heart damage due to the blood-clot and the degree to which a patient suffers. Some individuals seem to suffer pain more than others; and these will feel more keenly the severe anginal pain. "Pain" here is a rather vague word. The "pain" of angina pectoris is a "strangling," as Heberden reported; there are also burning, compressing sensations. The patient feels he is about to die. If the attack is mild, the pain usually goes away in five minutes. Angina itself is not a disease: it is only a symptom of a disease. Thus, the pain may serve to warn the individual that he needs to see a physician.

Myocardial Infarction

The heart muscle is composed of three layers, the endocardium, the myocardium, and the pericardium. By far the largest section of the

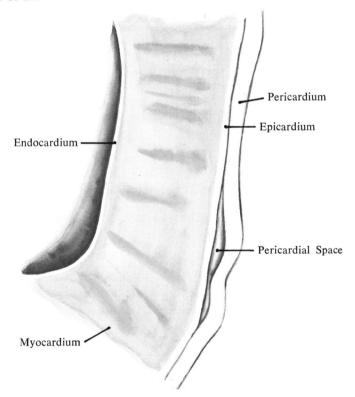

FIGURE 3. *Layers of the heart*

heart wall, the myocardium is the one best supplied with arteries and veins (Fig. 3). It needs to be, for its exertions require the oxygen and foods that the heart turns into pump energy.

Blood attempting to push through a narrow coronary artery may suddenly form a clot. Chances of blood forming a clot in atherosclerotic vessels are even greater. Once the clot is formed, the coronary arteries further on "downstream" are dried up. Unlike other organs, the heart cannot tolerate an "oxygen debt." Other muscles can work overtime for a short while; they can exhaust themselves

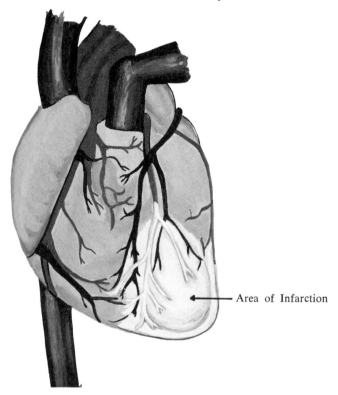

Area of Infarction

FIGURE 4. *Coronary circulation with coronary occlusion*

of food or oxygen. But the heart muscle must be nourished continually; it must not get behind. If an area of the heart is suddenly cut off from its oxygen, that area will "die." This death of a block of starved tissue is called "infarction" (Fig. 4). Hence the name "myocardial infarction" for the loss of working heart muscle. Naturally, the pump damaged by infarction becomes less efficient. Collateral vessels must form around the area of infarction, which will heal by scar tissue, and feed the heart tissue beyond the infarction.

The sudden attack of angina pectoris occurs usually after exertion. Attacks of coronary thrombosis and myocardial infarction happen more frequently at rest, making them unexpected and more frightening. A person will wake up in the middle of the night with a throbbing chest pain which soon parallels the crushing sensation of angina. The pain radiates to the shoulders through the neck to the jaws. But, while the pain of angina lasts only for minutes, the pain of myocardial infarction lasts for hours and morphine may be needed to allay it.

Causes of Atherosclerosis

The debate has not subsided, but most research scientists incriminate fat—either fat in the diet or some wayward aspect of fat metabolism—as one of several factors directly related to atherosclerosis.

Up to five years ago, almost all the evidence supporting this relationship had been obtained by direct experiments with animals. Research, concluded a half century ago, first showed that feeding cholesterol to rabbits could lead to the development of typical lesions in their arteries. In recent years, this has been extended to other animals, up to the monkey. Such experiments, however, still fall short of the critical animal, man.

Because of the obvious difficulties posed by this last and most crucial experiment, the evidence in man has been sought indirectly, through large-scale population studies. Some experiments have led to undeniable proof that groups of patients with sound clinical evidence of coronary artery disease have higher blood lipids (in general, fats) than comparable groups of normals. This is certainly true for Americans, a well-fed people, and it appears to be valid for some other population groups as well. In the study of populations on a world-wide basis, it is also strongly suggested that the nature of the diet is correlated with the lipid levels in the plasma (the fluid portion of the blood) and the incidence of atherosclerosis. Tentative conclusions indicate that diet is more important than, for example, race.

Most of these studies have concentrated upon the amount, others upon the kinds of fat eaten by one group as opposed to another. They have succeeded in demonstrating that populations eating larger amounts of animal fat seem to have more atherosclerosis. The studies have not yet proved a cause-and-effect relationship and have not attempted to rule out all other variables—even in the diet.

Finally, although most advances have been made in correlating the metabolism of lipids by the body with atherosclerosis, there are other areas, some unrelated, of progress. There is now convincing statistical evidence that hypertension (high blood pressure) accelerates the development of atherosclerosis. Internal injury and other local effects have been demonstrated to be of importance; and various aspects of the blood-clotting mechanism, especially the blood platelets, are being given increasing attention.

It is often pointed out that death from atherosclerosis among the Bantus of South Africa is rare, the reason being their low-fat diet—17 percent of the total caloric intake. In western Europe the caloric intake of fats is about 35 percent, and in America well over 40 percent. In these areas of the world atherosclerosis is now the major killer. Moreover, the serum-cholesterol level in the blood of a Bantu is a mere 150 milligrams per 100 c.c. of blood plasma as compared with the 225 to 250 in the European and American adult. The measurement of blood fats, like cholesterol and triglycerides, constitutes a worthwhile clinical test for screening patients who may have a greater tendency for atherosclerosis. Yet, while blood lipid measurements certainly do help single patients prone to an accelerated development of atherosclerosis, every physician is aware that many patients may still have severe atherosclerotic coronary arteries with blood lipid values well below the considered upper limit of "normal" for our population.

Lipoprotein Measurements

All the fats in the blood circulate bound to protein. The cholesterol, phospholipids and the triglycerides are present in the blood plasma in combinations of fat and protein called "lipoproteins." The lipoproteins contained in the plasma of a normal human may be considered for convenience in two great groups, arbitrarily called the "low-density" and the "high-density" lipoproteins. Each group contains several subspecies of lipoproteins.

The low-density lipoproteins in a group of patients with coronary arterial disease are significantly higher than in a group of similar age and sex who are free of clinical evidence of atherosclerosis. Strictly speaking, measurements of plasma cholesterol and plasma low-density lipoproteins are not the same. With the lipoproteins one also indirectly obtains a measurement of other lipids, particularly the triglycerides, which make up more of the lipoprotein molecules of lower density. About two-thirds of the cholesterol normally present in plasma is carried in the low-density lipoproteins. For reasons only poorly understood, it so happens that an elevation in plasma cholesterol usually expresses itself in a raised concentration of some or all of the low-density lipoproteins. Hence measurement of cholesterol does give a rough index of low-density lipoprotein levels.

Diet and Atherosclerosis

The exact relationship between dietary fats, cholesterol in the blood, and atherosclerosis is still a large and unsolved problem. Large-scale population studies suggest a relationship between the dietary fat and atherosclerosis. On the basis of sound experimental research, a relationship between dietary fats, plasma cholesterol and lipoproteins likewise seems to be established. Yet not enough evidence exists to be absolutely certain that these three factors are sequentially related—that dietary fat is related, through the amounts of cholesterol and glycerides in plasma, to the development of atherosclerosis. The evidence necessary to forge this crucial link in the chain is still unfound.

There are several aspects of the diet under scrutiny in the "hunt through the kitchen" for causes of atherosclerosis. One is the amount of cholesterol (relatively high in egg yolks, meats, milk) that is eaten. Probably the amounts of cholesterol *per se* that can be found in the American diet directly influence the cholesterol level in the plasma. Recent years have seen emphasis extended to the triglycerides or esters of fatty acids and glycerol, which make up most of the body and dietary fat. These dietary constituents have also been shown to affect plasma cholesterol in experimental studies in man.

The triglycerides consist mainly of fatty acids which may differ chemically in several ways. One important difference is the degree to which hydrogen has saturated the bonds linking the carbon atoms in the fatty acid chain. Acids containing double bonds are called unsaturated acids, because they can absorb more hydrogen at these linkages. When a hydrogen atom replaces one bond of the double bond, the linkage becomes "saturated." The saturated acids have *no* carbon-to-carbon double bonds (Fig. 5).

Unsaturated   Saturated

FIGURE 5. *Diagram of a saturated and an unsaturated compound*

With the exception of one vegetable fat, cocoanut oil, most saturated fats are of animal origin, such as milk and egg fats, and many meat fats. Most *unsaturated* fats, such as olive, peanut, cottonseed, corn, soybean and safflower oils, come from plants, and yet, some of the most unsaturated fats, such as the fish oils, may be animal in origin. Commercially, hydrogen is added to many naturally unsaturated fats to protect against rancidity and alter their textures for various purposes.

Good evidence, based so far on experimental diets, indicates that there is a very real difference between the effect of certain dietary fats on cholesterol in the plasma. When given in large amounts (50 to 100 grams per day) the more saturated (and cholesterol-rich) animal fats will raise the plasma cholesterol. When these fats are replaced by large amounts of unsaturated fats, such as corn oil, the cholesterol level is lowered. There is no question about these experimental facts at the present time, although it is still not certain how much relative importance to give the cholesterol content as opposed to the degree of saturation of the glycerides.

Is, then, vegetable fat (oleomargarine) healthier than animal fat (butter)? The answer is unknown. Oleomargarine usually consists of a mixture of naturally unsaturated cottonseed and soybean oils. However, partly because the housewife may not like her spreads to run at room temperature, and for other reasons too, oleomargarine is partially hydrogenated. While few if any studies have been made using oleomargarine as the *only* source of fat, extensively hydrogenated vegetable oils tend to behave like the more saturated animal fats in their effect on plasma cholesterol. Hence the origin of fat is probably less important than the subsequent handling, if it includes hydrogenation.

No one knows yet for sure whether altering the fat in the diet will reduce in any way the amount of atherosclerosis. Even on the basis of what we now know, many nutritionists are reluctant to recommend sweeping changes in the diet for everyone. Also, it is not known if radical changes in the diet in human beings will cause atherosclerotic lesions to regress or to disappear.

The way calories of any kind are used is also important—hence one of the arguments for exercise. The sedentary man needs to worry more about what he eats than the heavy laborer. One's genes also have a great deal to do with how much one's lipoproteins are affected by the food one eats. Oddly enough, there are some middle-aged, overweight people, often with a family history of diabetes, who develop higher levels of some lipoproteins and glycerides on high carbohydrate (sugar and starch) diets than on high fat diets. For some people, dietary instruction from their physician is in order. The best working hypothesis today is based on the observation that high levels of fats and lipoproteins in the blood are related in some way to atherosclerosis, and that these blood components can be affected by diet. The modifications in diet necessary to produce presumably desirable changes in blood lipids appear to be relatively safe as long as the diet remains balanced for essential food factors and is designed for proper weight control. This leaves out "fad diets." Probably when all the factors involved become clearer, it will be necessary to modify the diet in young people, for changes in middle age may be too late. This may be the only sober thought one can entertain on fats.

Estrogens

Women are more durable than men. And one of the reasons is that they suffer far less than men from heart disease. Myocardial infarction is far less common among young women. For every woman who suffers a heart attack before the age of 50, there are 20 men. At every age men seem to suffer more from atherosclerosis; 4 men per 1,000 will suffer some form of coronary heart disease at age 30; by age 70, the prevalence will be 115.5 per 1,000. Women at age 30 suffer 1.6 per 1,000; and at 70, only 79.0 per 1,000. Nonetheless, the women begin losing their high immunity after menopause, and this seems to indicate that female hormones play an active role in preventing atherosclerosis.

Research scientists have been studying estrogens, which are female sex hormones, for over 15 years, but as yet they are unsure how the hormones may reduce the frequency of atherosclerotic plaques in arteries. Some argue that the estrogens actually prevent the synthesis of cholesterol, others that estrogens increase the amount of cholesterol that becomes synthesized to bile acids. Or, perhaps, estrogens carry cholesterol out of the blood stream, where it does the most damage, to other parts of the body.

In any case, the weight of evidence points to estrogens as possible lipid-lowering drugs.

1. Castrated male rabbits were fed massive amounts of cholesterol for four months. They were also injected with ethinyl estradiol, an estrogen. The cholesterol and phospholipid levels in the plasma were lowered.
2. Rabbits feeding on alfalfa, rich in natural estrogens, were found to have low levels of serum cholesterol. When they were given a nutritionally-equivalent, but alfalfa-free diet, the levels of serum cholesterol suddenly rose.
3. The livers of female rats oxidized radioactive cholesterol somewhat better than did the livers of male rats.
4. Ovarectomized women showed a marked increase in coronary heart disease compared with normal women in the same age group.

Estrogen therapy, however, has some annoying side effects in men. Introducing a female hormone into a man leads to feminization:

testicular atrophy, loss of libido and potency, enlarged breasts. For many, the side effects are far worse than the disease. Thus far, the dosage of all estrogenic preparations must be pushed to the point where the patient has the usual unsatisfactory side effects before appreciable changes in blood lipids are observed.

There are, at present, several long-term studies in progress on the effect of the estrogens on the longevity of patients surviving myocardial infarctions. They have not yet established conclusions. The use of estrogens in patients with abnormally high concentrations of fat in the blood, but without other complications, is still mainly experimental. For women, especially under 50, they are unneeded. For men, they seem to decrease atherosclerosis in direct proportion to their inducing feminization. Unless an estrogen-like drug can be found that will produce the desired effect and not have the bad, estrogen therapy will probably never be applicable on a large scale.

Nicotinic Acid

Scientists at the University of Saskatchewan conducted experiments on the formation of cholesterol fifteen years ago. In 1955, they announced that nicotinic acid (niacin) reduces the level of cholesterol in the blood plasma. A dose of 3 to 6 grams daily was enough to lower the levels of cholesterol to the "normal" range in patients whose levels were 15 to 30 percent higher than average.

There have been several major studies on the use of nicotinic acid. In one, adults suffering from hypercholesterolemia (high level of cholesterol in the blood) lived on a diet of alternately saturated and unsaturated fats, for anywhere from four to six months. Lower serum concentrations of cholesterol, phospholipids, and total esters were measured when the diet contained chiefly unsaturated fat or after doses of nicotinic acid were given. As might be expected, the lowest levels were obtained when the diet was high in unsaturated fats and when nicotinic acid was being administered at the same time.

In another study, a group of hypercholesterolemic patients were observed for periods from 12 to 44 months. The following results of nicotinic acid therapy were obtained:

(a) In 80 percent, a reduction to "normal" serum cholestrol and β-lipoprotein cholesterol.

(b) In 18 percent, both levels reduced, but not to normal.

(c) In 2 percent, no reduction of any significance.

Another study was made over a period of six years. Daily doses of 4 grams of nicotinic acid were given to patients with atherosclerosis and hyperlipemia (milky blood due to high concentrations of glycerides), or with other evidence of abnormal metabolism of fats. In general, nicotinic acid sharply reduced the cholesterol levels in the blood plasma.

No one yet is sure how nicotinic acid prevents high levels of cholesterol from building up in the plasma. An amide of nicotinic acid is used against the vitamin deficiency disease—pellagra. But this amide vitamin does not lower cholesterol, and hence the roles of the vitamin and of the drug do not appear to be related. While it is possible that nicotinic acid may interfere with the formation of cholesterol, it may also affect the distribution of it. One noteworthy action of nicotinic acid is its ability to block the mobilization of fat from the depot stores in the adipose (fatty) tissue. This may be the reason the drug seems to be particularly effective in lowering elevated levels of blood glycerides. Although the drug disturbs certain enzymatic functions of the liver, these effects are neither serious nor persistent after the drug is stopped. Today, nicotinic acid is one of the drugs of choice for lowering cholesterol, especially when the blood glycerides are elevated as well.

Sitosterols, Heparin, Dextrothyroxine

Sitosterols are cholesterol-like substances found in plants. Careful experiments have shown that daily ingestion of large amounts of sitosterols can lower serum cholesterol. Some experimentalists believe that part of the vegetable oil effect on serum cholesterol may be due to the presence of sitosterols. The sitosterols are not absorbed, but they interfere with absorption of cholesterol in the intestine, both that coming in from the diet and that made in the body and secreted into the intestine. Generally, sitosterols will cause about a 10 to 15 percent reduction in plasma cholesterol, but this is not consistently obtained. A major problem, as with all drugs, is the necessity of continued administration for continued effect. This, plus the considerable bulk of the drug required, limits enthusiasm for wider use of sitosterol preparations.

There are two possible rationales for using heparin. One is its anticoagulant effect, to be dealt with later. The other is the interesting fact that heparin causes the release into the blood stream of a "clearing factor," or "lipoprotein lipase," an enzyme that catalyzes the break-up of the triglycerides. Such enzymatic activity may change hyperlipemic blood from a creamy to a clear state. Heparin is being used in several large experimental studies. It has been reported to increase the longevity of patients, following myocardial infarction. If this is true, it is still unknown whether this is due to the anticoagulant effect or to the effect on the clearing enzyme. Chronic use of heparin is expensive; it has to be given by injection and its use must be closely supervised by a physician. Long-term clinical trials with heparin in patients surviving myocardial infarction are continuing. Its use in patients with abnormal blood lipids but without coronary artery disease is still experimental.

Hypothyroidism (deficiency) and hypercholesterolemia (excess) often occur simultaneously; conversely, individuals with overactive thyroid glands usually have low cholesterol levels in their plasma. As a result, research scientists have attempted to find a drug that will imitate these effects of a thyroid hormone without inducing the usual effects of the hormone, an increase of body metabolism and weight loss. Such a drug is dextrothyroxine, a chemical "isomer" of the natural hormone. It is believed to be able to lower cholesterol without increasing body metabolism. The drug has to be used very cautiously in patients with angina, however, for it may make this condition worse, a price too high for a lower level of cholesterol.

The search goes on for an anti-cholesterol drug. The problem consists largely of side effects. Scientists want to interfere with the complex synthesis of cholesterol at the right point. If they interfere with the synthesis too early, needed hormones and lipids will be strangled in the embryonic stage. Yet if they interfere with the synthesis of cholesterol too late, an excess of some similar genetic agent may accumulate. Everyone agrees that the interference with cholesterol synthesis is a valid method of attack. The point is where?

Some drug companies were recently prosecuted for failure to submit to the Food and Drug Administration full details on toxicity associated with the anti-cholesterol drug, triparanol. This is an effective blocker of cholesterol-synthesis at the last stage in the long chain of synthetic reactions leading to its formation. As a result, desmosterol (cholesterol with one extra double-bond) accumulated in the blood and tissues. This was associated with side effects, such as temporary loss of hair, dryness of the skin, cataracts in some people; some of the hundreds of thousands who took the drug in the early 1960's were affected. Triparanol represents a sobering example of how difficult it is to devise a drug that regulates the synthesis of a vital body component effectively and safely.

Nitroglycerin and Anticoagulant Drugs

Long-term treatment of angina pectoris and coronary atherosclerosis may well take into account both diet and some anti-cholesterol drug. But when an attack of angina occurs, the patient needs immediate relief. One such drug, capable of doing this, has been in use since 1879; this is the well-known explosive, nitroglycerin. The drug is so rapid in its action that a patient who can anticipate an attack of angina can actually prevent the attack by taking a pill. The drug's effects last for about ten minutes and then quickly disappear.

There are currently two hypotheses about the action of nitroglycerin. The first one contends that the drug induces the coronary arteries to dilate, and thus to increase the blood supply to the heart and muscle. In an experiment on dogs, nitroglycerin was shown to increase the flow of blood in the heart, although blood pressure and heart rate were constant. It is still an open question whether the hardened atherosclerotic arteries in the heart have enough elasticity to dilate at all. In any case, in coronary thrombosis the collateral vessels seem to be opened up more quickly upon contact with nitroglycerin.

Another hypothesis holds that nitroglycerin lowers the oxygen requirement of the heart. It is known that the drug affects chiefly left ventricular function (the side pumping blood to the body, as opposed to the lungs). Nitroglycerin reduces arterial blood pressure in the same manner as an anti-hypertensive drug. All in all, nitroglycerin is like aspirin, another invaluable old drug; very little is known about its action at the cellular level.

Another way to combat a heart attack lies in altering the coagulability of the blood. Here the body's defenses are strengthened, as it were, before the attack can materialize. Arteries severely roughened by atherosclerosis may trick the platelets in the blood stream into acting as if there were an open wound, thus triggering the clotting mechanism. The anticoagulants prevent the formation of a clot by tampering with the clotting mechanism. Administering too much of an anticoagulant drug to a patient, of course, results in a condition simulating hemophilia; the blood cannot clot at all. But there should be some amount, varying with the individual, which could prevent a clot from forming in a coronary artery (coronary thrombosis), a cerebral artery (stroke), or an extremity (gangrene). Doctors are far from agreement about the value of using anticoagulants to prevent the conditions which may derive from atherosclerosis.

In an extended study, Drs. Kurt Iverson and Michael Schwartz observed 1,400 patients who suffered from heart disease. Among those taking an anticoagulant, 40.9 percent died within four years. 30.9 percent of those who were *not* taking an anticoagulant died in the same period. The evidence clearly does not suggest that anticoagulant therapy will increase the life expectancy of those who have had a myocardial infarction.

Yet there are other statistics to the contrary. In another study of anticoagulant drugs, 80 patients who had suffered from myocardial infarction were given the anticoagulants, heparin and bishydroxycoumarin; 100 patients were used as a control and were not treated with either drug. In this study anticoagulant treatment reduced the incidence of further thrombosis from 20 percent in the control group to 5 percent in the anticoagulant group, and deaths were reduced by 15 percent. In an early study supported by the National Heart Institute of Bethesda, Maryland, 1,000 patients were observed in 16 hospitals. Six hundred of these were treated with a standard anticoagulant. The scientists concluded that the proper use of anticoagulant therapy was strongly advisable. And in yet another study of bishydroxycoumarin, deaths were reduced a full 20% among patients who had suffered acute myocardial infarction.

One must not be too impatient with the difficulty of resolving contradictions in the apparent value of anticoagulants. Each patient with a myocardial infarct represents a complicated situation, too complex to be considered as a simple experimental variable. His physician's first consideration is—quite properly—saving the patient's life in an acute and perilous situation. Even after the acute phase, each patient's course is an individual one and drug trials may require many hundreds of patients before any conclusions can be reached.

There are other difficulties with this class of drug. The relationship between coagulation and atherosclerosis has not yet been determined. Moreover, an abnormal tendency to coagulate may not exist in the blood, except minutes—even seconds—before the blood actually clots. Finally, excessive doses of anticoagulants can lead to easy bruising and, occasionally, internal hemorrhage. In fact, it was on the basis of hemorrhage that the first oral anticoagulant was discovered in 1941 by Dr. Karl P. Link in Wisconsin. Cows which had been feeding on sweet clover hay had died of internal bleeding. Dr. Link discovered that a substance, a derivative of coumarin, found in spoiled sweet clover, was the cause of hemorrhaging. Derivatives of coumarin lower the blood content of prothrombin, the circulating precursor of thrombin. Thrombin and calcium act together to convert another circulating protein, fibrinogen, to fibrin. Blood clots consist mainly of strands of fibrin. The dose of the coumarin drugs is regulated by following the prothrombin content of the blood. An overdose can be quickly corrected by giving vitamin K.

The oldest anticoagulant, and it is still in use, is heparin. Heparin acts differently than coumarin, affecting the clotting mechanism at an earlier and different stage. The coumarin drugs take several days to be effective, heparin acts at once. Hence patients with a coronary thrombus are usually given both a coumarin drug and heparin. After a few days, when the coumarin has become maximally effective, heparin is stopped. Heparin is the drug used during open-heart surgery to keep the blood in the heart-lung machine fluid.

After the operation is over, protamine, an antagonist of heparin, is given quickly to return the clotting mechanism to normal and also to prevent undesirable hemorrhage during convalescence.

Most recently, drugs which dissolve clots already formed— the so-called fibrinolytic drugs—have become available in limited supply. The blood-clotting process is more complex than was just described. Floating in the blood plasma along with red and white corpuscles are the platelets. Whenever the platelets run up against a torn blood vessel—or even a rough inner surface such as in an atherosclerotic artery—they stick together and undergo other changes that set the blood-clotting mechanism into operation. Out of the platelets comes thrombokinase, an enzyme, which accelerates the clotting process.

Streptokinase, an enzyme, comes from a strain of the bacterium streptococcus that does not cause disease in man. When administered, this enzyme combines with a circulating protein to produce another protein, fibrinolysin. Fibrinolysin attacks the fibrin in clots and breaks it down, allowing the products to be washed away in the bloodstream. Unfortunately, streptokinase is a foreign agent in the body, and can sometimes produce allergic reactions. The body may also build up resistance to the drug, making it less effective over long periods of time.

From human urine another fibrinolytic drug, urokinase, is extracted, and this is not foreign to the body. The drug, only recently under investigation, is receiving considerable attention as a possible agent for treating patients with a coronary thrombosis or with a tendency to form clots in other parts of the body. Since it is present in the urine only in minute amounts, the procedures for isolating and purifying it are very tedious and costly.

Atherosclerosis is what scientists call an "iceberg." Although all of us have it to some extent, it may lie "beneath the surface" for 50 to 60 years unexposed, until angina pectoris, myocardial infarction, or blockage of blood flow in another part of the body occurs. At present, there are no easy tests to determine the degree to which an artery is thickened. X-rays of blood vessels made after filling them with radio-opaque liquid can be diagnostic, but these methods are not fool-proof. And even severely constricted arteries may be as durable as the wonderful one-horse shay.

SUPPLEMENTAL READING

Dietary fat and human health. Publication 1147, National Academy of Sciences, National Research Council, 1966.

The Coronary Spectrum, Journal of Rehabilitation, March–April, 1966.

Special Communication: Dietary fat and its relation to heart attacks and strokes. JAMA *175*:389–391, 1961.

Fredrickson, D. S.: Current attitudes about atherosclerosis. G. P. *18*: 102–106, 1958.

Blakeslee, A., and Stamler, J.: Your Heart Has Nine Lives. Pocket Books, Inc., New York, 1963.

Chapter 5

Digitalis for the Failing Heart

The foxglove, one by one,
Upwards through every stage of the tall stem,
Had shed beside the public way its bells,
And stood of all dismantled, save the last
Left at the tapering ladder's top, that seemed
To bend as doth a slender blade of grass
Tipped with a rain-drop.

Wordsworth *The Prelude* VIII

Foxglove is a tall flowering plant, sometimes rising to a height of five feet. The crimson bell-shaped blossoms open up and down the stalk during July and August. Then they drop off slowly, until the stalk is quite denuded—perhaps explaining why in the Middle Ages the plant was used as an emblem for the motto "Pride goeth before a fall." The flower grows wild all over western Europe, particularly in dry and hilly lands, by roads, in rocky semi-shaded places. Dark purple blossoms denote the species *purpurea,* but botanists have included even white varieties in the same species; other species of the plant may have differently colored flowers. When the flowers die, the dull green leaves become more apparent. They are elliptical in shape, like fingers. In fact, in southern Scotland, the plant is called "bloody fingers," in Wales "elf's gloves," in Germany *Fingerhut.* Possibly for this reason the Bavarian botanist Leonhard Fuchs, in his Latin herbal *De Historia Stirpium* published in 1542, gave the genus the name "like a finger," *Digitalis.* (Fig. 1.)

Brown Waters

For hundreds of years, peasant women in Shropshire, England, and probably elsewhere, gathered the finger-shaped leaves of the foxglove in flower, pounded them, and collected the gray-green powder. Taken with water, this was a cure for dropsy. "Dropsy" is an archaic term meaning the collection of fluid under the skin; water accumulates in body cavities and in the intercellular spaces of the tissues, causing swelling of the abdomen, the knees, and the ankles. Edema, as it is called, is commonly related to a heart ailment. In the second chapter of George Eliot's *Silas Marner* (1861), Silas gives "a simple preparation of foxglove" to a cobbler's wife who is suffering from dropsy. He says it is a remedy from a lore he

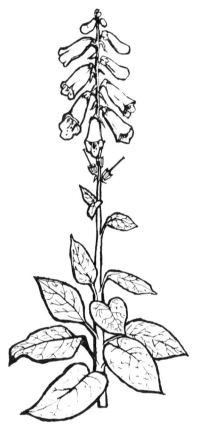

Digitalis purpurea

FIGURE 5. *Foxglove*

learned from his mother. Its success, where other concoctions had failed, raises Silas in the esteem of his new customers:

> The fact of her having found relief from drinking Silas Marner's "stuff" became a matter of general discourse. When Doctor Kimble gave physic, it was natural that it should have an effect; but when a weaver, who came from nobody knew where, worked wonders with a bottle of brown waters, the occult character of the process was evident.

William Withering first noted the effects of foxglove on the heart in the last quarter of the eighteenth century. In Shropshire, where he practiced for a time, he noted that farm wives were using the leaves for dropsy. He was particularly interested in the recipe of "an old woman of Shropshire" who had sometimes made cures after more regular practitioners had failed. In 1776, he borrowed her recipe, a compost of herbs in which he determined the active ingredient to be foxglove, and he carefully described the course of his medication.

"On the 25th of July I was desired to meet Dr. Darwin at the lady's house. I found her nearly in a state of suffocation; her pulse extremely weak and irregular, her breath very short and laborious, her countenance sunk, her arms of a leaden colour, clammy and cold. She could not lie down in bed and had neither strength nor appetite, but was extremely thirsty; her stomach, legs, and thighs were greatly swollen; her urine very small in quantity, not much more than a spoonful at a time, and that very seldom. It had been proposed to scarify her legs, but the proposition was not acceded to. She had experienced no relief from any means that had been used, except from ipecacuanha vomits; the dose of which had been gradually increased from 15 to 40 grains, but such was the insensible state of her stomach for the last few days, that even those very large doses failed to make her sick, and consequently purged her. In this situation I knew of nothing likely to avail us, except Digitalis: but this I hesitated to propose, from an apprehension that little could be expected from anything, that an unfavorable termination would tend to discredit a medicine which promised to be of great benefit to mankind, and I might be censured for a prescription which could not be countenanced by the experience of any other regular practitioner. But these considerations soon gave way to the desire of preserving the life of this valuable woman, and accordingly I proposed the Digitalis to be tried; adding, that I sometimes had found it to succeed when other, even the most judicious methods, had failed. Dr. Darwin very politely acceded immediately to my proposition, and, as he had never seen it given, left the preparation and the dose to my direction . . .

"The patient took five of these draughts, which made her very sick, and acted very powerfully upon the kidneys, for within the first twenty-four hours she made upwards of eight quarts of water. The sense of fullness and oppression across her stomach was greatly diminished, her breath was eased, her pulse became more full and more regular, and the swellings of her legs subsided." On the 26th of July he writes triumphantly of "our patient thus snatched from impending destruction."

Withering continued to experiment, and in 1785 published a medical classic, *An Account of the Foxglove and Some of its Medical Uses.* He warns that the drug which "has a power over the motion of the heart to a degree yet unobserved in any other medicine" should not be applied without "some instruction, however imperfect, from my experience." It was, he believed, essential that people heed his instructions on the use of "a medicine of so much efficacy," otherwise the "lives of men [would be] hazarded by its unguarded exhibition . . . and [the drug] condemned and rejected as dangerous and unmanageable."

Withering receives credit for the first scientific use of digitalis, one of the few classical drugs that has continually grown in use until today it is the leading heart drug. In the painting by Carl Frederik von Breda, Withering is portrayed with two short, flowering foxgloves in his left hand. In the Edgbaston churchyard foxgloves still bloom, descendents of the shoots he planted; from the flowers of this churchyard, the plant was brought to America where it is now widely cultivated. Significantly enough, in the Old Edgbaston Church at Birmingham, England, where he lies buried, a foxglove is carved on a tablet set up to his memory.

Congestive Heart Failure

Many patients with different kinds of heart ailments may develop congestive heart failure sooner or later. In this disorder the heart cannot carry its pumping load. The heart loses its effectiveness, for example, when it beats irregularly (arrythmia), or is beating too quickly (tachycardia), or when its valves are faulty, or the heart muscle (myocardium) is damaged by a disease, or has its load markedly increased as with high blood pressure (hypertension). Before observing some of these diseases more closely, let us look at the heart as a pump, an engineering marvel of considerable endurance (Fig. 2 and Fig. 3).

In the rest period, or diastole, blood enters the right atrium (auricle) of the heart from two large veins, the superior and inferior venae cavae, which drain respectively the upper and lower areas

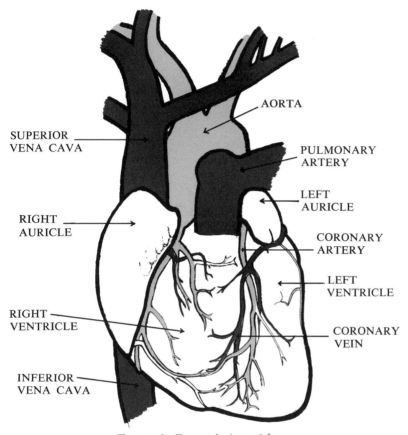

AORTA

SUPERIOR
VENA CAVA

PULMONARY
ARTERY

LEFT
AURICLE

RIGHT
AURICLE

CORONARY
ARTERY

LEFT
VENTRICLE

RIGHT
VENTRICLE

CORONARY
VEIN

INFERIOR
VENA CAVA

FIGURE 2. *External view of heart*

of the body. Impelled by the force of the contracting right atrium, the blood flows through the tricuspid valve into the right ventricle. The filled ventricle contracts in the phase called systole, the energy-expending period of the heartbeat, briefer than diastole, in which the muscle relaxes. From the right ventricle blood is pumped via the pulmonary arteries into the lungs where it is oxygenated. Then it returns via the pulmonary veins and enters the left atrium of the heart. This chamber empties into the left ventricle. This ventricle, more muscular than the right one, supplies the greater or "systemic" circulation with freshly oxygenated blood. The blood leaves the left ventricle by way of the body's largest artery, the aorta, whose branches go out to all tissues of the body. Both ventricles contract at the same time, the left being activated ever so slightly sooner than the right. Systole and diastole are repeated about seventy times a minute, for a lifetime, over two and one-half billion times for the individual who reaches the age of seventy.

The normal function of the heart requires a dependable rhythm of the beat and an efficient degree of contraction. The heart is of course really two pumps working side by side. If the right-sided pump breaks down, congestion develops in the veins that normally pour their deoxygenated blood into the right atrium. Blood is not speedily removed from the right ventricle and backs up. Pressure builds up in the veins, and thus fluid in the intercellular spaces is less able to drain into the veins against this pressure. As a result, "fluid" accumulates in the body.

If the left-sided pump breaks down, the pulmonary veins cannot as readily spill their blood into the left atrium. Now fluid accumulates in the lungs, causing shortness of breath and pulmonary rales, which are abnormal respiratory sounds. Left-sided heart failure frequently results from high blood pressure. The inefficiency of the heart becomes a vicious circle. When one pump is ineffective for a long period of time, it causes the other to overwork, so that in time it breaks down too.

The heart's efficiency can be more clearly illustrated by drawing an analogy between a living organism and a physical machine. The efficiency of a machine is related to the amount of energy required to do a given amount of useful work. Heart work (W) may be considered as the product of the blood pressure (P) times the volume of blood (V) which is moved during a beat, the "stroke volume":

$$W = P \times V$$

In heart failure, the heart actually requires *more* oxygen than it does under normal conditions. That is, the same amount of work requires more oxygen, an increase of energy input, while the efficiency of the heart is markedly decreased. As the heart loses its efficiency, it strains to do its work and enlarges; this adds to its requirement for more oxygen and thus a greater blood supply. There are two types of enlargement: increase in muscle mass is called cardiac hypertrophy; increase in size of the chambers, owing to the lengthening of muscle fibers, is called dilatation.

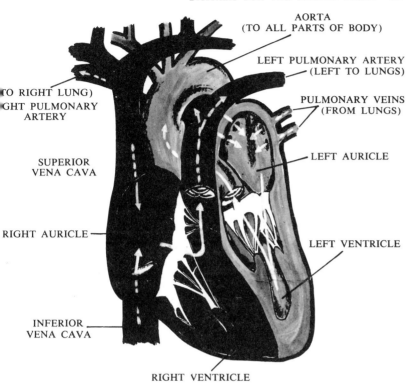

AORTA
(TO ALL PARTS OF BODY)

LEFT PULMONARY ARTERY
(LEFT TO LUNGS)

TO RIGHT LUNG)
GHT PULMONARY
ARTERY

PULMONARY VEINS
(FROM LUNGS)

SUPERIOR
VENA CAVA

LEFT AURICLE

RIGHT AURICLE

LEFT VENTRICLE

INFERIOR
VENA CAVA

RIGHT VENTRICLE

FIGURE 3. *The flow of blood through the heart*

There is an important rule about heart muscle work developed by a well-known physiologist. This is Starling's Law and according to it the energy of the contracting muscle increases as its length at rest is increased. Like a thick elastic, the larger it is and the further one pulls it, the more quickly it will snap back. Now when the heart is working under some difficulty, its muscle fibers will lengthen in an attempt to gain more energy to pump blood. This dilatation exacts a payment, however, for increased potential energy. A contracting, elastic sphere of small diameter can expel a given volume of its contents with less energy than if the diameter of the sphere were large. When the heart is small (the size of your fist), the pump works at a peak of efficiency. An enlarged heart alters Nature's carefully architectured design. As the chambers swell, their openings are distorted and the valves open or close less effectively. This either obstructs the outflow of blood or allows it to leak back into a chamber from which it has just been expelled.

The Action of Digitalis

Digitalis increases the force of contraction of the heart muscle and thus improves its efficiency. At the same time the drug can have a favorable effect on certain abnormalities of cardiac rhythm, changing a rapid rate to a slower one. The combination of greater force of ventricular contraction and a more normal rhythm increases the output of blood per beat. No other drug, besides the various glycosides of digitalis and related compounds, can simultaneously achieve these two vital improvements. Certain digitalis preparations, moreover, can take effect within an hour if administered by injection.

To combat the deficiency in the output of blood which results from congestive heart failure, digitalis acts directly on the ability of the muscles to flex themselves, forcing out more blood per beat. With a slower beating more time is allotted for the heart to fill up with blood. The systemic veins can in turn empty themselves, easing congestion and reducing "fluid" throughout the body. Likewise the pulmonary veins leading from the lungs to the left atrium, can drain off the backed-up "fluid" in the lungs. Besides, bodily tissues suffering in various ways from a deficiency of food and oxygen are relieved by a more ample supply of blood coursing through the arteries per minute.

Digitalis can change the heart rate by at least two mechanisms. It decreases conduction of the beat transmitted from the atria to the ventricles, markedly slowing heartbeat, i.e., rate of contraction of the ventricles. When the auricles are in one or another kind of excessively rapid rhythm like auricular fibrillation, this can be a very valuable effect. Also, digitalis irritates the ventricles themselves, and this irritation may trigger undesirable "extra-beats." Watching the heart rate and rhythm is essential for adjusting the dosage of this drug.

About one in five patients who are given digitalis in a general hospital suffer some kind of toxicity, but rarely of a serious nature. Part of the difficulty lies in the often-mentioned problem that the most effective dose is usually quite close to the amount causing toxic or other side effects. Dr. Withering was aware of this and commented upon it: "If inadvertently the doses of the foxglove should be prescribed too largely, exhibited too rapidly, or urged to too great length, the knowledge of a remedy to counteract its effect would be a desirable thing. Such a remedy may perhaps in time be discovered." Today, however, we are less likely to apply his cure for an overdose: "I have sometimes thought small doses of opium useful."

Perhaps when scientists learn how digitalis acts at the molecular level in the heart, they will learn how the heart fails to begin with. The action of this drug remains an enigma—after two hundred years of successful use. At present, several theories have been advanced to explain its effects on the heart.

Some biochemists believe that digitalis and its various glycosides may act directly on those proteins in the heart muscle that cause it to contract. Another theory sets the action of digitalis at the cell membrane; it suggests that digitalis affects the transport of certain salts, sodium and potassium, in and out of the cell. Digitalis, it has been thought, drives out some amount of potassium that was contained in the cardiac muscle. In some way this is associated with increased contractility. It has long been known that in a normal heart digitalis will decrease the concentration of potassium in the myocardium. Several scientists have experimentally observed a direct relation between the loss of potassium and the increase of contractility. And yet, some scientists still question whether the loss of potassium might be a side effect of digitalis, or is actually the reason for the drug's effectiveness. On the other hand, digitalis may increase calcium concentration in the heart. Several studies have set forth calcium as an essential in the increased ventricular contraction. Toxic doses of digitalis are known to result in high concentrations of calcium in the muscular membranes, but the sub-cellular mechanism by which calcium works on muscular fibers must be better understood before scientists can hope to understand how digitalis produces its effects. Thus far, no one theory has been universally accepted.

Derivatives of Digitalis

Today there are many different preparations of digitalis, although the basic actions of all are the same. Some last much longer in the body; some can be given intravenously if needed in a hurry.

The major digitaloids are still derived from dried leaves of the flowering foxglove, *Digitalis purpurea* and *Digitalis lanata* ("wooly foxglove"). The famous tablet, over one hundred fifty years old, has a dull gray-green color; it is taken orally and is absorbed in the gastrointestinal tract. It will not wear off for several weeks.

The crystalline digitoxin is derived either from *Digitalis purpurea* or *Digitalis lanata*. It is also taken by mouth, but is about 1000 times more potent by weight than digitalis. Deslanoside and digoxin are both derived from the species *lanata*. These various drugs are highly purified by chemical methods, unlike the natural powdered digitalis leaf, and in some patients they are less likely to cause irritation in the gastrointestinal tract or to induce nausea or vomiting. Ouabain is a glycoside obtained from another genus, *Strophanthus gratus*. This drug has to be administered intravenously, but its speed of action makes it preferable in the treatment of severe and sudden failure. Digoxin is its fast-acting oral analogue. It spends little time in the body and its effects are shorter-lived than digitalis leaf or digitoxin. Now there are drugs being developed that act on the heart within minutes; but they have not been released for general use.

Drugs as powerful as digitalis do not merely restore health, they help maintain a quality of life. To a person suffering from a failing heart, digitalis increases confidence and raises morale. A man stricken in his early fifties can take this drug or one of its analogues and expect that his heart will endure a good many years. In time, the taking of the pill will become such an ordinary part of his life that he will probably forget about its importance.

SUPPLEMENTAL READING

Harrison, T. R., Some unanswered questions concerning enlargement and failure of the heart, American Heart Journal *69*:100–115, 1965.

Gorlin, R., Recent conceptual advances in congestive heart failure, JAMA, *179*:441–449, 1962.

Braunwald, E., and Klocke, F. J., Digitalis, Ann. Rev. Med. *16*:371, 1965.

Braunwald, E., Mason, D. T., and Ross, J., Jr., Studies on the cardio-circulatory actions of digitalis, Medicine, *44*:233, 1965.

Chapter 6

Diuretics: Control of Body Fluids

Of the first philosophers, then, most thought
the principles which were of the nature of
matter were the only principles of all things.
That of which all existing things consist, the
first from which they come to be, the last into
which they are resolved (the substance remaining, but changing in its modifications),
this they say is the element and this the
principle of things, and therefore they think
nothing is either generated or destroyed since
this sort of entity is always conserved . . .
Thales, the founder of this type of philosophy,
says the principle is water (for which reason
he declared the earth rests on water), getting
the notion perhaps from seeing that the nutri-
ment of all things is moist . . . and from the
fact that the seeds of all things have a moist
nature, and that water is the origin of the
nature of moist things.

Aristotle   *Metaphysics*   983b

The Greeks thought that life came from the sea. They were not wrong, but perhaps they did not realize that animal life never left the sea. Such life simply encased the ocean inside its tissues and moved ashore. Today, human beings still encase a milieu of salt water. It is not as salty as a present-day ocean; it is weaker, like the weak saline solution that filled the primordial ocean. This solution inside us bathes the cells and lubricates all tissues. For its variety of functions, water is the ideal medium because more things dissolve in it than in nearly anything else. Moreover, hydrogen and oxygen, the components of water, are given off in a number of chemical processes going on in the body all the time, and this adds to the milieu. As a medium, it is a fine lubricant and an effective heat insulator. There is a comparatively large range of degrees between its freezing point and its boiling point. Water also permits many chemical processes to go on within it, and at low temperatures at that; many chemical reactions in solutions other than water would require higher temperatures—too high for life to go on. Small wonder that Nature took advantage of this substance to the hilt, filling the body to about two-thirds of its weight with water. Only a few strange bacteria have learned to live without it.

Diuretics are drugs that are used to regulate the amount of salt and water present in the various fluid compartments of the body. Diuretics are given to patients afflicted with congestive heart failure, a disease in which the heart is unable to pump blood at a rate that is adequate for normal functioning of cells and tissues. The delicate mechanisms that control the salt and water content of the body fail and, as a result, dietary intake soon exceeds losses from the body. The victim literally drowns in his own salty sea. The lungs become so waterlogged that oxygen cannot exchange readily for carbon dioxide.

It is excess salt, as we shall see, that causes this waterlogging or "edema." Fluid accumulates in the ankles and the legs, in the abdomen, and the arms. Although the blood volume may actually increase in congestive heart failure, the cells actually receive less oxygen and food because the failing heart has to work even harder to pump the extra blood; and the heart just is not up to the job. Sometimes, if the congestive heart failure patient is in an early phase of the disease, cardiac glycosides (see chapter "Digitalis for the Failing Heart") alone will correct the condition by improving the pumping ability of the heart, but often it is necessary in addition to rid the body of excess salt and water. This calls for the use of diuretics. In order to understand how diuretics work, we will have to consider the function of the kidney, the organ that has primary responsibility for maintaining a proper balance of salt and water in the body.

The Kidney

Most of us know and recognize the fact that urine is a waste product. Dissolved in it are many substances, end products of metabolism or unwanted dietary constituents, that would injure the body if they were not discharged by some means. Obviously the production of urine is one of the important tasks of the kidney. But the production of urine is more than simply a way of removing noxious substances from the body. The volume and composition of body fluids is dependent ultimately on what the kidney puts into the urine and on how much urine is excreted. If we consider volume alone, we can express this as a simple equation as follows:

dietary intake of water = loss of water (e.g. respiration, sweat, tears, and urine)

Final adjustments necessary for maintaining equality of intake and output are made by the kidney. On a hot day, when there is much sweating, urine flow decreases; when intake of fluids is large, as during a beer party, urine flow increases. Under all conditions the amount of salt present in urine reflects the need either to excrete or conserve salt. As we shall see the kidney does not accomplish its tasks alone but is assisted by hormones that modify its capacity to excrete salt and water.

It is the pumping action of the heart that initiates the process of urine formation. As blood is pumped through the kidney, pressure within the small blood vessels causes fluid to pass through their walls. This fluid contains all soluble elements of blood plasma except large molecules such as the plasma proteins. The blood vessels are surrounded at the point where fluid is pressed out by claw-like projections of renal tubules. The fluid passes into the hollow centers of the tubules, traverses the entire length of each tubule, and finally drips into a funnel-like organ (renal pelvis) that carries it out of the kidney. It is somewhat surprising but nevertheless a fact that less than one percent of the fluid that enters tubules will end up as urine. The reason for this is that cells comprising the walls of the renal tubules take back or "reabsorb" more than 99 percent of the fluid and salts as they pass through the hollow spaces of the tubules. In order to do this the cells must expend energy. In actuality the energy is used to push salts across the cells and back into blood vessels. Water passively follows salts, but the actual amount of water that does so is in part regulated by a hormone, an antidiuretic hormone, produced in the hypothalamus of the brain (see chapter "Hormones and Drugs"). Large amounts of the hormone, for instance, are produced when there is need to conserve water; under such conditions urine flow diminishes but the concentration or amount of waste products present in this urine is of course very high. The sex hormones and some of the hormones produced in the adrenal gland increase reabsorption of salts. Thus it is not unusual during pregnancy or periods of the human menstrual cycle, when large amounts of female sex hormones are circulating, to have excessive retention of salt and water in the body. Diuretics are often used to get rid of the extra salt and water present during premenstrual tension or edema of pregnancy.

In each of the two kidneys in the human, there are approximately one million individual units called nephrons. Each nephron comprises a filtering surface where much of the fluid and dissolved substances in the blood are pressed out of capillaries into the hollow space of a tubule, and the tubule proper which reabsorbs the bulk of the filtered fluid and substances present in the fluid. Nephrons vary in length from about one to two inches. About 42 gallons of fluid are filtered through the kidneys during a 24 hour period and less than one half gallon is excreted as urine (Figure 1).

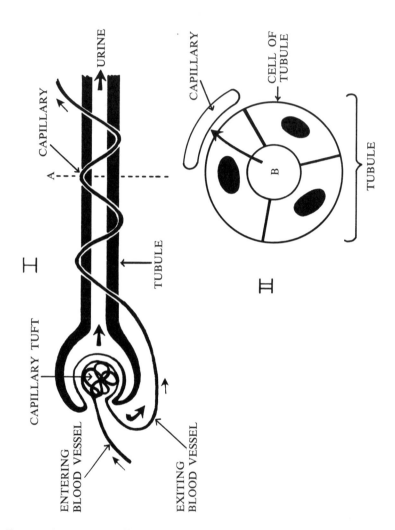

FIGURE 1. *Diagram illustrating process of urine formation in a single nephron. Process begins when fluid and salts are filtered through walls of vessels of the capillary tuft (I). Fluid and salts pass through hollow space A but, during passage, are reduced in amount because of reabsorption shown above (II). Diuretics interfere with reabsorption. There are approximately 1,000,000 nephrons in each human kidney*

Mercurial Diuretics

All effective diuretics act on the kidney and, even though the precise biochemical reactions in which the various classes of diuretics participate differ, all of them in the final analysis affect the same process. They simply interfere with the capacity of renal cells to reabsorb sodium chloride (table salt). The rate of formation of urine increases in order to keep pace with the increase in excretion of salt. The person who is carrying extra amounts of salt and water in his tissues gets rid of it quickly, and the first sign of this is usually a rapid loss of weight. Thus the patient in congestive heart failure may lose several pounds or even more the first day he is given a diuretic. Diuretics of course do not cure any of the diseases that cause retention of salt and water but they do alleviate many of the symptoms. The drugs must be given repetitively in order to keep the patient at his best weight (i.e., free of extra salt and water). Often it is necessary to take a diuretic every day.

Many plant substances have been known for centuries to have weak diuretic effects and were prescribed by physicians before the time of Christ. In the sixteenth century the Swiss scientist Paracelsus prescribed calomel (mercurous chloride) as a diuretic. Guy's Hospital, at which John Keats studied and earned his apothecary's and surgeon's license, produced pills that were famous throughout the nineteenth century; they contained inorganic mercury and digitalis. The modern era of diuretic therapy did not begin until the end of World War I.

The first safe and effective drugs were the mercurial diuretics, organic compounds containing carbon, to which the element mercury was attached. From the time of their discovery by Viennese physicians, at the end of World War I, until 1950, the mercurials were the only dependable diuretics. The mercurial diuretics had many favorable characteristics. Dosage could be adjusted to get the right amount of diuresis. When they were used properly there were few attendant side actions or undesirable effects, but there were a few drawbacks. In the first place mercurials were not very effective when given orally. Absorption from the gastrointestinal tract was incomplete and much of the mercury remained in the tract itself. For this reason mercurials had to be injected intramuscularly or intravenously. Moreover, mercurials could not be injected daily because it took several days for the body to rid itself of mercury; and mercury poisoning could develop if injections were not properly spaced. Typically, a patient would remain free of edema for a short period of time after receiving a mercurial but would then begin to reaccumulate salt and water in his tissues before another injection of the mercurial could be given. Physicians were acutely aware of the need for a diuretic that could be given by mouth and as often as necessary to maintain patients in proper salt and water balance. The active search for new diuretic agents continued. Efforts of the major drug houses in the United States first centered on discovery of better mercurial compounds but finally shifted to compounds that did not contain mercury.

Acetazolamide and the Thiazides

The first significant advance was the development of a drug called acetazolamide (Diamox). The story of the development of acetazolamide is too complicated and full of abstruse information to retell here. Although it does not possess the dynamic and sensational overtones of the discovery of penicillin, the discovery of acetazolamide was an equally remarkable achievement. Suffice it to say that at least four separate, difficult pieces of basic research had to be completed before the makers of acetazolamide, Lederle Laboratories, could devote any efforts to its synthesis.

Acetazolamide became available for clinical use in 1950. It was orally effective and could bring about a substantial diuresis. Unfortunately, there were limitations to its clinical use and these became apparent in short order. Patients on acetazolamide excreted large quantities of sodium bicarbonate, an alkaline salt normally present in all body fluids. With insufficient amounts of alkali remaining in the body, the body fluids inevitably became acidic. Although in most instances acidosis could be tolerated, once it had developed acetazolamide was no longer effective. Nevertheless, the drug was still useful, for it could be given alternately with mercurials, and could thus help to extend the edema-free intervals obtained by administration of a mercurial.

The most important thing about acetazolamide was the fact that it pointed the way to better diuretics. And, fittingly, clinicians have found other uses for it. Many people with epilepsy or glaucoma now rely on acetazolamide day by day.

The most important diuretics used today, the thiazides, owe their existence to acetazolamide, because they have in common with it one particular chemical grouping. Research chemists and pharmacologists working in the pharmaceutical industry spend much of their time with chemical groupings. Most had lost faith in the grouping that conferred diuretic activity on the acetazolamide molecule, but the workers at Merck Sharp and Dohme persisted. We can be glad they did, for the result was a new drug, chlorothiazide, that is a diuretic *par excellence*. Chlorothiazide is probably one of the most innocuous drugs ever used in clinical practice and yet it is one of the most valuable. It is orally effective and can be used daily without loss of activity. One of its relatives, hydrochlorothiazide, is the most widely-used diuretic in existence. The only serious drawback to its use is the fact that some patients excrete excessive quantities of potassium when given the drug. In most instances this can be handled by simply instructing them to eat foods that contain large quantities of potassium.

An added bonus is the fact that chlorothiazide and its relatives can reduce blood pressure in patients who have high blood pressure but not in those whose pressure is normal. Thus the thiazides have multiple uses. Most patients who require diuretic therapy can be treated adequately with thiazides. Others require periodic injections of mercurials coupled with daily administration of thiazides.

Needless to say, there are and always will be those who are more seriously afflicted and whose water and salt balance cannot be controlled adequately. This is why the search for more effective diuretics and for diuretics that do not increase excretion of potassium continues. Two new drugs are in the offing.

One of them is a so-called "non-mercurial mercurial", an orally effective drug that does not contain mercury but has a similar mechanism of action. A drug of this type, ethacrynic acid, is now available. The drug is remarkably effective, its overall effect clinically being potentially greater than that of mercurials. The risk of potassium depletion, reminiscent of thiazides, persists. Ethacrynic acid is a valuable drug chiefly for two reasons: 1. It is a "broad-spectrum" diuretic. Dosage may be adjusted to suit needs of any particular patient—the sightly edematous patient with mild to moderate congestive heart failure or even the severely edematous patient with cirrhosis of the liver. 2. The drug appears to be especially useful in patients who do not respond to thiazides or mercurials.

The other new diuretic presently available is the compound furosemide. This drug was modeled after the thiazides but the structure was altered sufficiently so that the resultant compound cannot structurally be considered a thiazide. Furosemide appears to have all the properties of the thiazides except that it is a much more effective drug and rivals ethacrynic acid in effectiveness. It too may be considered a "broad-spectrum" diuretic. There is reason to believe that most side reactions to furosemide will be the same as those to thiazides. If this proves to be the case the drug will have singular advantages in that one may rely upon the record of safety of thiazides when using furosemide, providing he takes into account the exceptional diuretic activity of furosemide as a possible cause of serious side effects. The objective of diuretic therapy is to rid the body of excessive salt and water—not to deplete the body of salt and water.

Recent scientific advances have yielded new products of great use to the practicing physician. The exemplary properties of the mercurials and thiazides serve to stimulate progress in the field of diuretic research. We now look to furosemide and ethacrynic acid as precursors of even more selective diuretics, perhaps some that will spare potassium. The pharmacologists, of course, hope to provide drugs that will work in every situation. We are close to this objective but have not yet achieved it.

SUPPLEMENTAL READING

Welt, Louis G., Disorders of Hydration and Acid-Base Equilibrium, 2nd ed., Little, Brown and Company, Boston, 1959.

Smith, Homer R., Principles of Renal Physiology, Oxford University Press, New York, 1960.

Pitts, Robert F., The Physiological Basis of Diuretic Therapy, Charles C Thomas, Springfield, Illinois, 1959.

Chapter 7

The Nerves that Control Automatically

As a general rule drugs do not actually start new processes in the body. Their action is supportive, regulative or suppressive. This principle can be illustrated in no better way than by examing the effects of drugs on the nervous system. By learning to manipulate a set of signals, doctors have been able to police many of the nerve messages in the body—speeding them up, slowing them down, or bringing them to a full stop. Little will be said of drugs in this chapter. However, by considering closely a few basic principles about autonomic activity, one will find the substance of the next chapter more meaningful. Here we are concerned with theory; there, with practice.

The Autonomic Nervous System

Many of the functions of the body are regulated through nervous activity, but in an involuntary or autonomic way. The heart, for the simplest example, beats slowly when we are at rest. When we exercise, however, it speeds and contracts more vigorously to pump more blood and therefore more oxygen and nutrients to the muscles and other tissues. The response of the heart to exercise is an autonomic or involuntary one. It happens without our consciously willing it. This is in contrast to the consciously directed events in muscle activity involved in walking, talking, or playing the piano.

The changes in the size of the pupils in response to light or dark are brought about by nerve-mediated contraction and relaxation of the two sets of muscles of the iris. Increased intestinal activity that follows a meal is caused by nerve-induced contraction of the muscles of the intestines. The increased formation and secretion of saliva as a response to the aroma of roast beef is due to nerve-mediated stimulation of the secretory cells of the salivary glands. All of these are examples of autonomic nervous activity.

105

The nerves that bear messages from the brain to the various organs for autonomic regulation are anatomically distinct from those that innervate our sekeletal or voluntary muscles. Collectively these nerves are designated the autonomic nervous system (ANS), sometimes called the involuntary nervous system, or the vegetative nervous system. In man, structures that are so innervated include the secretory glands such as the sweat, tear, and salivary glands, smooth muscle fibers in many organs such as the intestine, the bladder, and the blood vessels and the heart. In this chapter only the motor part of the ANS will be considered: the nerves carrying impulses to activate or to alter the function of peripheral organs. These nerves leave the central nervous system and may link up (or *synapse*) outside the central nervous system (brain and spinal cord) with another nerve, which ultimately innervates a given organ.

The ANS is composed of two major parts, the sympathetic and the parasympathetic nervous systems. The sympathetic nervous system is a series of nerves originating in the thoracic (chest) and lumbar (abdominal) portions of the spinal cord (see Fig. 1). Within a short distance after emerging from the spinal cord, these nerves (preganglionic) terminate in close proximity to the cell bodies of other nerves (postganglionic). The term "postganglionic" derives from "ganglion," designating a collection of the terminals of nerves that originate in the spinal cord. The postganglionic nerve cell bodies send out fibers that travel varying distances to various organs and tissues such as the heart, blood vessels, intestine, or the iris of an eye.

The outflow of parasympathetic nerves is both from the brain and from the lowermost part of the spinal cord, the so-called sacral spinal cord. These preganglionic nerves travel to the organs innervated where they form junctions with short postganglionic fibers which innervate the tissues. To understand how drugs act on the autonomic nervous system, it is necessary to understand the manner in which nerve impulses are transmitted *across* junctions, both the ganglionic junction or synapse (between two nerves), and the neuro-effector junction (between a nerve and the tissue or organ affected by it). The impulse is transmitted across these synapses by chemical messengers. A nerve impulse, which can be thought of as an electrical wave passing down the nerve fiber, causes the release of a chemical

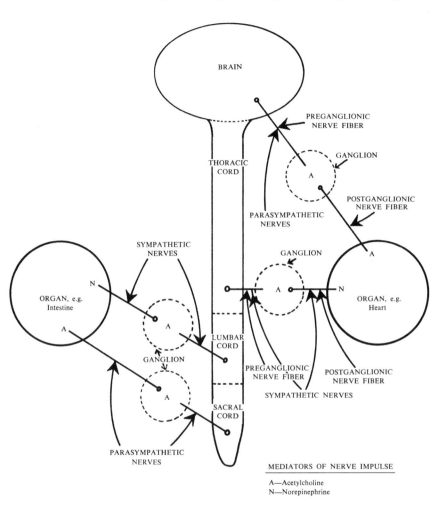

FIGURE 1. *Schematic representation of the Autonomic Nervous System*

substance at the nerve ending. This substance, called a neurohumoral transmitter or mediator, diffuses across the short distance to the next nerve or cell in line (Fig. 2). The chemical substances that are released from the nerve endings vary in type with the location and the anatomical division of the autonomic nervous system.

There is an increasing amount of evidence supporting the concept of neurohumoral or chemical transmission. Scientists posit that the nerve impulse must release a transmitter from the nerve terminals. The transmitter is then stable for a sufficient time to diffuse and to react with the next cell in line. But the transmitter substance must also be capable of being rapidly inactivated so that its action on the receiving cell is of limited duration. There are two primary modes of inactivation of the chemical mediators: one, by metabolic (chemical) alteration so that the transmitter is no longer physiologically active; and two, by uptake into a cell and binding within the cell to specific binding sites. In some instances the cell that binds the nerve mediator is actually the cell that released it. Although all the steps in the process have not yet been determined, the concept of neurohumoral transmission has allowed a rational explanation for a crucial aspect of nerve activity. However, transmission along a nerve fiber is still best described in electrical terms, although certainly the electrical changes are of chemical origin.

There are two established chemical mediators involved in autonomic nervous system transmission: one is the cholinergic mediator, acetylcholine, and the second is the adrenergic mediator, norepinephrine (known as noradrenaline outside of the U.S.). Acetylcholine is released from all nerve terminals in the parasympathetic division of the autonomic nervous system—both from the terminations of preganglionic nerve fibers and from the terminations of the postganglionic nerve fibers (see Fig. 1). Acetylcholine also mediates transmission at all ganglionic junctions in the sympathetic nervous system. However, the chemical mediator released from most of the postganglionic sympathetic neurons is norepinephrine. Acetylcholine is released from a few specific sympathetic postganglionic fibers.

Little is understood now about the processes of release of mediators, although it is known that there are substances which will inhibit release of mediator, as well as substances which will inhibit the synthesis of the mediator. Upon release, the mediator

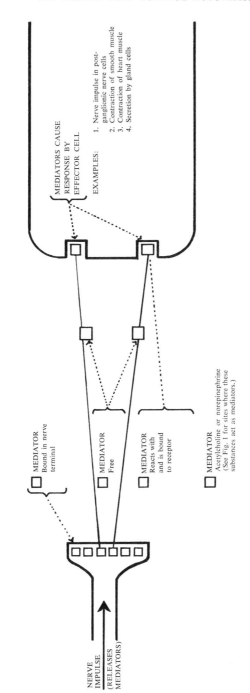

FIGURE 2. *Diagrammatic concept of neurohumoral transmission, i.e., chemical transmission of the nerve impulse*

EFFECTOR CELL
1. A postganglionic nerve
2. or a smooth muscle
3. or a heart muscle
4. or gland cells

MEDIATORS CAUSE RESPONSE BY EFFECTOR CELL

EXAMPLES:
1. Nerve impulse in post-ganglionic nerve cells
2. Contraction of smooth muscle
3. Contraction of heart muscle
4. Secretion by gland cells

NERVE TERMINAL

NERVE IMPULSE (RELEASES MEDIATORS)

☐ MEDIATOR Bound in nerve terminal

☐ MEDIATOR Free

☐ MEDIATOR Reacts with and is bound to receptor

☐ MEDIATOR Acetylcholine or norepinephrine (See Fig. 1 for sites where these substances act as mediators.)

diffuses across the extremely short distance—less than two one-millionths of an inch—between the cell releasing it and the next cell. The mediator then reacts with this next cell, the effector cell. When the mediator is released from a preganglionic terminal, the effector cell is just another neuron (nerve cell) in the chain. The effector cell that responds to the chemical mediator released from a postganglionic neuron is a nonnervous cell: a heart muscle cell, a smooth muscle cell, or a gland cell.

The Receptor Site

An important corrolary to the concept of neurohumoral transmission is the concept of specific receptor sites on the cells. Mediators are specific chemical compounds, synthesized and stored in the nerve terminals, and released upon signal (the nerve impulse); they react with specific components, called receptors, on the receiving cell. The receptors have not yet been identified either biochemically or anatomically. Although they are still termed hypothetical entities, they are undoubtedly real. They can be described by their response or failure to respond to a variety of drugs. In fact, the concept of specific receptors largely underlies much of the action or knowledge of the action of drugs on the autonomic nervous system.

The specific receptor can be considered as the part of the receiving cell that reacts with the mediator. This reaction triggers the change in the activity of the cell. For instance, the smooth muscle of the intestine, that muscle which provides the rhythmic activity for the mixing and propulsion of food contents in the intestinal tract, is caused to contract by acetylcholine. When a nerve impulse goes down the vagus nerve (a parasympathetic nerve), which has its origin in the brain stem, it reaches a ganglionic junction in the wall of the intestine. Here the nerve stimulus releases acetylcholine. The acetylcholine diffuses to the next neuron in line, and reacts with a cholinergic receptor on the postganglionic neuron. The reaction between receptor and acetylcholine is the triggering event in a series of cellular reactions that initiate the nerve impulse in the postganglionic nerve. This impulse then travels down the fibers of the postganglionic neuron. Upon reaching the terminations of the postganglionic neuron, the impulse again induces the release of acetylcholine that diffuses across a gap to the receptor, again a cholinergic type of receptor on the smooth muscle cell of the intestine. This reaction between the smooth muscle receptor and acetylcholine serves once again as a triggering event leading to an alteration of intracellular processes, ultimately bringing about contraction of the smooth muscle. The smooth muscle returns to its original state (relaxation) when the acetylcholine is destroyed.

Several types of receptors have been identified, each definable by their responses either to various pharmacologic agents, to the neurohumoral mediators, or to antagonistic drugs. The cholinergic receptors, for example, are of three distinct types, two of which are in the autonomic nervous system. One type is found on the effector cells—the gland, smooth muscle, and heart cells. A second type is the cholinergic receptor which is found on the postganglionic nerve cells of all ganglia, both parasympathetic and sympathetic. A third is the cholinergic receptor found on the skeletal muscle cell. All three of these receptors appear to react readily with acetylcholine to which they are equally sensitive. Yet they differ with respect to location, function, and response to antagonistic drugs. Drugs that will block or antagonize the effects of acetylcholine at one location may be relatively ineffective at another. The concept of pharmacological blockade will be covered in the following chapter.

Among the adrenergic receptors there are two types which have been designated by the Greek letters *alpha* and *beta*. These two receptor types are not distinguished by their locations but by the variations in responses of tissues to inhibitory drugs. The *alpha* adrenergic receptors are those which generally mediate rapid responses such as the contraction of the smooth muscle in the blood vessels, the contraction of the dilator muscle of the eye's iris, and the contraction of the small muscle at the base of the hair follicle. This latter contraction causes the hair to rise in response to cold or fright, the so-called goose pimples. The *beta* adrenergic receptors, for the most part, take care of or serve slower responses within the sympathetic nervous system. These include some metabolic changes within the cell, such as the increased breakdown of glycogen and fat tissue. *Beta* receptors also function in the heart. When stimulated by the adrenergic mediator, the cardiac *beta* receptors initiate increased rate and force of the heartbeat. On a functional basis the distinctions among these receptors are based upon their various reactivities to different types of drugs which are closely related to norepinephrine. More importantly, as with the cholinergic receptors, the differentiation comes on the basis of blocking drugs, about which more will be said in the next chapter.

Thus, acetylcholine is a primary mediator at all autonomic nervous system ganglionic junctions (both parasympathetic and sympathetic), at the parasympathetic postganglionic neuroeffector junctions and at the few sympathetic "cholinergic" postganglionic neuroeffector junctions. Acetylcholine also mediates the transmission at the skeletal or voluntary neuromuscular junction. In contrast, norepinephrine is a mediator only at the sympathetic postganglionic adrenergic neuroeffector junctions.

The Fate of Transmitters

In order to understand the actions of drugs on the autonomic nervous system we must consider the fate of the mediators. That is, how they are inactivated once they have been released from nerve terminals and have reacted with the receptors. Acetylcholine is inactivated by an enzyme known as cholinesterase, which exists in the areas of the nerve terminals and in the cells where acetylcholine is released. Cholinesterase breaks acetylcholine down into acetic acid and choline (both nearly inactive) so rapidly that the nerve or the cell which is stimulated by acetylcholine recovers immediately. There is no evidence that acetylcholine is inactivated by binding to nerve terminals.

Norepinephrine is inactivated by several mechanisms. Two enzymes, monoamineoxidase (MAO) and catechol-O-methyltransferase (COMT), contribute to its metabolic destruction. A large and important component of inactivation of norepinephrine is the rapid rebinding of the intact molecules by the nerve terminals. Both methods of inactivation, i.e. enzymatic alteration and binding, rapidly lower the amount of free mediator available to stimulate the receptors.

Now, here is a brief review of what we have considered of the anatomy, physiology, and chemistry of the autonomic nervous system. It should be stressed that we have only been concerned with the motor aspects of the autonomic nervous system—impulses travelling outward from the central nervous system and serving to bring about involuntary motor responses, either changes in smooth or cardiac muscle activity or glandular function, and in correlation with these, metabolic changes. The autonomic nervous system is comprised of two main parts, the parasympathetic and the sympathetic divisions. These divisions are based upon the anatomical locations of the fibers that leave the central nervous system. The parasympathetic nerves leave the central nervous system in two widely separated places—from the brain stem, and from the lower end of the spinal cord, the sacral or caudal region. The sympathetic nerves leave the central nervous system from portions of the spinal cord in the chest or thoracic region and in the lower back or lumbar region. In both instances the fibers that leave the central nervous system have their cell bodies within the central nervous system. The fibers leave the central nervous system to join other neurons. These junctions—between the nerve fibers emanating from the central nervous system and the peripherally placed neurons—are called ganglionic junctions or ganglia. In the sympathetic nervous system these junctions constitute in many instances discrete swellings that can be seen; the word "ganglion" derives from a Greek word meaning "swelling."

In the sympathetic nervous system a collection of nerve junctions—the nerve terminations and nerve cell bodies—are found in a segmental or regularly-occurring distribution up and down the spinal cord. These are known as the paravertebral ganglia. A similar cluster of ganglia, the prevertebral ganglia, are found anterior to the vertebral column. The medulla or inner portion of the adrenal gland is comparable to the ganglia. In fact, it is innervated by sympathetic preganglionic fibers. The junction here is with a medullary cell. This is a cell in the adrenal medulla, the central portion of the adrenal gland. In the adult animal this is not a nerve cell, though in the embryonic period it did in fact start out as a nerve cell. These cells, moreover, started out as nerve cells with the potential of synthesizing and releasing norepinephrine; but in the adult adrenal gland they are specialized as hormone cells, releasing norepinephrine or epinephrine into the bloodstream upon stimulation of the preganglionic fibers (see Chapter 19). Since the ganglia in the sympathetic nervous system are relatively close to the spinal column, the postganglionic fibers travel long distances to come to terminations near or in the walls of the organs which they innervate.

The mediator from preganglionic fibers to postganglionic neurons is acetylcholine. This includes the mediator in the adrenal medulla from the preganglionic fiber to the adrenal medullary cells. The mediator released from postganglionic neurons in the sympathetic nervous system is believed to be norepinephrine, although closely related chemical compounds may be released from certain terminals. When released from the preganglionic fiber, the mediator acetylcholine reacts with a type of cholinergic receptor on the postganglionic neuron. This reaction gives rise to the development of an impulse in the postganglionic cell. The impulse then travels down the postganglionic fiber. At the terminal, it elicits the release of norepinephrine, which then excites the effector cell, causing it to respond in a characteristic manner.

In the parasympathetic system the preganglionic fibers are very long; the preganglionic fibers travel, for instance, from the brain stem in the head down to the middle part of the intestine. And there are no discrete ganglia in this system. Fibers are rather diffusely arranged, usually in the walls of the organs that are innervated by networks of nerves. The postganglionic fibers having their origins in the organ which is innervated, are therefore very short. The mediators in the parasympathetic nervous system are acetylcholine at the ganglionic junctions, and acetylcholine at the postganglionic nerve fibers. As if it were not doing enough, acetylcholine is also the mediator in the skeletal neuromuscular system—but this is a voluntary system and does not conern us here.

It sounds quite complex, and it is. However, in the course of evolution Nature took several billion years to attain this complexity, and it has taken a few minutes to read about it. In view of the context of the following chapter, one could do worse than read this chapter over again.

Chapter 8

Mimickers and Blockers of Nerve Action

D rugs can step up action in various parts of the autonomic nervous system, and drugs can block this action. Consequently, they are termed mimetic agents or mimickers and blockers. More specifically, they are designated by that part of the autonomic nervous system upon which they act. Agents, for example, that simulate action of the sympathetic nerves in the heart are called sympathomimetic drugs because they mimic sympathetic nerve stimulation. Drugs that block the chemical transfer of impulses from a preganglionic nerve to a postganglionic nerve are called ganglionic blocking agents. Many diseases involve disturbances of the autonomic nervous system or depend for their effective treatment on alteration of the activity of some part of this system. If the physician can correctly diagnose the disease, chances are there will be a highly specific drug that can affect the parts controlled by those nerves.

Types of Autonomic Drug Action

Physicians prescribe these agents either to mimic or to block the effects of neurohumoral mediators. These mediators, one recalls, are natural body chemicals that provide a crucial link in the communication of nerve impulses. The mimicking of a nerve impulse can be accomplished by three possible mechanisms:

1. Drugs can act upon nerve endings to cause the release of the neurohumoral mediator, the released mediator then acting in its usual manner.

2. They may inhibit inactivation of the natural neurohumoral mediator at the neuroeffector junction, so that the transmitted impulse will keep firing. If the supply of mediator is low, this method takes maximal advantage of the mediator.

3. They may react with the receptors on the effector cell to cause the same response as that elicited by the normal

117

neurohumoral mediator. In this instance the mimicking drugs are usually very closely related in chemical structure to the neurohumoral mediator itself. Note that in two mechanisms drugs increase the concentration of the endogenous or normal mediator, one by causing the release of the mediator, the other by inhibiting its inactivation. In the third mechanism the drug reacts with the receptor itself; the receptor is fooled into accepting the drug as the mediator.

Drugs antagonize or block the effects of neurohumoral mediators in several ways. First, they can act on nerve terminals to inhibit either the synthesis, the storage, or the release of the mediator. Secondly, drugs can react with the receptors, occupy them, and thus prevent the mediator from reacting with the receptors. Some blocking drugs, for example, may initiate a cellular response; then, by firmly adhering to the receptor, they prevent any further response to the mediator. In other instances the blocking drug may react with and occupy the receptor without initiating a cellular response. Both mimicking and blocking actions of the various types may occur wherever a junction between two nerves or a nerve and an effector cell (smooth muscle, cardiac muscle or gland cell) occurs in the autonomic nervous system. While a drug (mimicker or blocker) may act by one or more of the mechanisms described, any one drug does not usually possess all such actions.

How do autonomic drugs affect functions of the body? An agent that mimics the effects of sympathetic nerve stimulation (a sympathomimetic drug) generally will increase the heart rate and blood pressure, perhaps dilate the pupil (providing the dose is large enough), and cause some central nervous system reactions such as anxiety and a fine tremor of the hands and fingers. Measured effects of such a drug on metabolism would probably show higher levels of blood sugar and free fatty acids (the breakdown products from fat stores). Intestinal activity would be slowed down. According to the famous American physiologist Walter Cannon, the sympathetic nervous system rallies so that an animal is best prepared for *fight or flight*—to stand and fight for life or to flee the danger with which he is faced. This physiological reaction occurs in civilized man, but it may become distorted. To the animal in a situation requiring fight or flight, however, it is essential that the amount of blood pumped to the muscles be increased. Blood pressure must be raised to do this, and blood vessels in the muscles themselves must dilate to increase the volume of food and oxygen. Even the pupils dilate, for better vision during the stress. Moreover, certain physiological functions, such as intestinal activity which is not vitally necessary in the moments of "excitement," must be inhibited. All these reactions can be rather consistently reproduced by the injection of a sympathomimetic drug such as epinephrine. Also, many of these reactions, e.g. anxiety-induced reactions, can be antagonized by the injection of sympathetic blocking drugs.

Drugs that mimic the effects of stimulation of parasympathetic nerves (parasympathomimetic drugs) tend to increase the motility or activity of the intestinal tract, cause contraction of the bladder, lower blood pressure, slow the heart rate, constrict the pupils, and induce sweating. Drugs that block the actions of parasympathomimetic nerves, that is cholinergic blocking drugs, will produce an opposite effect. They elevate heart rate, decrease intestinal activity, inhibit urinary bladder contraction, dry the mouth (inhibited salivary secretion), blur the vision, and cause photophobia. Impaired vision is due to paralysis of the small muscles within the eye which control the convexity of the lens, in turn controlling accomodation for near vision. The photophobia is due to the dilated pupils which cannot constrict in response to light.

Drugs that Mimic Stimulation of Parasympathetic Nerves

Muscarine. Muscarine is found in *Amanita muscaria,* the fly mushroom, major type of poisonous mushrooms. It is a substance that reacts with the cholinergic receptors on the various effector cells. It produces violent gastrointestinal aberrations, marked slowing of the heart rate, a fall in blood pressure, salivation, and other effects that are common in parasympathetic stimulation. Although muscarine has little or no clinical value today, it is used experimentally.

Pilocarpine. Pilocarpine is a material obtained from the leaf of a South American shrub known as *Pilocarpus jaborandi.* This plant was chewed by native Indians of South America, presumably for certain effects such as profuse salivation and altered consciousness. It was not until the latter part of the nineteenth century that the parasympathomimetic effects of pilocarpine were discovered. Today this drug is used primarily in ophthalmology.

Derivatives of choline. Certain compounds closely related chemically to the normal parasympathetic mediator acetylcholine are used in medicine. These include such drugs as methacholine (Mecholyl), carbachol (Doryl) and bethanecol (Urecholine).

Cholinesterase inhibitors. Another type of parasympathomimetic drug antagonizes or inhibits the enzyme cholinesterase, responsible for the inactivation of the neurohumoral mediator acetylcholine. This type of biological activity was first found in the plant *Physostigma venenosum,* native to West Africa. The ripe seeds of this plant are called Calabar beans, and the active chemical in them is a substance known as physostigmine or eserin. "Eserin" is derived from the fact that the bean also was called the Esere Nut or the bean of Atu Esere. Certain tribes of West African natives referred to the bean as "ordeal bean" because of its use as a poison in ordeal trials for witchcraft. In these trials, Calabar beans were fed to the suspect. Innocent persons who had nothing to fear were supposed to eat them rapidly. Since a large dose produces vomiting, the material would be expelled and poisoning would not occur. Guilty people were supposed to be reluctant to eat them fast, fearing poison. So, in hope of slowing down or mitigating the effect, they would nibble at the beans. The poisonous substance would then be absorbed and retained, and as a consequence there would be a fatal reaction.

The essential ingredient of the ordeal bean and the nature of its action on the parasympathetic nervous system was discovered in the latter part of the nineteenth century. This substance, physostigmine, was the forerunner of a large series of synthetic compounds capable of inhibiting cholinesterase. The most notable of those compounds related to physostigmine is neostigmine (Prostigmin). More recently, a large number of so-called organophosphorus anticholinesterase agents have been developed. These are the so-called nerve gases and have been widely employed as insecticides—they are among the more highly potent and lethal agents of this type.

Parasympathetic Blocking Drugs

Atropine is the grandfather of all these drugs. It is present in *Atropa belladonna,* a poisonous plant with red bell-shaped flowers and bright black berries, native to Western Europe (Fig. 1). Known as the "deadly nightshade," the plant was sometimes used for the sake of beauty, and sometimes murder. Atropos, was one of the three Fates, the one who cut the thread of life. *Belladonna* (from

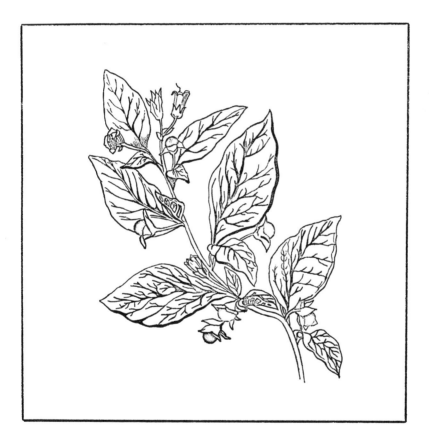

Figure 1. Atropa belladonna

the Italian for "beautiful lady") was assigned as a species name because women had long applied a preparation of the plant topically to the eyes to dilate the pupils. To have widely dilated pupils was a mark of beauty among the ladies of the Middle Ages and the Renaissance. For Lucretia Borgia belladonna probably had more than one use.

A number of substances in *Atropa belladonna* are biologically active. Except for minor variations, all these materials work because they block the cholinergic receptors on effector cells. They do not initiate a cellular response in this reaction. However, they do react in some way, occupy the receptor for long periods of time in a slowly reversible way, and prevent access to the receptor by the mediator acetylcholine. Thus they block effects of the parasympathetic nervous system. The results should be obvious; dryness of the mouth from inhibited salivation, a dry hot skin from reduced sweating, decreased intestinal motility even to the extent of constipation, inhibition of bladder contraction with consequent retention of urine, increased heart rate from antagonism of the slowing effect of the vagus nerve. The effects—only a few have been listed—vary from mild to severe, depending upon the size of the dose.

Numerous compounds that resemble the basic structure of atropine have been synthesized in the laboratory. These are available under a variety of trade and generic names. More will be said about them later.

Ganglionic Blocking Agents

Acetylcholine acts as the neurohumoral mediator at both parasympathetic and sympathetic ganglia. Doctors consider it neither clinically useful nor desirable to stimulate these ganglia. However, one of the most widely consumed agents in the world today, nicotine, has a very specific effect upon the receptors of the postganglionic nerve cells. In fact, the physiologist John Newport Langley (1852–1925) provided our initial understanding of the function of ganglia by experimenting with the tobacco alkaloid. Many of the characteristic responses to nicotine, such as nausea, intestinal discomfort, and vomiting in the novice, are due in large measure to this ganglionic stimulant action that occurs at low dosage.

Of most importance to medicine are drugs that block the receptors on postganglionic nerve cell bodies. It is noteworthy that atropine, which blocks the responses to acetylcholine on the smooth muscle, cardiac muscle and gland cells, does not block the effects of acetylcholine on nerve cells in the ganglion. A large group of synthetic drugs, however, will block these receptors. Hexamethonium, like most drugs in this class, is a highly charged molecule, and consequently it is poorly absorbed from the intestine. Mecamylamine is unusual among the ganglionic blocking agents in not being a highly charged molecule, and hence is readily absorbed after oral administration.

These drugs, like atropine, react with the receptor without causing a response, occupy the site for long periods of time, sometimes several hours, and thereby produce a persistent antagonism. Blockade at this level virtually cuts off all effects of the autonomic nervous system. Blood pressure drops, because the sympathetic nerves, primarily responsible for maintaining blood pressure, are blocked at the ganglia. Moreover, since the motility of the intestines is largely under vagus nerve control, and since the ganglia of this major nerve are blocked by these drugs, there is marked inhibition of intestinal activity and, as a result, constipation. For similar reasons, the urinary bladder loses its tone, or may even become paralyzed.

One of the unfortunate side effects of ganglionic blockade is a situation known as orthostatic or postural hypotension, a response to rapid change from a sitting or reclining position to an upright position. In the normal individual, reflexes maintain blood pressure at normal levels by producing constriction of the blood vessels in the more dependent portions of the body, thus preventing the pooling of blood from the effects of gravity. But in an individual taking a ganglionic blocking drug, this reflex response through the sympathetic nervous system is impaired. When the patient stands up, there is no compensatory vasoconstriction in the lower portions of his body. Consequently the blood remains in the feet and legs, and in the intestinal blood vessels. Return of blood to the heart and output of blood from the heart becomes inadequate. This results in decreased blood flow to the brain, with insufficient oxygenation and subsequent fainting.

Drugs that Mimic Stimulation of Sympathetic Nerves

There are two main types of sympathomimetic drugs:

1. Drugs that are chemically related to the neurohumoral transmitter norepinephrine, i.e. they so closely counterfeit the structure of norepinephrine that they can activate norepinephrine receptors.

2. Drugs that act indirectly, either by causing the release of the natural mediator, or by inhibiting inactivation of the mediator. The drugs that stimulate the release of the mediator are numerous and, for the most part, exhibit a close chemical resemblance to the mediator. Some of these, in addition to releasing the mediator, also act directly on the receptor.

The more prominent drugs acting directly on the receptor include norepinephrine (the mediator substance itself), epinephrine, isoproterenol, and phenylephrine. The indirectly acting drugs include such agents as metaraminol (Aramine) and ephedrine.

Sympathetic Blocking Drugs

A physician can prevent stimulation of sympathetic nerves, but that is more complex than blocking responses to parasympathetic nerves. There are drugs which can inhibit the synthesis of the mediator norepinephrine within the nerve; others that can prevent the accumulation or storage of norepinephrine within the nerve terminals; others that can prevent or block the release of norepinephrine within the nerve terminals; and still others can prevent or block the release of norepinephrine from the nerve terminals in response to the nerve impulse. These drugs are commonly considered antisympathetic drugs. All of them act by impairing, in one way or another, the release of norepinephrine. Thus they prevent the effect of norepinephrine on the effector cells. Furthermore, by acting upon the nerve terminals, these drugs spare the receptors. As a result, sympathomimetic drugs, which act directly on the receptor, can remain effective.

Another way of antagonizing the effects of sympathetic nerve stimulation is to block the receptors themselves. In a similar manner, atropine blocks the effects of acetylcholine on the effector cells. Within the sympathetic nervous system there are, as mentioned previously, two types of adrenergic receptors. Briefly, those sympathetic receptors which cause contraction of smooth muscles in the blood vessels, in the eye to produce dilatation of the pupil, and on the hair follicles to cause goose bumps, are referred to as *alpha* receptors and are activated primarily by norepinephrine. These reactions are rapid and are blocked selectively by a group of compounds known as *alpha* adrenergic blocking drugs, a rather diverse class of chemical compounds. It includes such substances as derivatives of ergot, the fungus which is a parasite to rye, and a number of unrelated synthetic compounds, e.g. phentolamine (Regitine) and phenoxybenzamine (Dibenzyline). The physiologic effects of blockade of *alpha* receptors are a fall in blood pressure, decrease in heart rate (a reflex response to the fall in blood pressure), increased activity of the intestine, orthostatic or postural hypotension as described for ganglionic blockade and impotence in men.

The other sympathetic receptors, the *beta* receptors, are found in such organs as the heart, in the smooth muscles of the bronchioles (small tubules in the lungs), and in certain blood vessels, particularly those which are in the skeletal muscles throughout the body. Activation of *beta* receptors causes dilatation of blood vessels and increased blood flow through the muscles. Many of the metabolic effects of sympathetic nerve stimulation result from activation of *beta* receptors. These include an increase of sugar, free fatty acids, and lactic acid in the blood.

Alpha and *beta* receptors have been distinguished most clearly on the basis of their responses to various blocking drugs. *Alpha* blocking drugs such as phenoxybenzamine, phentolamine and ergotamine (an ergot drug) do not antagonize the effects of sympathetic nerves on the *beta* receptors. Conversely, *beta* blocking drugs have no effect on *alpha* receptors. Blockade of the *beta* receptors slows the heart rate and reduces the force of the heart's contractions without affecting the blood pressure. In some persons suffering from asthma, constriction within the bronchial tubes occurs.

Beta blocking drugs were first introduced only ten years ago. The early ones were not clinically useful because, upon administration, they first stimulated *beta* receptors, greatly increasing the heart rate, an effect both uncomfortable and potentially dangerous. More recently, other drugs of this type have been developed which do not have such stimulant activity. The most prominent of these is propranolol or Inderal. This drug is currently undergoing clinical trials, but has not been released for general use.

Uses of Autonomic Drugs in Medicine

When the intestinal tract and urinary bladder lose their tone, the *parasympathomimetic drugs* are often administered. Loss of tone and activity in the intestine results in distention and a failure to propel the contents along the tract. Similarly, with loss of tone the bladder becomes distended and cannot contract to expel the urine. A specific example of a situation in which such drugs are useful is the condition called postoperative ileus. This is a general paralysis of the intestinal tract, accompanied by urinary retention from paralysis of the bladder. These two conditions are more apt to occur following an abdominal operation, but may be present after any type of anesthetic procedure. For these conditions the physician might use methacholine or a cholinesterase inhibitor such as neostigmine.

A complex disorder of heart rhythm called paroxysmal atrial tachycardia usually requires a parasympathomimetic drug. In this disease the atria (upper chambers) of the heart begin beating at very rapid rates, as if they had escaped control of the vagus nerve (a parasympathetic nerve). The administration of a parasympathomimetic drug, e.g. methacholine, may restore the heart rhythm to normal.

Another important use of parasympathomimetic drugs lies in treatment of glaucoma, a disease of the eye. In this condition the fluid in the eye, the aqueous humor, cannot sufficiently drain off, causing increased pressure within the eye. Applying a parasympathomimetic drug topically to the eye will, under appropriate circumstances, improve the drainage of aqueous humor and reduce pressure. More recently, one of the organophosphorus cholinesterase inhibitors, disopropyl fluorophosphate (DFP), has been used and found effective. It will be remembered that these compounds inhibit the breakdown of acetylcholine by the enzyme cholinesterase, and thus mimic the effects of parasympathetic nerve stimulation. Because these organophosphorus anticholinesterase agents have a rather persistent action, there is less need for frequent administration of the drug.

The mechanism by which these drugs act to promote drainage of fluid from the eye is admittedly rather complex. Suffice it to say that eye structures affecting drainage are under the influence of parasympathetic nerves, and whatever mimics the action of these nerves will promote the removal of fluid from the eye.

Finally, parasympathomimetic drugs, specifically the cholinesterase inhibitors, can be used in the diagnosis and treatment of myasthenia gravis. In some unknown way, this disease afflicts the junctions between nerves and voluntary muscles. Although this is not a part of the autonomic (involuntary) nervous system, the same general principles hold. Acetylcholine is first released from the nerve endings to the skeletal muscles; it transmits the impulse of the nerve to the muscle. The receptor here is a cholinergic one, that is, it is stimulated by acetylcholine. But it differs from those on ganglion cells or the effector cells supplied by parasympathetic nerves. The receptors on skeletal muscles are blocked neither by ganglionic blocking agents, nor by parasympathetic blocking drugs. However, they can be blocked by a class of drugs exemplified by curare, the South American arrow poison. Myasthenia gravis is a condition resembling the effect that would be produced by curare, i.e., severe muscle weakness. To relieve a patient of myasthenia gravis, a physician might administer neostigmine; by inhibiting cholinesterase at the junction between nerves and voluntary muscles, neostigmine allows acetylcholine to accumulate and may produce a remarkable recovery of muscles function. While the effect of neostigmine is not long lasting and is accompanied by many side effects, it has proved useful in the treatment of this serious and puzzling disease.

Parasympathetic blocking drugs are used to relieve spasm or hyperactivity of the stomach and intestinal tract, e.g. an irritable colon or the hyperactivity that is believed to accompany peptic ulcers. Administration of atropine, or one of the large number of related synthetic compounds, reduces intestinal activity by blocking the parasympathetic receptors on the smooth muscle in the intestine. These compounds are now standard agents in the therapy of peptic ulcer. Their use in this disease is based on the assumption that hyperactivity adds to the pain, or even the perpetuation of the ulcer. Such drugs may be administered in tablet form for antispasmodic action, although side effects are sometimes prominent and disturbing. These

include blurring of vision, dryness of the mouth from inhibited salivation, and palpitations of the heart. This last effect arises from a
blockade of the vagus nerve, which regulates the rhythm of this
organ.

In a recent textbook of medical pharmacology, twenty-six
synthetic antispasmodic drugs are considered. As in many fields of
pharmacologic agents, there is, so to speak, an embarassment of
riches. In actual practice, however, there seems to be very little difference among them.

Preparing a patient for surgery normally requires drugs in
the atropine family. One recalls that such drugs inhibit the para-
sympathetically induced secretions of the salivary glands and the
mucous glands of the respiratory tract. These effects, usually considered side effects, can in certain instances be considered the major
effects. Before an operation, an anesthesiologist usually prefers to
"dry" a patient's respiratory tract. Under anesthesia, during which
coughing and clearing of the respiratory tract is not possible, danger
arises from saliva and secretions from the mucous glands in the
larger air passages. If these secretions drop down into the lungs,
they can plug the tinier air passages, possibly causing pneumonia.
If a patient is treated with atropine or a related compound prior
to administration of the anesthetic agent, secretion by the glands
is inhibited. Scopolamine might be employed here. It is a naturally
occurring material closely related to atropine, found in the same
plant, *Atropa belladonna*. Besides the parasympathetic blocking
effect, scopolamine exerts a slight tranquilizing action on the brain.
Anesthesiologists consider this desirable.

A third major use of these drugs lies in ophthalmology. The
application of an atropine solution to the surface of the eye will
produce marked dilatation of the pupil. This makes it possible for
the ophthalmologist to see the interior of the eye, and to examine
the network of blood vessels and certain other anatomical features.
At the same time that atropine produces pupillary dilatation, it pa-
ralyses the muscles of accommodation. When these small muscles
contract, they change the shape of the lens, allowing for the appropriate adjustment for vision at close range. These muscles come
into play when sight is turned from a distant object to an object
within a few inches from the eyes, such as a book. By blocking

the effects of the parasympathetic nerves on these muscles, atropine impairs our ability to accommodate and produces blurred vision. Paralysis of accommodation is sometimes necessary to the ophthalmologist when he has to determine the refractive index of the eye. Such information is needed to prescribe eyeglass lenses.

There is danger in using a drug such as atropine to dilate the pupil because it might initiate an acute attack of glaucoma, either in a patient known to have the disease, or in a patient who has the disease but in whom it has not been recognized. Therefore, in patients with a history of glaucoma or in older persons generally, it is unlikely that any member of this class of drug will be administered for routine eye examination. The mechanism by which an attack of glaucoma is precipitated by parasympathetic blocking drugs is the opposite of the mechanism by which parasympathomimetic drugs are effective in the treatment of glaucoma. Marked pupil dilatation and paralysis of accommodation impair the drainage of the aqueous humor from the eye. In a normal eye, however, there is little likelihood of precipitating an attack of glaucoma.

Finally, parasympathetic blocking drugs are used in the treatment of two types of poisoning. The first, not too common, is poisoning from ingestion of the fly mushroom *Amanita muscaria,* mentioned earlier, and related substances. This mushroom contains large amounts of muscarine. The site of action of muscarine is primarily restricted to those receptors that are effectively blocked by atropine and its derivatives. Consequently, such poisoning can be readily treated by administering any one of these drugs.

A more frequent type of poisoning is due to inhibition of the enzyme cholinesterase, particularly by insecticides such as parathion and similar agents used as sprays on farms and in fruit orchards. These compounds prevent destruction of the mediator acetylcholine, thus allowing it to reach very high levels, high enough to cause death. Atropine can inhibit many of the effects of acetylcholine in the peripheral tissues, and is an important drug in the treatment of this kind of poisoning. These insecticides also produce toxic effects in the brain. Again, such toxicity is presumably caused by accumulation of acetylcholine. In this case, however, atropine does not block acetylcholine's action and other measures have to be employed.

Ganglionic blocking drugs are almost exclusively employed

in the treatment of high blood pressure. Blockade of sympathetic ganglia inhibits the transmission of impulses along autonomic nerves which are primarily responsible for determining the degree of constriction of blood vessels. If no impulses are allowed to pass down these nerves, the smooth muscles in the blood vessels relax and blood pressure falls. These drugs do not cure essential hypertension or any other forms of hypertension, but are given on a well established rationale that lowering of the blood pressure prevents many harmful effects of sustained hypertension (damage to the kidneys, eyes and heart, and hemorrhages in the brain).

High concentrations of nicotine were shown long ago to be capable of blocking ganglia, but toxicity precluded clinical use. Not until the middle 1940's when Acheson and Moe described the effects of tetraethylammonium, did a clinically useful ganglionic blocking drug became available. This work led to the synthesis of a large number of drugs, most of which are highly charged molecules that are poorly absorbed from the intestinal tract. Variable degrees of effectiveness may thus be expected when they are taken orally. While these agents effectively lower blood pressure, they also produce a number of unpleasant side effects such as orthostatic hypotension, reduction of the heart's output of blood, inhibited activity of the intestinal tract, and loss of tone in the bladder. Mecamylamine, which is not a highly charged molecule, and hence better absorbed, produces similar side effects; moreover, higher doses of this drug may cause tremors, mental confusion, and even convulsions.

Sympathomimetic drugs are among the most widely used therapeutic agents in medical practice. Their one most extensively applied action is constriction of blood vessels, brought about by activation of the *alpha* receptors on the smooth muscle of these vessels. One of the more well-known uses in this regard is to shrink the engorged vessels in the nasal mucosa when congestion results from such diseases as hay fever or colds. Here the sympathomimetic is applied directly to the nasal mucous membranes in the form of drops or a nasal spray. The drug is absorbed through the membranes, comes in contact with the receptors on the smooth muscles of the blood vessels of the mucosa, and causes them to constrict; this reduces the amount of blood flowing into the tissue and thereby shrinks it. Certain disadvantages follow from chronic use of these agents;

prolonged reduction of blood supply can cause the death of some nasal tissue. Upon cessation of drug use a rebound phenomenon is common, that is, a greater swelling of the mucosa and a more obvious obstruction of nasal passages. This causes the patient to use more nose drops than before, again affording temporary relief which is followed by rebound congestion.

Formerly, one of the better known uses for a sympathomimetic drug, such as epinephrine, was for treatment of shock. Many cheap novels and third-rate movies played upon the effects of Adrenalin on a person in shock and his dramatic recovery. Unfortunately this was more fiction than fact. The rationale for using epinephrine, norepinephrine and related sympathomimetic agents in the treatment of shock has been based on their effects on blood pressure. In a state of shock, blood pressure is usually low. Higher pressure is required to force blood through the vessels; a sympathomimetic drug constricts blood vessels, and consequently the pressure is raised. But this rationale is no longer considered to be a good phsyiologic one in all cases, and considerable harm may be done to a person by the injudicious and excessive use of such drugs.

There are, however, certain instances when generalized constriction of blood vessels is desirable. The fall in blood pressure associated with spinal anesthesia can be checked by an injection of a sympathomimetic drug. A physician might employ a local analgesic which contains some epinephrine, a sympathomimetic, in order to constrict vessels and to prevent the analgesic from being quickly washed away in the bloodstream. These examples are discussed more fully in Chapter 9, "Localized Pain Control."

From the previous chapter one may recall that some sympathomimetic drugs activate *beta* receptors. These receptors are primarily found in blood vessels supplying skeletal muscles, where activation of the *beta* receptors produces dilatation. Some drugs of this class have been used for the treatment of certain diseases, e.g. Buerger's disease, in which these vessels are constricted. A more recent use of these agents, particularly isoproterenol, is for treatment of circulatory shock. The actions of these drugs on the heart are assuming increasing importance in modern therapy. One salient example lies in treatment of cardiac arrest (stoppage of the heart), in which the ventricles (lower chambers of the heart) cease beating.

Slow intravenous infusion of a drug such as epinephrine or isoproterenol will stimulate the lower pacemaker, where the heartbeat originates. The pacemaker, which lies in the ventricles and drives the heart, is ordinarily inactive because of the dominance of the main pacemaker in the atrium (upper chamber of the heart). However, by administration of these drugs the ventricles can be at once stimulated and regulated—to contract rhythmically, thereby providing a consistently adequate supply of blood to nourish the body tissues.

Bronchial asthma is a disease characterized by intense constriction of the bronchioles (smaller air passages) of the lungs, impairing a person's ability to breathe. The smooth muscles in these bronchioles, as has been mentioned previously, can be relaxed by the action of sympathomimetics on the *beta* receptors. One such drug is ephedrine, a compound occurring naturally. It can be taken by mouth, and has a longer duration and a slower onset of action than epinephrine (Adrenalin), another drug used for treatment of asthma. The latter drug is administered by injection under the skin. Given by this route it produces fairly prompt relief of the asthmatic attack—an effect that may last up to fifteen minutes. The abortion of an attack of asthma may be all that is necessary; that is to say, the attack may not recur immediately after the administration of the epinephrine. A more convenient form of therapy is inhalation of the sympathomimetic drug in the form of an aerosol. To reduce deterioration of the drug in solution, technologists have devised small pressurized cans filled with a solution of either epinephrine or isoproterenol in an inert medium or propellant, in most instances a liquid or a gas such as Freon. By an appropriate built-in control the right dose of sympathomimetic drug can be administered, providing very prompt relief of asthma. Although aerosol therapy relieves a patient for a shorter time, its convenient self-administration renders it more advantageous.

Allergic reactions, such as those produced by bee stings or ingestion of foods to which one is allergic, can be treated in part by the administration of sympathomimetic drugs. At its worst, an allergic reaction known as anaphylaxis may occur, a condition characterized by a fall in blood pressure, hives, constriction of the bronchi similar to that occurring in the asthmatic patient, and collapse of the circulatory system. Even death may occur. Allergic reactions may, of course, assume less severe forms—hives, itching, a tightness in the chest, and difficulty in breathing. Injection or inhalation of epinephrine is very beneficial in these instances. It dilates the bronchi and thus allows a patient to breathe with ease. By constricting the blood vessels, epinephrine raises blood pressure. Hives are reduced, presumably by decreasing blood supply to the areas where they occur. The use of epinephrine in allergic reactions like this takes advantage of the dual action of epinephrine on the two types of sympathetic receptors. The dilating effect on bronchi results from activation of *beta* receptors; the constriction of blood vessels is due to an effect on *alpha* receptors.

In ophthalmology, sympathomimetic drugs that act on the *alpha* receptors are used to dilate the pupils. One can dilate the pupils by relaxing the constrictor (circular) muscles or by causing a contraction of the dilator (radial) muscles of the iris. The pupillary dilatation induced by sympathomimetic drugs is different from the dilatation by parasympathetic blocking drugs such as atropine. Atropine produces pupillary dilatation by paralysis of the constrictor muscles. Sympathomimetic drugs cause the same dilatation by an active contraction of radial (dilator) muscles of the iris. Because it is not supplied with sympathetic nerves, the muscle in the eye involved in accommodation for near vision is not affected by sympathomimetic drugs. Hence, no blurring of vision occurs when the pupils are dilated by these drugs. Furthermore, these drugs do not interfere with drainage of fluid (aqueous humor) from the eye, and therefore can be used without danger in patients with glaucoma. One of the more common sympathomimetic drugs used to dilate the pupil is phenylephrine, also known as Neo-synephrine.

Many sympathomimetic drugs—amphetamine is among the most prominent—have some effects on the central nervous system. Their actions on the brain are considered in Chapter 11, "The Psychiatrist and Drugs."

Of drugs that block receptors for the sympathetic mediator norepinephrine, the selective blockers of *alpha* receptors will be considered first. Theoretically, these drugs would be useful in any condition where blood vessels are excessively constricted because of overactivity of the sympathetic nerves. Such drugs have been tried for a variety of vascular abnormalities and have been most successful in the condition known as Raynaud's disease, in which severe vascular constriction occurs primarily in the fingers, hands and toes, particularly upon exposure to cold. The condition is always painful, but with prolonged vasoconstriction the tissues may actually die. Physicians treat Raynaud's disease with an *alpha* blocking drug. Unhappily, success is not uniform.

In a condition known as pheochromocytoma, a tumor develops in the medulla of the adrenal gland, an organ atop the kidney. These tumors produce large amounts of epinephrine and norepinephrine. The disease is characterized by episodic bouts of hypertension, tremor, anxiety, headache—many of the signs that one would expect from injections of large doses of epinephrine or norepinephrine. One way of diagnosing this condition is by the administration of an *alpha* blocking drug, usually phentolamine (Regitine). The compound is injected into the patient, and the change in blood pressure is observed. If the blood pressure falls in excess of a certain level, a presumptive diagnosis of pheochromocytoma is established. What is the rationale for this test? The high blood pressure is due to excessive amounts of epinephrine and norepinephrine in the bloodstream. These substances act upon *alpha* receptors on the smooth muscle cells of blood vessels, cause them to contract and thus raise the blood pressure. *Alpha* blocking drugs prevent the circulating epinephrine or norepinephrine from reacting with the receptors, and thus reduce the degree of constriction of blood vessels, lowering blood pressure. The sympathetic nervous system controls the degree of vasoconstriction which, in turn, is closely correlated with the level of blood pressure in normal individuals. Hence, an injection of an *alpha* blocking drug will lower blood pressure in the normal individual to some extent. Consequently, the presumptive diagnosis of pheochromocytoma must be dependent upon an excessive fall in blood pressure. The margin of error is obviously wide, and the use of these drugs in the diagnosis is only one of several measures used. *Alpha* blocking drugs may also be used in preoperative management of pheochromocytoma, or in the treatment of patients for whom operation is considered unsafe.

A relatively new use for *alpha* blocking drugs lies in the treatment of certain forms of circulatory shock, in which a profound fall in blood pressure occurs due to widespread dilatation of blood vessels. The rationale of the use of these drugs is simply to prevent excessive and damaging blood vessel constriction which occurs as a compensatory reaction in response to the fall in blood pressure.

The *beta* blocking drugs are also largely experimental. At the present time the foremost drug of this type is propanolol or Inderal, now considered to possess some value in operations for the removal of pheochromocytomas. During surgery, manipulation of the tumor before excision may cause a sudden expulsion of epinephrine and norepinephrine into the bloodstream. These substances may adversely affect the heart during anesthesia, producing disturbances of rhythm or excessive increases in heart rate. Blockade of the *beta* receptors in the heart by a drug such as propanolol will control or prevent these effects. Such drugs are also being tried for the treatment of various disturbances in the rhythm of the heartbeat. Disturbances due to excessive sympathetic nervous activity would appear to be prime targets for successful treatment by these drugs.

Propanolol is being tested in a third major disease, angina pectoris. Angina pectoris, one recalls from Chapter 4, is a condition in which chest pain occurs upon exertion or in states of anxiety. It is a manifestation of a disease of the coronary arteries, in which there is some narrowing of coronary vessels. The pain is presumably the result of transient periods of poor oxygenation of areas of the heart muscle. Standard treatment of angina pectoris lies in the use of drugs which dilate blood vessels (see Chapter 4). Dilators open up the coronary blood vessels and allow greater circulation of blood to the heart muscle. The rationale for the use of *beta* blocking drugs is based upon the fact that there may be a component of excessive sympathetic activity in angina pectoris. The results of therapy with these agents are still inconclusive. *Beta* blocking agents are not without side effects—the danger of precipitating a depression of the heart muscle, heart failure, or an attack of bronchial asthma in a patient with a known history of this disease.

Another class of sympathetic blocking agent interferes with the nerve terminal's release of norepinephrine to stimulate the effector cells. All adrenergic nerve terminals are affected, whether the organ is innervated by *alpha* or *beta* receptors. These blocking drugs may be grouped under three headings. The first may be exemplified by a drug called methyldopa (Aldomet). This compound theoretically blocks the enzymatic formation of norepinephrine, and therefore should prevent formation of norepinephrine in the nerve terminals. Hence, there should be little or no norepinephrine for the nerve impulse to release. Aldomet also lowers blood pressure, but it is not certain whether the lowering of blood pressure is related to the inhibited synthesis of norepinephrine, or whether there is some other subtle mechanism at play here.

There are two drugs which do not interfere with synthesis of norepinephrine in any way, but appear to prevent the responses of an organ to sympathetic nerve stimulation, presumably by blocking the release of norepinephrine from sympathetic nerve endings. One of these is guanethidine (Ismelin). At first, it blocks completely the responses to nerve stimulation without reducing the amount of norepinephrine in the nerve terminals. As time passes, however, the amount of norepinephrine is diminished. Bretylium (Darenthin) is similar to guanethidine in producing a block without depleting stores of norepinephrine in sympathetic nerve endings. Unlike guanethidine, it does not deplete norepinephrine with time.

All of these drugs which act on sympathetic nerve terminals are used primarily for one condition, high blood pressure. They block the constricting effects of sympathetic nerves on the blood vessels. Their main virtue lies in their specificity, for, unlike the ganglionic blocking drugs, these agents act only on the sympathetic nervous system. They possess no blocking effect on the parasympathetic nervous system. Some side effects arise from blockade of the sympathetic nerves, effects such as increased intestinal activity, postural hypotension, and even some degree of impotence. Although the uses of these drugs are limited, they are a valuable part of our armamentarium in the treatment of hypertension.

Chapter 9

Localized Pain Control

$$T$$he coca shrub grows wild in the Andes Mountains. For centuries the Indians of the Inca Empire chewed and sucked on coca leaves—before battle to sustain their endurance, on their wounds to kill pain, after dinner to bring on a state of euphoria. Spanish conquistadors who invaded Peru in the sixteenth century found that the Incas cultivated the plant for use in religious rituals as well. The natives still take coca, some twenty million pounds annually, but the "cocaine market" has considerably widened in the past seventy years.

Sigmund Freud was naturally interested in any drug that had a psychosomatic effect. In 1884, long before he began mapping the precincts of the mind, he published an essay on cocaine in which he considered its psychological effects:

> [Cocaine produces] exhilaration and lasting euphoria, which in no way differs from the normal euphoria of a healthy person . . . In other words, you are simply normal, and it is soon hard to believe you are under the influence of a drug. Long, intensive mental or physical work is performed without any fatigue . . . The result is enjoyed without any of the unpleasant aftereffects that follow exhilaration brought by alcohol.

Freud concluded by pointing out possible uses: "The capacity of cocaine or its salts when applied in concentrated solutions to anesthetize cutaneous and mucous membranes suggests a possible future use, especially in cases of local infections." Later, Freud accidentally discovered that cocaine has addictive properties, and in fact, he broke a morphine addict of the habit by using cocaine as a drug, at the expense of making a cocaine addict.

An associate of Freud, Carl Köller, looked at cocaine from a different point of view. In the summer of 1884 he applied cocaine topically to the eyes of a frog, a rabbit, and a dog, and finally to his own. In each case the drug anesthetized the area thoroughly

139

Köller's applications are considered to be the first rational use of a local pain-killing drug in medical history.

Medical use of cocaine spread rapidly, but the drug was too dangerous to be given (like Novocain) under the skin. It is in fact so potent that it can perform its action merely by being applied to the surface of the skin.

Like many drugs, cocaine seems to be a sword with a double edge. It has the advantage of constricting the blood vessels, and this of course prevents excessively rapid elimination from an area. Yet when cocaine used to be injected directly into the bloodstream, vessels all over the body would constrict in a matter of seconds. The heart would have to pump much harder to force the blood through the narrower vessels. This raised the blood pressure and heart failure commonly resulted. Now applied to the surface of the skin, cocaine only constricts blood vessels in a small area. Here at any rate, constriction is desirable, for cocaine does not leave or desert its pain-relieving duties too quickly. And more importantly, the constricted vessels reduce the blood flow in the area, permitting only a little cocaine to enter the bloodstream at a time. With only small amounts of cocaine in the bloodstream at any one time, the liver is given enough time to inactivate the drug, and toxicity is thereby minimized.

Local Analgesics

Cocaine may have been the first successful local analgesic (pain-relieving drug) in modern medicine, but there have been others in the past. Ice and snow, for instance, were quite commonly used. Half an hour in an ice-cold shower will benumb the toughest hide. Today the search continues for a local analgesic that will last for days, even weeks—a painkiller to prevent postoperative and other kinds of pain—which will not damage body tissues and nerve fibers. Meanwhile, physicians have a wide variety of anesthetics from which to choose (Figure 1).

Some people should be awake during anesthesia. For these people there are the local anesthetics, or more properly, the local analgesics. These drugs do not induce unconsciousness, but only suppress pain in a particular locale of the body. Although the precise

DIAGRAMS OF BASIC FEATURES OF
LOCAL ANALGESICS

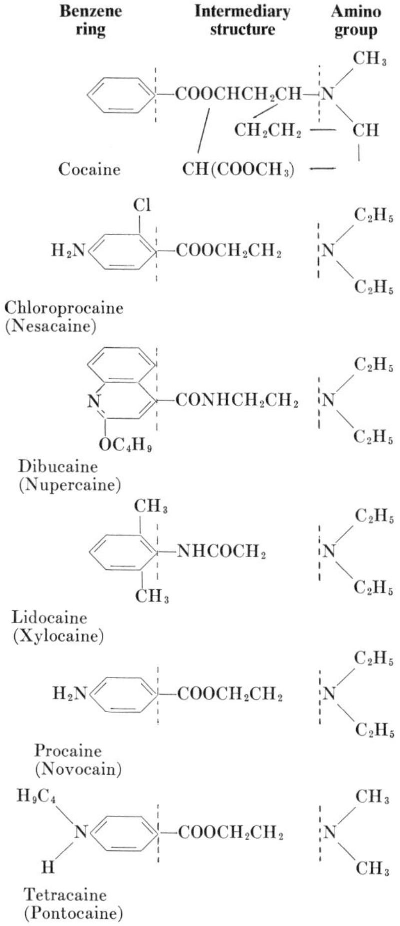

Benzene ring	Intermediary structure	Amino group

FIGURE 1. *Some commonly used local analgesics. These share certain basic features. All have a benzene ring, an intermediary structure, and contain nitrogen usually in the form of an amino group.*

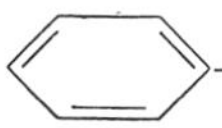

—benzene ring

C—carbon
H—hydrogen
O—oxygen
Cl—chlorine
N—nitrogen

manner in which local analgesics act is not completely known, it is fairly well agreed that the nerves become paralyzed in the vicinity of the application.

Local analgesics can be externally applied or injected. Many commercial ointments and jellies contain some local analgesic that is absorbed by the skin. This can quickly deaden local pain. The drugs may also be injected under the skin—though not into a blood vessel. In dental work, procaine (Novocain) is usually injected into the gum or into the inner lining of the cheek. By not injecting the drug into blood vessels, a doctor prevents it from being washed away too quickly, and so lengthens the time for an operation. Some local analgesics *are* administered directly into a blood vessel. To anesthetize the entire foot, for instance, a doctor might inject lidocaine (Xylocaine) into an artery above the ankle. The procedures must be considered carefully, since the analgesics must be kept away from the heart and brain. A high concentration of a foreign substance in the bloodstream may lead to poisoning. Thus, if the drug cannot be rapidly inactivated, it may inflict damage elsewhere in the body.

There are about 10 billion nerve cells or neurons in the body. Some of these transmit thought into action; some relay sensations of warmth and cold; others sense touch and pain. These sensory nerves lie all over the surface of the body, but they are more numerous in areas where their presence is of special value. Touch a pin lightly to any point on the fingertip and there will be a nerve to transmit the event. But touch a pin with the same light pressure to the back of the neck and most probably you will not feel anything. Yet if the pin is drawn even an inch across the neck, a nerve will soon be hit upon and pain will be felt.

Consider a single nerve cell that registers pain. Say it is touched gently but it does not fire a sensation of pain. If it is hit with a hammer, however, it fires and sends a tiny pain sensation to the brain. Somewhere between the touching it gently and the hitting it hard, the nerve cell has what is called its "threshold." The threshold equals the amount of pain it takes to cause a painful sensation to be *felt*. Every nerve cell fires only at a certain discrete level, its threshold, no matter what the degree of stimulation. The *amount* of pain is measured by the number of times the single nerve cell fires in a given period of time, or by the number of single nerve cells involved in a sensation of pain at the outset. A wound to the finger, dense with nerves, is far more painful than a wound to, say, the upper arm.

Thus nerves fire like a succession of bullets from a machine gun. Either the trigger is pulled all the way and the gun goes off, or not at all. There are no half-bullets, nor quarter-bullets. But continual pressure on the trigger will send out a steady stream of bullets, just as the inflicted pain will not go away after the nerve cell fires the first time. Pain is usually thought of as qualitative. Actually it is quantitative—at least to our nerve cells.

A local analgesic drug acts by raising the threshold of sensation in the sensory nerve cells—the ones that detect pain, heat, cold, and pressure. It takes a much greater stimulus to fire the nerve cells in their benumbed condition—so much stimulus in fact that it rules out the possibility of firing altogether. Smaller nerve fibers are blocked by the analgesic first, because the proportion of their surface to their mass is highest. It takes longer for the larger nerve trunks to be affected.

Nerve Block

In regional anesthesia pain is suppressed by cutting off the conductivity of a sensory nerve trunkline. This does not mean that the individual loses all sense of feeling in the area. He may retain touch, heat and cold, but he loses the sensation of pain. A hand so anesthetized can be placed on a hot stove and no pain will be felt—until the local anesthetic wears off.

Nerve block is a form of regional anesthesia in which a local anesthetic is injected around or directly into the nerve or nerves supplying the area. It can be performed just about anywhere on the surface of the body. It all depends, of course, on the nature of the operation, the comfort of the patient, and the convenience of the surgeon. Once a "local" is decided upon, the physician proceeds to map out strategically the area around the target. He may need to deaden nerves on the spot itself; perhaps he can knock out communications farther on up the line. Field block, another form of anesthesia, creates, as it were, a blockade of defenses around the field of operation.

Local anesthesia is used most for operations on teeth. Upper teeth are innervated by the superior alveolar nerves; these are branches of the larger maxillary nerve. A simple local infiltration— not a nerve block—will suffice to any one of the upper teeth. The drug is injected on both the inner and outer side of the tooth. Lower teeth are more difficult to anesthetize. The mandibular nerve supplies the lower teeth with inferior alveolar nerves. The gum, however, is supplied by the lingual nerve; this nerve serves the floor of the mouth and the front two-thirds of the tongue. A local infiltration will not anesthetize the area, because the bone of the lower jaw is too thick to permit the injection to spread to the teeth. Hence, nerve-block techniques must be employed, and the physician blocks the inferior alveolar and lingual nerves at the ramus of the mandible (the lower jawbone).

If a small cyst must be removed from the chest, a local anesthetic might well be used. Here the physician may attempt to block one of the intercostal nerves. These nerves run along the lower edge of each rib. Lidocaine (Xylocaine) is often used for this kind of operation, but a muscle relaxant is usually a necessary supplement.

Many women who may remain alert safely during childbirth receive a form of nerve block called caudal anesthesia (a type of spinal anesthesia in which the drug is injected into the lowest part of the spinal canal). Anesthesiologists believe in general that caudal anesthesia kills pain, yet at the same time allows for uterine contractions. This is because the motor supply to the uterus comes from higher up, above the tenth thoracic segment of the spinal cord via the splanchnic nerves; sensory nerves come from lower branches, however, and these are the nerves paralyzed in caudal block. Anywhere from 5 percent to 20 percent of caudal anesthesias fail. Most of the difficulty seems to be that the sacrum is a very anomalous piece of Nature's handiwork, and an injection must be precisely on target to be successful.

The choice of local anesthetic depends on the nature of the operation. Lidocaine (Xylocaine) and mepivacaine (Carbocaine) offer advantages in blocking sensory conduction in peripheral nerves and are major drugs in this form of anesthesia. First, their effects last long enough to be useful and adequate for most procedures. The delivery of a child may be delayed for hours and analgesia with these drugs appears to offer more advantages and comfort to the mother without damage to the child. Also, in the event of operative emergencies that require longer anesthesia these provide it safely. These drugs also produce lengthy postoperative analgesia which reduces the total amount of opiates or other drugs necessary. Thus, complications are few and can be managed by an anesthesiologist in attendance.

The thought of procaine (Novocain) calls up a dentist's smiling face intent upon the extraction of a tooth. This occasional event will never be one of pleasure, but procaine deadens all traces of pain a few minutes after injection. Ever since the drug was synthesized in 1905, until recently, it has been considered the ideal local analgesic. Depending on the dose, procaine will anesthetize a small area for thirty minutes to an hour. It leaves few unpleasant aftereffects, although people always seem to remember where the needle went in, perhaps for another reason. Because procaine paralyzes the motor nerves as well as the sensory ones, it has the further advantage of relaxing muscles while killing pain.

One persistent concern with procaine and many similar drugs is the speed with which the blood washes them out of the area. Even if the drug is not injected into a blood vessel, sooner or later the bloodstream will come in contact with the drug. The blood bathes the nerve cells as it would any other cells, and so the procaine is removed from the area. Moreover, procaine unfortunately causes blood vessels in the area to dilate. This opens the area to more blood per unit of time, thereby hastening the removal of the drug.

To delay the rate of departure of the analgesic, the dentist may choose to use a blend of procaine and a blood-vessel constrictor such as epinephrine. Epinephrine constricts the local blood vessels, enough at least to cut down the rate of blood passing through the tissues without damage to their food and oxygen supply. For difficult and time-consuming dental work, such as grinding down teeth for a bridge or extracting several well-rooted molars, the nerves might need to be paralyzed for at least an hour or more. Fearing excessive toxicity, the doctor prefers adding a small dose of epinephrine rather than upping the dose of procaine. There is only one danger here. Epinephrine stimulates the heart muscle, and thus it might not be given to patients with a heart ailment. Some doctors feel, however, that unallayed pain is more dangerous to the heart than a miniscule amount of epinephrine. Purely anatomical problems must also be considered in combining epinephrine with a local analgesic. Epinephrine should not be used with procaine on a finger, for example. For its size, a finger has a very large number of blood vessels—required, of course, to supply with food and oxygen the numerous nerves in this highly sensitive area of the body. Constriction of blood vessels here might lead to gangrene.

Swedish scientists introduced the local analgesic called lidocaine (Xylocaine) in 1948. More potent than procaine, lidocaine can be applied on the surface of the skin for quick anesthetization. Lidocaine is more prompt acting, longer lasting, and produces a more intense effect than procaine. One unaccountable aftereffect is sleepiness, but this may be desirable after a minor operation. For all these reasons (and others, such as its low toxicity), lidocaine has surpassed all other local analgesics used in dentistry, in the past ten years.

If wisdom teeth have become impacted and abscessed, there are compelling reasons why an oral surgeon will choose a general anesthetic rather than a local analgesic. When an injection of a drug is pressed into the tight spaces beneath the skin, it drives the liquids that are present in all directions from the site of the injection. (Incidentally, this is how the analgesic defines its "site of action.") If the area is infected with pus, the injection drives the pus further from the abcess, thus spreading the infection into new tissues.

Spinal Anesthesia

A spinal anesthetic is injected into the region just within the bony canal surrounding the lumbar region of the spinal cord. There the analgesic comes into direct contact with the nerves as they emerge from the cord. This spinal injection soon deadens every nerve with which it comes in contact. Anyone undergoing an operation involving a procedure below the waist—for a hernia or prostate—is likely to consider having a spinal. Ever since 1899 when Dr. Karl G. A. Bier performed the first "spinal," as the practice is called, this form of anesthesia has been popular—and controversial. The popularity is undoubtedly due to the fact that for some people the "fear of going to sleep" is avoided. The controversy arises over the possibility of permanent nerve paralysis caused by this method.

Administration of the spinal anesthetic requires an anesthesiologist, and a skillful one at that. He will choose his drug depending on the length of the operation: all-purpose procaine lasts an hour, tetracaine two hours, and dibucaine three hours or longer. The injection is made between the second and fifth lumbar vertebrae—roughly described as the small of the back. The drug is injected into the delicate lining of the spinal cord, and great care must be taken that the puncture of the cord's sheath is small and neat, like a pinprick. If the hole is too large, spinal fluid will leak out of the cord, a major cause of paralysis. Improper performance of the injection is thought responsible for 90 percent of the complaints after a spinal—complaints including headaches, weakness, backaches, and pains.

A few minutes after injection, a patient actually *feels* the numbness coming on. Heavier per unit than spinal fluid volume, the drug diffuses *downward* and thus benumbs the lower extremities. The upward diffusion of the anesthetic affects the respiratory and circulatory systems. Since these side effects are among the most frequent causes of death, an anesthesiologist must be ready to ventilate the lungs artificially with oxygen, and he must be alert for signs of heart flutter or other abnormalities of rhythm. Surprisingly, his task becomes more difficult in spinal rather than general anesthesia. No longer does the anesthesiologist have that close contact with the heart and lungs through the ingenious airways, monitors, and recording instruments.

Most patients, moreover, grow tired after an hour or two on the operating table. Their arms and the chest and head muscles stiffen in a major operation. Random movements to alleviate discomfort frustrate the surgeon. He must cope with a patient's other problems as well; he has to encourage him, for example, and this can interfere with his more important work; this tends to lengthen operations and to exacerbate the problem further. For these reasons "spinals" are rapidly going out of fashion, among doctors and patients alike.

Advancements in the field of local anesthetics should not

obscure some ancient records. In the first century A.D., the Greek physician Dioscorides wrote that rose oil applied to the eye or to the mucous membrane of the mouth would allay pain, and his observation has been experimentally tested and upheld in this century. One might wonder all the more at the plant that Homer (900 B.C.?) mentions at the close of the eleventh book of the *Iliad*. This book is teeming with heroes and battles, with wounds and death. And death would have its day, had not Homer concluded with these fitting lines on the art of healing:

Patroclus held the shepard in his arms and carried him
To his hut. A servant saw them and spread oxhides on the ground.
He set him down on these, then cut the pointed arrow out,
Tearing through his thigh; and then he bathed the running dark
Red blood with warm water, while his hands rubbed in the juice
Of bitter roots, the roots that took away the bitter pain,
Ending all anguish. So the blood stopped and the wound dried.

SUPPLEMENTAL READING

Ritchie, J. M. and Greengard, P., Mechanism of Action of Local Anesthetics, Annual Review of Pharmacology, *6,* 405, 1966.

Green, N. M., Physiology of Spinal Anesthesia, Williams and Wilkins, Baltimore, November, 1958.

Long-term follow-up of patients who received 10.098 spinal anesthetics.
J.A.M.A., *156,* 1486, 1954,
J.A.M.A., *161,* 586, 1956,
J.A.M.A., *172,* 1483, 1960,
Surgery *38;* 463, 1953.

Moore, D. C., et al, Block of the Upper Extremity, Arch Surgery, *90,* 68, 1965.

Peridural Block: Analysis of 3637 Cases and Review, Anesthesiology, *18,* 723, 1957.

Chapter 10

General Anesthesia

When a patient undergoes anesthesia, he surrenders himself to a set of drugs and a stranger. He gives up all that we know of life—consciousness and feeling. But for most people anesthesia is only a minor aspect of surgery. On the way to the operating room the patient may drop off to sleep casually and wake up several hours later when the ordeal is over. Anesthesia is quite simply taken for granted.

Long and careful planning has gone on to insure that those hours of unconsciousness will be safe and painless. To begin with, the anesthesiologist will drop by the patient's hospital room the night before. He will chat with the patient, check his health charts, decide what drugs can and cannot be used for the operation. Most of all, he will assess the mental preparedness of the patient for anesthesia and the operation. Then he will instruct the nurse to give a mild sedative that night, or a stronger one the next morning. By the time the patient is reading the sign on the operating room, he is drowsy; soon he is asleep. This sleep will soon be deepened by the anesthesiologist to lower and lower states of being.

During the course of the operation the anesthesiologist is no interloper on more serious affairs. He serves as the guardian of the patient's life, and his task proves to be as important to the patient's well-being as the surgery itself. In fact, difficult surgical operations could not be performed without anesthesia. It was not until a dentist, Dr. Thomas Morton, had successfully demonstrated anesthesia in Boston in 1846 that surgery, as we know it today, could be developed. Moreover, a surgeon cannot work on a patient who is not perfectly anesthetized. If muscles are twitching in jerky rhythms, the operation will be longer and more dangerous. So when the nurse taps the patient on the cheek to wake him up in the postoperative recovery room, the patient may never realize what he owes to the anesthetic drugs, or to the stranger-friend.

151

General anesthesia has many objectives in any operation. At the outset there must be a mental tranquility, a decrease of muscular activity, and, if possible, a sense of well-being or euphoria. A mild sedative usually will accomplish this. Then begin the stages of anesthesia proper. The first of these is analgesia, which is the loss of pain sensation. Deeper anesthesia brings on the loss of memory or amnesia. Finally we are at the blank bottom, unconsciousness, but there are even lower stages. After the purposeless movements abate, the body loses control of eyelid reflexes and the pupils dilate. Loss of all feeling follows. The word anesthesia itself is derived from the Greek word meaning "insensibility." In the lowest stages, the lungs do not work efficiently.

The heart, now retarded, still has strength to beat on its own. Besides the blood, it may be the only visibly moving thing during deep anesthesia. The patient who slowly descends these steps of anesthesia may seem to have come to the door of death. Indeed, one aim of anesthesia is to simulate lifelessness. In this period the surgeons ply their tasks while the anesthesiologist, somewhat like a guardian angel, maintains safety and life for the patient and watches over him.

The Anesthetic Drugs

Nearly all anesthetics are gases or volatile liquids. Many kinds of machines have been invented to regulate the amount of anesthetic in a given mixture. Liquid anesthetics must, of course, be vaporized first, and this problem has been met in several ways—for instance, by bubbling oxygen through them to saturate the gas with anesthetic vapor. The anesthesiologist creates an atmosphere out of the various gases and liquids he will use, each specific for a desired end such as loss of pain or muscle relaxation. Eventually the anesthetic mixture, containing life-sustaining oxygen, is inhaled. In deep anesthesia where the patient has no respiratory control, the lungs must be artificially ventilated. In order to bring the anesthetic into closer contact with the blood that will carry the gas molecules, an airway is funnelled down through the mouth and down the trachea or windpipe into the lungs. Made usually of synthetic rubber or plastic material, the airway maintains an air tunnel for the anesthesiologist, should obstruction the patient's throat suddenly impede the air supply. Thus, the patient can be placed in many positions for the operation, while the anesthesiologist retains constant control over his breathing.

The blood absorbs the gaseous mixture in the air sacs of the lungs. These gases are soluble in the blood in different amounts, and the degree of that solubility in blood will be important to consider in deepening or raising the state of anesthesia in the course of an operation. For example, those vaporized gases which are liquids at room temperature go into solution in the blood stream more readily than the other gases. By controlling the amount of any one gas from a tank, the anesthesiologist can cause the blood to absorb more of one gas than another.

It is mistakenly thought that the anesthesiologist uses one all-purpose drug, ether. This volatile liquid has become the most famous anesthetic, and for good reasons. The first anesthetic drug, it was the preferred drug for over a hundred years. But ether irritates the bronchial tubes. Using ether takes too long to produce sufficient depression in a patient, and too long to wake him up afterwards. Etherized patients may suffer from nausea and vomiting. Besides, ether is explosive, and this is a problem not only for the anesthesiologist but also for the surgeon and the hospital officials.

There has never been a *single* anesthetic drug which could do everything. Each drug has many desirable characteristics in itself, but may be incomplete for ideal clinical use. For this reason, in the past twenty years anesthesiologists have employed systems of drugs, some administered by inhalation, but others intravenously. Gases are often preferred because the anesthesiologist can more rapidly alter the concentration of gas in the blood than he can a liquid. A simple decrease in the amount of gas inhaled, for example, and the gas will leave the blood through the lungs. It is like taking the cap off a coke bottle. But liquid anesthetics will not bubble out as readily; hence their concentration in the blood cannot be so closely controlled.

A mixture often used for anesthesia combines nitrous oxide, oxygen, thiopental and curare. Nitrous oxide, sometimes referred to as "laughing gas," would be an ideal anesthetic drug if it were a stronger agent. Pain is suppressed and amnesia induced only when a mixture of at least 35 percent nitrous oxide is inhaled. Often

65 percent nitrous oxide is used with 35 percent oxygen. The earth's atmosphere at sea level is roughly composed of 80 percent nitrogen and 20 percent oxygen. Usually the amount of oxygen given to a patient in an operation is higher than the normal 20 percent. Since nitrous oxide cannot bring on deep anesthesia without seriously limiting the percentage of oxygen, it is often strengthened by other drugs. Its advantages are its relatively minor toxic effects, and it is nonexplosive.

Thiopental (Pentothal) is given intravenously to enhance the less potent but safe nitrous oxide. A barbiturate, thiopental blocks the part of the brain which controls waking. The speed with which the drug acts is strongly in its favor. About forty seconds after the drug is injected into the blood stream, one tenth of the dose is at work on the brain. Thiopental has no ability to deaden pain, however, and it could never be used without nitrous oxide and oxygen or another set of analgesics. But it does reduce postanesthetic excitement and vomiting, provides a quiet respiration, and is nonexplosive. There are few aftereffects.

The final drug in this mixture, curare, relaxes the muscles. The history of the drug is outlined elsewhere, but its ability to induce paralysis has been taken over by modern science for anesthesia. Curare breaks down the relation between the nerves and the muscles. The nerves cannot give commands in an orderly fashion. As a result of the confusion, the body becomes flaccid and relaxed.

Another common system of anesthesia reinforces nitrous oxide and oxygen with halothane, a volatile liquid. Halothane has been in use for about ten years. It is not explosive or flammable, and produces deep anesthesia even though it is only a small percentage of the total gaseous mixture. For patients suffering from asthma or bronchial diseases, halothane is a choice drug because it relaxes the bronchial tubes and slightly dilates them. It is sometimes damaging to the liver, however, and high concentrations depress the action of the heart muscle.

Great care is necessary in managing this type of anesthesia. Muscle relaxants, succinylcholine (Anectine) and curare, paralyze the muscles, including the muscles of breathing. The anesthesiologist must be skillful to maintain even, level anesthesia, and must "breathe" for the patient either by squeezing the breathing bag by hand or with a mechanical respirator at proper intervals. The anesthesiologist literally becomes his brother's breather. Muscle pain has been a complication after succinylcholine, and it lasts for several days if patients are allowed out of bed too soon.

What is the ideal anesthetic? There will probably never be one all-purpose drug for the simple reason that all people are not the same. Each patient must be considered individually and the range of drugs evaluated for his needs. At least, however, there are some ideal values which most anesthetics should have. First, the drug should not discomfort the patient. The drug should be specific for a desired end, such as pain-killing, or muscle-relaxation, and have no side effects. Also, it should quickly induce anesthesia, and its effects should disappear soon after the operation is over. It should be nonexplosive, and, of course, if possible, it should be inexpensive. If the drug is a gas, it should be effective at 40 percent concentration or less. In this way, the anesthesiologist can maintain at least 60 percent oxygen if the heart requires it.

Danger Signals

The patient is now anesthetized, and the operation is in progress. What could happen if the patient has his mind paralyzed? Sleep relaxes one part of our mind, but it does not depress its total activity. Our bodies are still regulated by the brain, our hearts beat regularly, our diaphragms rise and fall automatically. But during deep anesthesia, these fundamental rhythms of life are controlled by a skillful anesthesiologist.

One danger is respiratory failure. It is recognized that anesthesia usually results in respiratory depression. The resulting problems are related to reduced airflow. This makes it more difficult to get anesthetic drugs into the lungs and to remove waste materials (such as gaseous carbon dioxide) from the body. All of these problems must be dealt with immediately. By means of the airway, an anesthesiologist can ventilate the lungs as required. The concentration of oxygen in the gaseous mixture is likely to be increased. Ridding the lungs of carbon dioxide requires effective assistance to breathing, and the procedure is now commonplace in modern anesthesia.

What if the heart begins to beat in irregular rhythms, an ailment known as arrhythmia? Arrhythmias have been observed with all commonly used anesthetics, and certain drugs appear to predispose the heart to this condition. Factors other than anesthetics, however, have also been found to be the immediate cause. Mechanical irritation of the airway or surgical manipulation during light anesthesia can initiate arrhythmias which are generally transient. The accumulàtion of carbon dioxide in the lungs, hypercarbia, can cause arrhythmias as well. A popular anesthetic, cyclopropane, may start the vicious circle by causing hypercarbia. Thus, if this anesthetic is being used and a patient's heart begins to beat irregularly, the anesthesiologist will lower the percentage of cyclopropane in the inhaled mixture and increase the breathing to eliminate carbon dioxide.

Anesthesiologists have importance beyond the walls of the operating room. One important function which they have only recently been called upon to fill is the resuscitation of potential suicides. These cases usually show the same danger signals apparent in the complications from deep anesthesia, and so the anesthesiologist treats these persons *as if they were anesthetized.* Most suicides from drug poisoning actually die from failure to breathe. The anesthesiologist supports the person's breathing by ventilating his lungs with a high percentage of oxygen. Or, the doctor will dialyze the person's blood, that is, strain it of the undesired chemicals. Persons suffering from coma due to other causes are also treated as if anesthetized.

Drugs in Obstetrics

In the nineteenth century, the dulling or relief of pain associated with labor was considered immoral for childbirth. But there were a few trailblazers, and among the greatest was Queen Victoria herself. Against the wishes of her court physicians, dauntless, she inhaled a general anesthetic, chloroform, to aid the birth of her eighth child in 1853. When her doctor, a Scot by the name of James Y. Simpson, was challenged by the Calvinist ministry, he pointed to the passage in Genesis on the birth of Eve:

> And the Lord God caused a deep sleep to fall upon Adam, and he slept: and he took one of his ribs, and closed up the flesh instead thereof:
> And the rib, which the Lord God has taken from man, made he a woman, and brought her unto the man.
>
> Genesis ii.21–22

In any case, the Queen was "grateful for the discovery of this means of alleviating and preventing pain," and Simpson was knighted for his service.

There will always be a cult of the "natural" childbirth. One might well question, however, what is "natural" about a childbirth with doctors and nurses and the latest medical equipment at hand? Most women now prefer the use of drugs. Although it may be a beautiful experience to witness the birth of one's child, there may be excessive risks involved. Analgesics and certain anesthetics strike and ideal compromise. The mother will be sufficiently alert to assist the obstetrician, yet pain will be suppressed.

Two British pharmacologists, Lawrence and Moulton, have outlined the drugs used during the stages of labor:

Early first stage of labor—mild sedatives (chloral, barbiturates) and mild analgesics (codeine).

End of first stage of labor—stronger analgesics (pethidine, also called meperidine) and then trichloroethylene, or nitrous oxide and air.

Second stage of labor—trichloroethylene, or nitrous oxide and air.

Pethidine, also known as meperidine or Demerol, is commonly used, and there is much clinical evidence in favor of it. It kills pain without causing sleep. With its use, a mother may take a more active role in the birth of her child (as if she were not doing enough). The machine which mixes the mild anesthetics, nitrous oxide and air, can then be operated and controlled by the hand of the mother as her pain increases or diminishes.

One danger with meperidine does not involve the mother but the child. Meperidine enters the placenta, the organ in the uterus which nourishes the fetus via the umbilical cord. Meperidine and narcotics like morphine spread to the placenta and are thus absorbed to some extent by the fetus. This may cause a certain amount of prenatal depression.

New Anesthetic Equipment

Considerable improvement has been made in the design of anesthetic appliances for safer and more physiologic conduct of anesthesia. The installation of the pin-index system to improve proper positioning of gas cylinders, and of devices to prevent inadvertent disconnection of gas sources, is now mandatory on all anesthetic machines. Another means has been designed to guard against the hazard of failure of oxygen supply. In this device all pressure regulators for anesthetic gases are controlled by oxygen pressure instead of the conventional spring-loaded valves—in the "master-slave" proportioning regulator system. If oxygen-line pressure falls, the line pressure of anesthetic gas will fall in proportion, so that the delivered mixture will contain the same percentage of oxygen. More importantly, the anesthetic gas will shut off automatically if the oxygen supply fails.

The dangers of respiratory depression during anesthesia and the effect of the accumulation of carbon dioxide in the lungs have led to efforts to minimize equipment causes of carbon dioxide retention. A number of directional valves that have a minimal external dead space and resistance to airflow have been designed. Elimination of carbon dioxide from the anesthetic circuit has also been made more efficient with the use of jumbo-sized lime canisters, which provide rapid absorption of the undesirable gas.

The need for a precision vaporizer to deliver a known concentration of a potent anesthetic vapor prompted the design of the "copper kettle." A known volume of oxygen is bubbled through a brass cylinder containing the anesthetic liquid. The design is such that the effluent mixture is saturated with the vapor. If the temperature and the vapor pressure of the anesthetic agent at this temperature are known, the exact volume of vapor may be calculated. Proper dilution of the mixture from the vaporizer with oxygen (or oxygen and some other gaseous mixture) will give a known concentration of vapor. Because of the high thermal-transfer efficiency of the system, the heat of vaporization can be supplied from the surrounding air so that with few exceptions (for example, high flow through diethyl ether) the liquid temperature changes little, and the volume of anesthetic vapor delivered remains constant over a long period. Even when considerable cooling occurs because of the high rate of vaporization, the output from this type of vaporizer is still predictable, assuming that the liquid temperature and the vapor pressure curve of the anesthetic liquid are known. These values are available for all commonly used volatile anesthetic agents.

Another type of vaporizer has been designed so that the vapor concentration can be adjusted with a dial. A portion of the carrying gas is directed through the vaporizing chamber and, laden with vapor, rejoins the main gas stream. Compensation for variations in total rate of gas flow and ambient temperature is provided so that a constant vapor concentration is obtained under usual circumstances. Similar vaporizers are available for other anesthetics—chloroform, trichloroethylene and methoxyflurane.

A third type of precision vaporizer utilizes the method of introducing a known volume of anesthetic liquid (with a liquid flowmeter or a liquid injection system) to a known volume of carrying gas. If provisions are made for complete vaporization, the vapor concentration in the final mixture may be predictable and constant.

These precision vaporizers have made it possible to conduct anesthesia with volatile anesthetic agents on a more quantitative basis. It should be obvious, however, that the patient's physiologic response to anesthesia is always more important than any values registered on flowmeters or dials.

The acuity of the anesthesiologist in sensing a patient's physiologic condition during anesthesia and operation can be improved with a variety of monitors. As yet, only certain monitors are practical and useful for day-to-day clinical practice. Furthermore, monitors do not take the place of the clinical acumen and judgment of a vigilant physician but only serve as his aid. The electrocardiogram serves well for the detection of irregular heartbeats but sometimes cannot indicate a total heart failure. The electroencephalogram can generally indicate the approximate depth of anesthesia and present an early warning for insufficient brain perfusion or oxygenation. The respirometer measures ventilatory volume. Its accuracy must be determined, and the anesthesiologist must decide what is the appropriate ventilation volume for a given patient. He can even gauge the adequacy of pulmonary ventilation by measuring blood carbon dioxide or acidity. However, some of the instruments for these measurements cannot yet be considered useful for routine clinical procedures.

A number of mechanical ventilating devices are available for use during anesthesia and for long-term respiratory support in cases of respiratory insufficiency. Generally, these ventilators can be classified into two groups: the pressure-limited, volume-variable ventilators; and the volume-limited, pressure-variable ventilators. Some have an arrangement for the patient to initiate a cycle so that they can be used to assist respiration at the patient's own rhythm. A good mechanical ventilator should be sturdy, dependable in its performance, able to deliver adequate ventilation under circumstances of changing pulmonary mechanics, relatively trouble free and easy to service. Above all, it should be simple and easy to operate. Few ventilators satisfy all these criteria. The anesthesiologist will decide which device is most suitable for his need and must be thoroughly familiar with its characteristics and limitations.

Theories of Anesthesia

The past thirty years have seen the introduction of many anesthetic drugs and as many theories of their action. One theory claims that certain anesthetics change the permeability of crucial nerve cells. Another advances that biochemical reactions lower the amount of oxygen in the brain, and thus turns it down but not out. In 1961, Linus Pauling, twice Nobel Prize laureate, advanced a proposal that inhaled anesthetics combine with water molecules to form crystals, infinitesimally small "icebergs." When the anesthetic wears off, these icebergs thaw and no damage is done to the nerve or brain cells. Thus far no one has devised a satisfactory theory of anesthesia. The reason is that the theory will have to tell us a good deal about consciousness and unconsciousness as well as the mechanism of the drug's action. And scientists are far from agreement as to what those baffling states are.

Whatever the theory, the practical benefits of anesthesia are here to stay. Of course, there have been fatalities in the past hundred and twenty years with the introduction of new drugs or the misuse of old ones. Part of the difficulty will always lie with the sickness of the patients. Sick people are a paradox to anesthesiologists. For one thing, their weakened state renders them more susceptible to an anesthetic. For another, they are more likely to suffer from side effects, and they are harder to bring out of anesthesia after an operation. Whatever the difficulties, Dr. Emanuel Papper, Chairman of the Department of Anesthesiology at Columbia University College of Physicians and Surgeons, has placed the proper emphasis: "It is so much more important to wake someone up, than to see to it that he loses consciousness."

SUPPLEMENTAL READING

Cohen, P. J., and Dripps, R. D., History and Theories of General Anesthesia, Pharmacological Basis of Therapeutics, Goodman, L. B., and Gilman, A., Eds. Third Edition, McMillan Company, New York, 43–49, 1966.

Ngai, S. H., and Papper, E. M., Medical Progress—Anesthesiology, New England Journal of Medicine *269*, 28, 83, and 142, 1963.

Vandam, L. D., Anesthesia, Annual Review of Pharmacology *6*, 379, 1966.

Papper, E. M., and Kitz, R., Uptake and Distribution of Anesthetic Agents, McGraw-Hill, New York, 1963.

Price, H. L., and Cohen, P. J., Editors, Effects of Anesthetics on the Circulation, Thomas, Charles C, Springfield, Illinois, 1964.

Severinghaus, J. W., and Larson, C. P., Respiration in Anesthesia, Handbook of Physiological Society II, Editors, Fenn, W. O., and Rahn, H., American Physiological Society, Washington, D.C., 1219–1264, 1965.

Chapter 11

The Psychiatrist and Drugs

Feare and *Sorrow* are the true Characters, and
inseparable companions of most *Melancholy,*
not all . . . In such obscurity, therefore,
variety and confused mixture of symptomes,
causes, how difficult a thing is it to treat of
severall kindes apart; to make any certainty or
distinction among so many casualties, dis-
tractions, when seldome two men shall be like
affected *per omnia.*

Robert Burton   *Anatomy of Melancholy*
Part I, Sect. 1, Memb. 3, Subsect. 1, 4.

The mind hovers over the joinings of molecules. A variety of notions have been, and still are, held about its workings. Less mysterious, though very complex, are the efforts of scientists to relate molecular events to certain critical operations that affect behavior in one way or another. In the treatment of psychiatric disorders, drugs affect physical processes in the body, but their practical importance stems from effects on behavior—the way a person thinks, feels, and acts. Such drugs work because they somehow modify excesses and imbalances in the way a person behaves. The "work" these drugs perform is remarkable; the "somehow" remains in large part an enigma.

As has often been the case in medicine, psychotropic drugs were for the most part discovered by accident. Incidental behavioral effects were recognized during the drug treatment of an organic disease. The antidepressant effect of the drugs known as MAO (monoamine oxidase) inhibitors, for example, was noted when occasional euphoria occurred as a side effect during their use for the treatment of tuberculosis. The MAO inhibitors were then tried by psychiatrists in schizophrenia to activate the sluggish patient; but the patient's condition was in fact aggravated. Only later were they finally tried in severe depression. The drugs now in use were developed from the first successful prototypes by chemical rearrangements of the parent compounds, and then refined by studies made on animals. Final evaluation of an effective drug, however, can be made only in *the* animal, man—and usually in man suffering from a specific disorder. Psychopharmacology, the study of drugs that affect behavior, began in the early part of our century and continues to expand. Scientists have just begun to chart the forest. Experts in biochemistry, physiology, psychology, and psychiatry must contribute to the great map-making.

165

Drugs or Psychiatry?

Many of the new drugs employed by the psychiatrist resemble, in whole or in part, certain body chemicals that affect human mood and behavior in still unknown ways. The present state of knowledge assumes that these drugs masquerade as chemicals already present in the body, thereby altering the normal (or abnormal) reactions already taking place. One might think of the drug and the bodily chemical it resembles as a set of twins. Outwardly, they appear to the cell to be virtually the same, but their individual actions can critically differ. The "foreign" twin gains access to the many pathways available to the body's natural chemicals, producing an altered effect on the body's chemistry and responses.

Eventually, psychiatrists may find specific aberrations in the body chemistry of mentally ill patients for which quite specific curative drugs can be administered. In fact, progress has already been made. A few children have been shown to be retarded because of failure of their metabolic systems to break down phenylpyruvic acid. This aberration (phenylpyruvic oligophrenia or phenylketonuria, known as PKU) can be corrected to some extent by dietary adjustment, and often the mental deficiency can be prevented. It is known that thyroid deficiency produces cretins while thyroid excess may result in a psychosis. Both of these can be aided by controlling the thyroid level with drugs. In cases of thyroid excess, the brain as an organ "superior" to the thyroid and participating in the chain of controls of that gland can be influenced by psychotherapy and the glandular excess often diminishes.

For most psychotic patients no specific chemical defect has been found, but there is good reason to believe such defects might occur in highly local portions of the brain's systems of cells. Furthermore, there is sound reason to expect that a number of widely different and interacting causes are at work in the patient. Accordingly, analysis of differential drug responses and the chemicals they affect may delineate some of the areas of the brain important for mental illness, but drug treatment alone will probably never be the whole answer. Research therefore continues into other methods of treating the mentally ill, i.e., by social and psychological procedures.

In fact, the results obtained from a drug are never limited

to its effect on behavior. All drugs act through a number of body cells and cell systems. The manner in which a drug may act to replace a body chemical has already been mentioned. Drugs act in a number of ways, essentially to inhibit, facilitate, block, or compete with the cell chemicals that normally regulate body processes. Moreover, when we look at the "effect" of a drug we see the end result of innumerable cellular actions and interactions with other cell systems. Thus the status of the cells, prior to administration of the drug, and the nature of the environment both determine the result that the doctor and the patient see. One recalls that in heart failure a desired goal of therapy is reduction of edema; but it is not the heart that secretes urine. Rather digitalis acts on the heart and causes it to beat more forcefully, and as a result, blood flow through the kidneys is increased and the patient loses water via the urine (see Chapters on Digitalis and Diuretics). Similarly, drugs affecting behavior act through a network of different systems in the brain, ultimately to affect the way we think, feel, and act. Drugs may even have an indirect effect on the social environment. A once-agitated patient who is made calmer is "rewarded" by the attention and good feeling of those around him. With the complexity involved, it is more useful to describe typical *patterns* of drug effect rather than to assign a single response to a single drug.

To call a drug an energizer, for example, is convenient; it describes the desired, but not the inevitable, or the only, effect. To call the barbiturate Amytal, "truth serum", is misleading. The drug does not compel one to tell the truth. It may merely relax the subject, allowing him to recall some painful memories.

Drugs must be considered in their relationships to the individual personality, the immediate situation, and the composition of the brain. The brain has certain cells that retard and other cells that facilitate motor activity. To create an imbalance in the activity, a drug can inhibit or excite either system. Thus, the same effect can be achieved by exciting one system or inhibiting an opposing system. With this in mind, drug effects which seem paradoxical can be understood. For example, in some excited people such an unusual balance might exist in the opposing systems that they fall asleep when given stimulants rather than becoming more excited. Moreover, the prior state may also determine the intensity of the drug's effect.

This may suggest why antidepressants usually have no mood-elevating effects on normal individuals—and, in fact, act as sedatives. The use of drugs to modify mental behavior is not new. Since ancient times, men have known that certain plant and animal products could do curious things to the mind. Primitives held faith in potions to induce love and hate. And long before our own time, opium and wine were used both to treat disease and to make life in general more bearable. The Asian Indians took rauwolfia, a "tranquilizer," as early as 1000 B.C. Shakespeare's Cleopatra calls for mandragora "that I might sleep out this great gap of time" that Antony is away from her. Shakespeare's Macbeth asks an attending doctor:

> Canst thou not minister to a mind disease'd,
> Pluck from the memory of rooted sorrow,
> Raze out the written troubles of the brain,
> And with some sweet oblivion's antidote
> Cleanse the stuff'd bosom of that perilous stuff
> Which weighs upon the heart?

Bromides, paraldehyde, and barbiturates—all common sedatives—were introduced between 1857 and 1903 and the latter two are still important in the treatment of certain psychiatric disorders. During the last forty years, most of the older drugs used in severe psychiatric disorders have, however, been replaced. In the 1930's insulin shock therapy was introduced. It was followed by electroconvulsive therapy (still used to treat depression of late middle life), then by lobotomy (largely abandoned now), and most recently by the new psychotropic (acting on the mind) compounds. Among such compounds are chlorpromazine and reserpine, introduced in 1952 and 1953. They tranquilize, that is produce sedation without "hypnosis," the pharmacologists' word for sleep. In 1957 iproniazid came into use as an antidepressant, and shortly thereafter, imipramine—a different kind of chemical—was introduced as an antidepressant. Following the initial discovery of tranquilizers much was heard about miracle drugs producing an amazing new cure for mental illness. The facts, of course, were not as dramatic.

Swallowing a neurochemical pill does not make obsolete the years of research into psychodynamics, a study largely initiated by

Sigmund Freud. In general, drugs are not a solution to nor do they eliminate normally troublesome human emotions. Emotional experience links one to civilization and to human relationships. To develop psychological strength and maturity, man needs to experience emotional tensions created by love, friendship, and grief, among many others. Neurochemicals help in more severe stress—not in the everyday miseries of life.

The psychoanalytic theories of Freud and his followers have contributed greatly toward understanding the development and treatment of neuroses. Neuroses have been defined as the maladaptive results of the conflict between unfulfilled desires and repressive tendencies. Psychoanalysts developed the technique of free association and candid reminiscence to reach the source of neurosis, usually a core of memories which lie buried under guilt and the naïve fears of childhood. Analysts who use the technique believe that recovering and reexamining these repressed memories allow the patient to come to understand his previously hidden source of confusion and tension; childish theories, habits, attachments and fears can be exposed to the reasoning mind of the adult. With the support of the doctor, old ghosts, old habits and outworn resentments can be laid gradually aside. Once this is done the patient can presumably better accept himself and life around him.

Quite obviously, drugs cannot give the kind of insight to the patient that psychotherapy can sometimes provide. Drugs simply cannot tell anyone how to "solve a problem." Yet one can question whether such insight is necessary for the patient to be helped. In one of their most important uses, drugs modify the emotional and mental state of the severely ill or anxious patient, making him more receptive to psychotherapy. An agitated manic patient can be calmed by chlorpromazine, or a depressed, withdrawn, patient aroused by imipramine to the point where both can communicate with a therapist, and also hear, see, act, and reflect in an atmosphere which is now— with pharmacological help—less fraught with tension, panic, and disorganization. Since the number of mentally ill precludes intensive psychotherapy for all who need it, psychopharmacology can become very valuable. It may also be valuable because psychotherapy for many disorders is of secondary importance to the intensity of disorder which is primary. The limitations are considerable, however. Drugs cannot directly influence the heredity, the family structure, or the socio-economic situation of the patient. They can modify his reaction to the environment and change the intensity and quality of his emotional and intellectual functioning. Ongoing behavior will still be largely determined, of course, by the welter of ongoing stimuli. So the problem remains: the causes of mental disease are obscure, as is the mechanism of drug action used to treat the disease. Although much is still obscure, the latest research in psychopharmacology is heartening, especially that work which tries to analyze the specific mechanisms of drug action. There are three areas in which research is proceeding at this level of analysis: (1) neurobehavioral studies, (2) biochemical studies, and (3) clinical studies.

Neurobehavioral Studies

In this area reserpine and the phenothiazines have been the most extensively studied. The compounds are screened with a series of laboratory tests and observations with animals. Among other things, scientists in the laboratory search for a drug which will induce catalepsy, or physical rigidity and immobility, for substances that will calm the rage produced in rats by brain lesions, and more generally, for drugs that affect motor and autonomic responses. In this last category, an animal's proficiency to perform a motor skill usually induced by pain is tested with drugs. But since no suitable analogue to human schizophrenia exists in animals, and since depression is difficult to induce, results of the experimentation cannot be completely satisfactory.

Finally, scientists in the laboratory have been testing the influence of drugs on neural systems that process and filter stimuli. Experimentation in this area is potentially very valuable. Drugs might be developed which could—even more than present compounds—create a period of delay between stimulus and response. This pause might help the patient organize his thoughts—an interposition that could be used to treat psychiatric disorders.

Biochemical Studies

Although neurochemical processes cannot comprehensively account for all drug effects, a number of the processes and their relationship to drug action have been identified. Psychotropic compounds have stimulated research into the mapping and evaluation of cellular components as they affect neural function. Thus far, little detailed knowledge exists about the relationship of a drug's action to metabolic or enzymatic processes occurring within the cell. In general, the attempt to link physical-chemical phenomena to bodily and behavioral response has centered upon critical "transducer" sites. One such site is the all-important synapse, an area in the neural system where information is transferred across a junction between cells.

The various amines—highly potent bioactive substances derived from the diet and present in neural tissues in minute quantities—seem to play key roles in the transfer of information. Microquantities of these highly active biochemicals can induce physiologic response in a wide range of tissues. Now it is known that psychotropic drugs act to affect the activity of brain amines at various subcellular sites. It is also known that alterations of brain amine metabolism are associated with certain excited or sedated states. A period of stress might involve a change in the uptake, binding, or release of amines.

Although it is not yet established how animes affect neural functions, some scientists think that amines might regulate and buffer certain states of excitation in the brain. When the biochemical equilibria of the amines are disturbed, intensified maladaptive response to normal excitation can occur. Thus, if a patient had some genetic or stress-induced condition which affected the uptake, binding, or release of amines or the enzymes concerned with their formation or inactivation, the individual might be chemically disadvantaged in the normal tug and pull of life. Drugs controlling these substances, it is agreed, could help him. At this point enough is known to say that biochemical regulations of overinhibited or overaroused behavior do exist and that psychotropic drugs, at least in part, act upon the mechanisms of this regulation.

Clinical Studies

Clinical studies have attempted to formulate an understanding of drug action at a descriptive level. From this perspective, drugs can be seen to raise the threshold to signals of pain or mental anguish. They produce a delay or indifference to certain situations and permit the patient to regulate the pace at which internal events occur. Seemingly the patient is given more time to think—and less intense internal and external milieu in which to think—allowing him to integrate his perceptions. In this condition he may be able to modify extreme behavior appropriately.

Drugs can usually help psychotic patients in therapy. But the way in which they help depends largely on the plan of treatment and the objectives. For many schizophrenic outpatients, a brief weekly or monthly (or even yearly) visit is common and practical. During the visit, the doctor can assess the medication as well as provide a focus for therapeutic support. This kind of therapy does not attempt to probe the motives or responses of the patient in the complexities of his personal life. While it can be argued that the technique is seemingly superficial, any other is often impossible. Psychiatrists are learning to be concerned with what is effective, whether this is "deep" or "superficial." The patient may in fact not need or well tolerate anything more than a monthly visit or he may not be able to afford more comprehensive treatment.

The Antidepressants

Sadness and depression are common human feelings. In most of us such moods pass; in others, they become rooted, horribly intense and pervasive, affecting thought and judgment. But because everyone has experienced these unhappy periods, understanding and sympathy for patients with depressive reactions should not be as difficult as is the case with the more bizarre schizophrenics.

Neurotics have exaggerated or prolonged responses to emotions that all of us have at one time or another. The neurotic response sometimes becomes incapacitating. These depressions are termed reactive and a precipitating factor can usually be identified. Other depressed people may have been so most of their lives, with no specific set of events precipitating the depression. Such people often have degrading images of themselves and tend to avoid social intercourse. Alcoholics and drug addicts commonly suffer from this kind of depression and seem to seek relief from such states through their drug intake.

Another type of depression has a definite onset, but the onset is apparently unrelated to external events. Termed endogenous depression, it occurs generally in older people. The depressions often come in cycles, with the nondepressed period sometimes being quite lengthy. The illness is characterized by retardation and feelings of guilt, associated with physical manifestations such as constipation, loss of weight, and early waking. In severe cases suicidal tendencies emerge. Here the endogenous depression is best called psychotic.

In the last ten years a great number of antidepressant drugs have appeared. One might assume from this that depressions are now easily controlled by drug therapy. Unfortunately, this is not true. Individual cases of depression tend to be idiosyncratic. So a case may often require a frustrating kind of trial-and-error empiricism. The classification of depression states is not as clear-cut as the various descriptive terms may suggest—primary and secondary, endogenous and reactive, neurotic and psychotic, and so on. And since depressions are episodic and the danger of suicide ever present, treatment is further complicated.

Psychiatrists will have to make finer distinctions within the various depressed, anergic (marked by lack of energy) and withdrawn states before they can know exactly how the antidepressants affect disease. Most commonly, depressions are differentiated by severity, by precipitating factors, or by an underlying biological disorder. Earlier we said that variation in mood is part of the human condition. Certainly it is not the psychiatrist's task to induce perpetual euphoria, thereby blunting genuine personal experience. Rather it is his function to blunt pathological distortions of these feelings.

Nevertheless, in the proper therapeutic surroundings, many depressions can be treated. Among the major proven antidepressant drugs are: monoamine oxidase (MAO) inhibitors; diabenzazepines such as imipramine, desipramine, and amitriptyline, and a number of minor antidepressants such as amphetamine and metamphetamines.

The Monoamine Oxidase (MAO) Inhibitors

The MAO inhibitors (Figure 1) comprise a group of drugs that can block the oxidative inactivation of naturally-occurring amines. The power to inhibit deamination is probably a major but not the sole source of their therapeutic action, and the exact relationship between such inhibition and the observed therapeutic value of these compounds is still obscure. One such MAO drug is iproniazid. It was first used in 1951 in the chemotherapy of tuberculosis. Since patients responded with hyperactivity, euphoria, and even toxic psy-

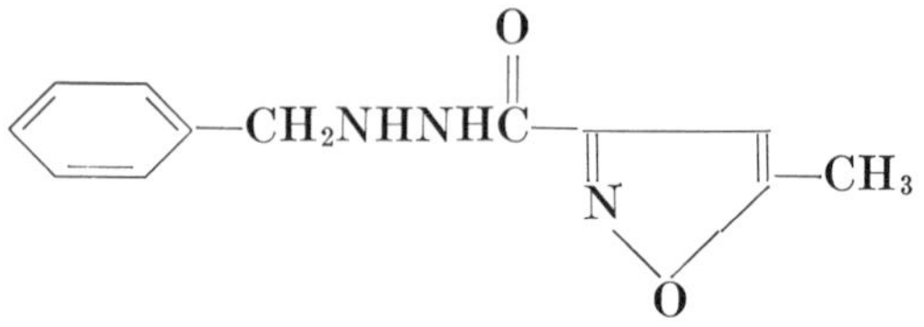

Isocarboxazid

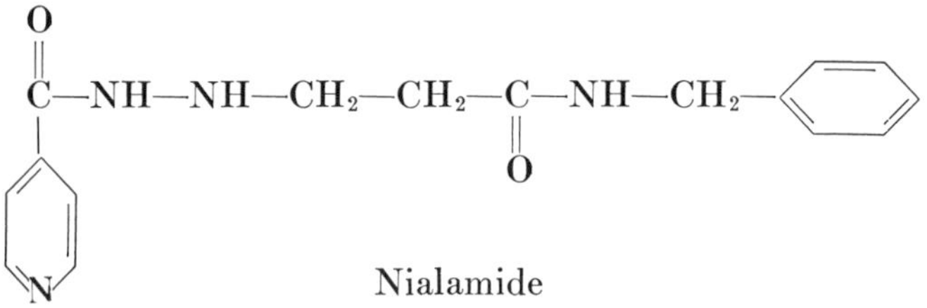

Nialamide

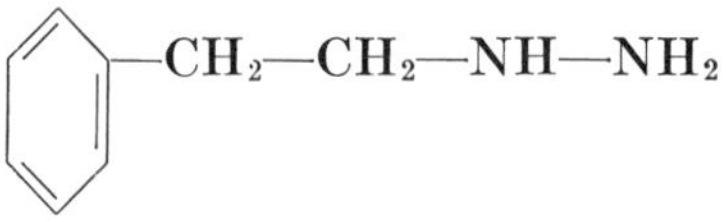

Phenelzine

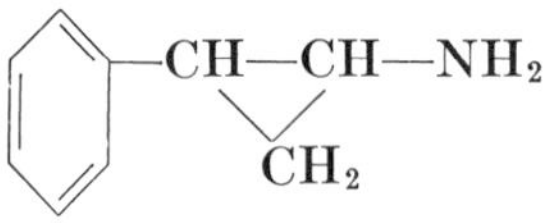

Tranylcypromine

FIGURE 1. *Some MAO Inhibitors*

choses, its use as an antitubercular drug was discontinued. In 1957, the drug was reintroduced into medicine, this time in psychiatry. Called a "psychic energizer," iproniazid was given to patients suffering from depression.

While the drugs produce an irreversible inactivation of MAO by forming stable complexes with the enzyme, this one property is not the limit of their pharmacological actions. What actually happens must be based on a more general principal; namely, these drugs interfere with a number of interrelated mechanisms governing the amines. Since MAO normally limits intracellular amine levels, amine concentration within the cell is increased by administration of a MAO inhibitor. To what extent this increased concentration plays a role in their therapeutic action is uncertain. But because of their ability to block other enzymes MAO inhibitors may produce problems by affecting the mechanism for detoxifying some other drugs. Thus, they prolong and intensify the actions of certain central depressant agents such as alcohol and barbiturates, of antidepressant agents, and of anticholinergic agents (see chapter on blockers of nerve action). Acute toxicity from an overdose of MAO inhibitors can be manifested by agitation, hallucinations, convulsions, hypotension, and hypertension. The drugs can also permanently damage the liver. Most interestingly, if a patient is taking a MAO inhibitor, eating ripe cheese (such as Camembert), herring, a variety of rich soups, and certain other foods, can cause hypertensive crises; these foods contain substances that release amines in the body. Once released, these amines are protected from destruction by MAO, and thus their effects are more pronounced and prolonged. Hence, diet must be watched by individuals taking MAO inhibitors.

MAO inhibitors are less frequently used today because of the availability of compounds that are both safer and more effective. Too often acute toxicity occurs from an overdosage of MAO inhibitors. As indicated previously, effects range from hallucinations and hypertension to convulsions. Also, these compounds tend to damage the liver in one way or another. The major compounds in current use are isocarboxazid (Marplan), which is less likely to produce liver damage, but has been known to precipitate seizures; nialamide (Niamid) and phenelzine, (Nardil) which are not particularly potent; tranylcypromine (Parnate) and pargyline (Eutonyl).

Dibenzazepine Derivatives

The drugs most widely used in the treatment of depression are the dibenzazepine derivatives, imipramine and amitriptyline. Their structures are shown in Figure 2. No one knows just how these drugs work to produce an antidepressant effect. It is thought that some forms of depression may be caused by excessive cholinergic activity in the brain, and the two compounds are known to have an anticholinergic action (see chapter on blockers of nerve action). In normal subjects, the drugs first produce a sense of alertness and well-being, followed by sedation and psychomotor retardation. The depressed patient does not experience the aftereffects. But toxic side effects of the drug can lead to pseudo-Parkinsonism, blurred vision and dry mouth, among other conditions. Imipramine cannot be used confidently immediately after a MAO inhibitor, as hypotensive deaths have on occasion resulted. There is one speculative explanation of

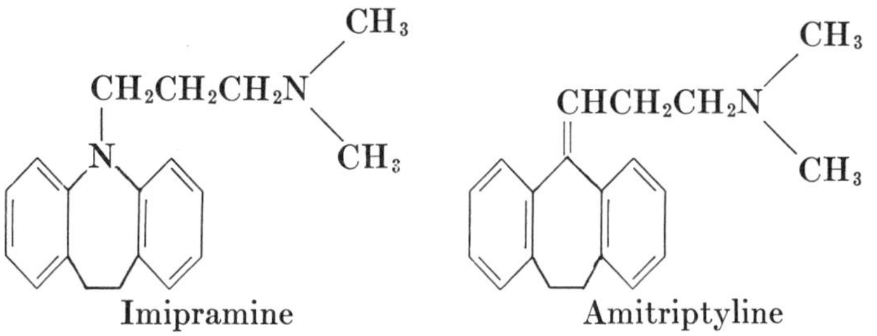

Imipramine   Amitriptyline

FIGURE 2.

its mode of action. As amines such as norepinephrine are taken up into the cell (from the blood) or manufactured, stored, and released, they "circulate" in and out of the cell and the orangelles within the cell. Imipramine in some way interferes with this circulation and quickly exposes the receptors to the newly-made amine. In this way it is thought, the receptors are "activated."

Minor Antidepressants

Amphetamines and piperidine derivatives, weak antidepressants, are not particularly effective in severe depression. They are sometimes taken with a sedative or tranquilizer to counteract side effects of somnolence and in narcolepsy (a compulsive seizure-like sleep occurring for moments during the day). They are tried in *petit mal* epilepsy, and are used as anorexiants, substances which diminish the appetite. They are taken alone when the patient is fatigued or when alertness is required in extreme situations. Amphetamines are, incidentally, useful in certain hyperactive (so-called hyperkinetic) children—sedating or calming them—an interesting example of the importance of "prior state" in therapy. They also can, when misused or taken improperly, lead to a toxic psychosis which even skilled psychiatrists have difficulty in distinguishing from schizophrenia.

Management of the Depressed Patient

Depressed patients make up a rather heterogeneous group. Consequently a variety of techniques are employed to cope with the problem. Methods include hospitalization, individual and group therapy, family counseling, electroconvulsive therapy, antidepressant drugs and sedation. The techniques are compatible and often several are used in concert. For nonpathological sadness and grief, the antidepressant drugs are of little value; antianxiety agents, sedatives or simple and appropriate attention and care are more effective for severe problems on occasions of grief. Many kinds of pathological depressions are recurring. Continuous or periodic antidepressant medication may someday reduce the severity of the episodes when they do occur, and lengthen the interval between attacks. Lithium ion, for example, is being cautiously tested now for such effects. Drug therapy may eventually find its greatest use against periodic mania and depression. Thus far, however, we have only treated the antidepressant drugs, and psychiatrists employ another class of drugs that exert different effects—the tranquilizers (see chapter "Altering Our Behavior with Drugs").

Without doubt there are moral considerations involving the degree to which the therapist should influence the patient's behavior by the use of drugs. The therapist's attitude regarding his right to influence the patient's way of life and his obligation to apply his knowledge is crucial. The important thing is that the patient be enabled to make psychologically sound adjustments to his life in order to fulfill the role which he has chosen for himself. By virtue of his training, it is hopeful that the psychiatrist would be able to help the patient without policing him. He undertakes a brief or prolonged dialogue with the patient, monitoring thereby his methods of treatment and the effects. The therapist is, after all, one who has been specifically trained in dealing with the maladjustments to life that plague the mentally ill. If the therapist is one who maintains his personal integrity and objectivity in his work, then he should be able, by virtue of his knowledge about drugs and their effect, to apply them with a certain degree of competence.

SUPPLEMENTAL READING

Solomon, Philip, ed., Psychiatric Drugs, Grune and Stratton, Inc., 1966.
Redlich, Frederick C., and Freedman, Daniel X., Theory and Practice of Psychiatry, Chaps. 5 & 6, Basic Books, Inc. N.Y., 1966.

Chapter 12

Altering Our Behavior with Drugs

And hence it cometh to pass that it is a hard
matter, and by many thought impossible, to
distinguish exactly between sense and dreaming.
For my part, when I consider that in dreams I
do not often nor constantly think of the same
persons, places, objects, and actions, that
I do waking, nor remember so long a train
of coherent thoughts, dreaming, as at other
times, and because waking I often observe the
absurdity of dreams, but never dream of the
absurdities of my waking thoughts, I am well
satisfied, that, being awake, I know I dream
not, though when I dream I think myself awake.

Thomas Hobbes   *Leviathan I., 22.*

Ne of the more imposing facades on the landscape of Aldous Huxley's *Brave New World* is the College of Emotional Engineering. The bleak building rises sixty stories on Fleet Street, London; and it is noteworthy that it houses the Bureau of Propaganda as well. Huxley's work may have seemed more fantastic than ominous when it first appeared in 1931. Now the brave new world has become more familiar, and some of Huxley's prophecies have been realized. If, however, we have caught up with his predictions, we may be missing the moral. One of the worthier characters in *Brave New World,* to the amazement of nearly everyone in that streamlined inferno, claimed "the right to be unhappy." Today, doctors proceed with considerate caution in attempting to alter behavior with the so-called "mind" drugs.

The Tranquilizers

One American commentator has said that "tranquilizers will soon make us a nation of zombies." This is simply an exaggeration. In the past ten years tranquilizers have not benumbed many of us at all. Psychiatrists and other physicians have, in fact, found tranquilizers to be very useful in helping people. These drugs not only prepare the way for meaningful and long-lasting psychotherapy, but they aid the severely ill in reorganizing their scattered thoughts and feelings and in sustaining their level of functioning.

Potent, yet generally safe, tranquilizers are a class of drugs that reduce tension without inducing amnesia, sleep or confusion; that do not impair normal impulses and that permit personal initiative. Commonly they are recommended for psychotic patients in mental hospitals. Here the drug may or may not aid the patient to return within the bounds of normality, but at least he will be calmer and better organized in his interaction with his fellow patients and with the personnel of the hospital. As a consequence, he can enter into more complex social relations and occupations with greater confidence, although he may or may not be able to turn his tranquility to insightful purposes. And while psychotherapy may not be greatly facilitated, the dampening of the extreme and disorganizing tension, the opportunity thereby afforded for reflection and for delay between impulse and action, the diminished hallucinations and primitive thought, lead nonetheless to better overall organization. The confidence given to the patient through such behavioral improvement makes the use of tranquilizers highly valuable.

Many relatively healthy people take tranquilizers to deal with everyday tensions. In these instances the drugs are less effective than with psychotic patients, but they still may be useful. One neurotic patient, for example, was a good wife raising a family. She was attractive and provocative, but also very intense. At times excitement and impulse boiled over and she would walk out of her house feeling murderously angry, with others and herself. Through psychotherapy she learned something about herself, her charming but childish sensitivities, and with the aid of a common tranquilizer she learned to pause, control and reflect on her impulses. In brief, with the proper use of pharmacotherapy she was able to consolidate herself.

Tranquilizers are generally divided into four categories on the basis of chemical structure:

1. Phenothiazines, e.g. chlorpromazine.
2. Rauwolfia derivatives, e.g. reserpine.
3. Propanediols, e.g. meprobamate (Equanil; Miltown).
4. Diphenylmethanes, e.g. benactyzine.

There is another group, a rather miscellaneous category usually employed as "safe" sedatives, that includes glutethimide (Doriden), methylparafynol (Dormison), and ectylurea (Nostyn, Levanil). Although rauwolfia root was used in India as long ago as 1000 B.C., nearly all daytime sedatives—drugs that with increasing dosage calm the patient by producing sleep or drowsiness—date from the mid nineteenth century. While the barbiturates were introduced as early as 1857, chlorpromazine was not introduced into psychiatry until 1952; reserpine, in 1953. Unlike the barbiturates these drugs produce calming without significant or sustained drowsiness. Both were initially used for patients who suffered from physical, not psychological, abnormalities. Chlorpromazine, derived from antihistaminics, was tested as an aid in anesthesia, and reserpine was—and is—used for hypertension. Astute empirical observation was responsible for their ultimate use as tranquilizers.

The mechanism by which tranquilizers act is still unknown. The brain is capable of a wide variety of states which can be graded into various levels of excitement or sedation. In the deeper-lying areas of the brain, neural nets discharge to glands, muscles and blood vessels, and to the cerebral cortex. Various body chemicals may alter this delicate balance. Hormones, for example, may ready the body, psychologically and physically, for a period of vigorous activity. Hormones elaborated by the medulla of the adrenal gland may spill into the bloodstream in response to significant visual stimuli. When one's car begins to skid dangerously on a snowy road, when an elevator drops too swiftly and suddenly, when one rides through a thunderstorm in an airplane, a variety of chemical and psychical systems come into play at once. The brain organizes and coordinates all these physical and mental responses. When we alter certain intrinsic rhythms, such as sleep, the chemistry and function of the brain may be upset.

Dr. Daniel X. Freedman, Chairman of the Department of Psychiatry at the University of Chicago Medical School, has commented on the neural basis for the action of tranquilizers and their role in revealing the function of various brain systems, many of them lying buried within the "primitive" brain that man shares with his animalian ancestors:

> By regulating the readiness with which distant sensory and motor neurones receive or discharge an impulse, these reticular systems affect the degree and duration of arousal both of consciousness, and its expression. They also may reflect the degree of motor and glandular response as well as psychological features such as tension, attention, and perception. Subtle chemical differences among tranquilizers are revealing both the paths by which brain systems are influenced and subtle differences in the organization of well-known behavioral states such as fear, attention, excitement and sleep.

Under the following headings, we shall treat the three major categories of psychopharmacologic drugs.

The Phenothiazine Derivatives

Phenothiazines as a class, and especially chlorpromazine, are among the most widely administered drugs in medicine. They are employed chiefly in treating patients with severe and disabling psychiatric disorders and in preventing nausea and vomiting. It is with the psychiatric uses that we are concerned here. At present, approximately one dozen phenothiazine drugs are used in the treatment of schizophrenia. Since the drugs bear so many similarities, chlorpromazine will be taken as a model.

The first report on the treatment of mental illness by chlorpromazine alone was made by French scientists in 1952. These researchers were convinced that chlorpromazine provided more than a symptomatic relief of anxiety; the drug acted to ameliorate basic neural functions affecting mental life. Moreover, they were able to distinguish between chlorpromazine's effect in the treatment of psychoses and those effects observed in "sleep therapy," a form of therapy then commonly used in the Soviet Union. The general mental confusion that resulted from use of hypnotics did not occur with chlorpromazine. Agitation and confusion alike were reduced by the drug.

Chlorpromazine was first used as a tranquilizing drug in the treatment of psychomotor excitement and manic states in 1954. The drug brought on sedation, relaxation, and slight hypothermia (subnormal temperature of the body). Clinical studies soon revealed that the drug was valuable in treating a range of psychotic states. Improvement in patients who were quite asocial or even violent was dramatic and impressive. For a time some doctors and journalists talked—rather overenthusiastically—about "emptying the mental hospitals." Although toxic effects, especially jaundice, were reported, the incidence was small and the liver malfunctions were not permanent. Most of the side effects on the motor system—tremors, restlessness of the limbs—could be controlled by adjustment of dosage or by drugs used in Parkinson's disease.

The chlorpromazine nucleus has a three-ring structure in

which two benzene rings are linked by sulfur and nitrogen. There are several crucial positions at which substitutions may be made. The addition of a group at position 2, for example, makes the pheno-thiazine nucleus asymmetrical and renders it more active (Fig. 1).

What is the sedative effect of chlorpromazine? After a high dose, the patient becomes motionless, often pale, and his eyelids droop. If he is questioned, his answers are slow and deliberate, de-livered in a monotone and with indifference. These answers are very

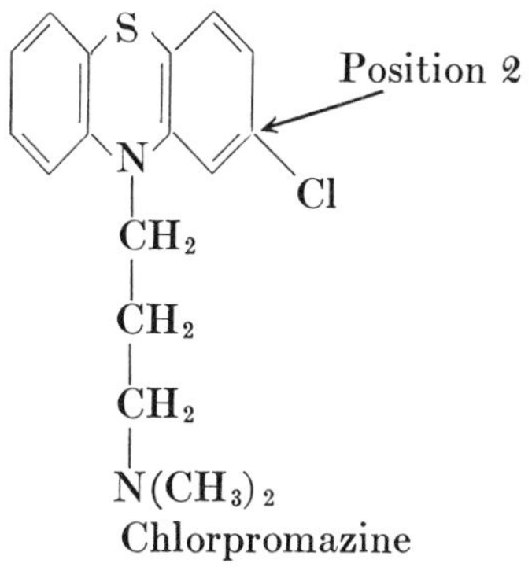

Chlorpromazine

FIGURE 1.

brief but fairly appropriate, showing that the patient is capable of attention and thought. Normally the patient will not initiate a ques-tion, nor will he express his desires or preferences. He is generally aware of his improvement from treatment, but does not enter into a state of euphoria. The apparent indifference, the slowing of re-sponses to external stimuli, the lessening of his initiative and anx-iety—without change in the state of waking and consciousness or intellectual faculties—constitute the initial psychological syndrome attributable to the drug. If the patient is in an environment encourag-ing responsiveness, he may be quite able to initiate conversation and to call up past memories. Tolerance develops rapidly to the obvious sedative action but not to the ameliorative effect on his behavior. Accordingly, many patients then resume their normal pace of thought and activity and can work or concentrate while taking the drug. We should point out that there is a considerable difference between the sedative effect of chlorpromazine and that of the barbiturates. Under chlorpromazine, a patient suffers little ataxia or incoordination and he may be easily aroused.

Another interesting aspect of chlorpromazine's action was discovered in examining its effect on conditioned responses in animals. Chlorpromazine impaired the ability of animals to respond to auditory cues that signaled the onset of punishing shock. The shock could be avoided by engaging either in a learned behavior pattern such as pushing a button, or by escape such as jumping a barrier to a safe area. While the conditioned (or learned) response was blocked by the drug, there was no effect upon the unconditioned or "escape" behavior in the actual presence of punishing shock. By contrast, barbiturates affected both responses equally, and only in doses sufficient to produce an hypnotic state.

The phenothiazines have proved to be remarkably safe agents when compared with previously used sedative and hypnotic drugs. They are nonaddictive, possibly because they do not induce euphoria. The doses usually employed may cause faintness, palpitation, nasal stuffiness, dryness in the mouth, and slight constipation. The most serious side effects, however, are those resulting from hypersensitivity reactions: jaundice, usually mild, rashes and other skin reactions are grouped in this category. Under increased dosage, Parkinsonian symptoms appear in nearly every patient. These take the form of involuntary muscle activity such as twitching or tremors. In general the toxic side effects of the phenothiazines are readily controlled by picking the right phenothiazine for the sensitive patient and by care in deciding upon the correct dosage.

Chlorpromazine has provided researchers a fulcrum with which to conduct major studies in the treatment of psychotic disorders. Prior to its introduction, the standard form of psychotherapy was available only to more affluent patients. Even now the extent to which psychotherapy is successful is quite variable and not clearly understood. The shock therapies, insulin and electric, as well as prefrontal lobotomy were among the physical treatments available for psychotic disorders. All these treatments have disadvantages, either being difficult to perform or producing undesirable side effects. Physical restraints were necessary for destructive patients. Now, however, many patients who would have had to be hospitalized can live at home and work productively; or they can live more useful lives within the hospital. The treatment involves little more than taking a pill. A definite ameliorating effect is exercised not only on excited or hyperactive psychotic patients, but on quiet, withdrawn, very tense patients. Combativeness and hallucinations disappear, while relaxation, organization and cooperativeness become prominent. Withdrawal diminishes and the patient begins to respond; this can lead in some patients to more evident worries or verbally expressed suspicions which then can be dealt with. Of course, while useful particularly in schizophrenia, the drugs are not specifically curative. They do offer a pathway for cure, either for reaching the patient, or for giving him the chance to "get hold of himself" and thereby to alleviate many of the symptoms of his illness.

Newer studies have shown that the phenothiazines tend to effect behavorial improvement both in relatively neglected and economically poor patients in large state hospitals, and in patients in the small, quite expensive, highly-staffed and psychotherapeutically-oriented hospitals. The difference lies in the discharge rate which is better for the relatively affluent who have a community obliged by custom to find a place for the improved patient. The readiness of many schizophrenic patients to accept an institution as a home and to drift toward minimal participation in group activities is a problem with social, economic and psychological aspects. The trend now is to involve the community (family neighborhood) in "aftercare." Because drugs have helped to improve the behavior and organizational ability of patients, the capacity to use other sources of aid in the environment is enhanced. Accordingly, physicians have become more inclined to use more flexible group, occupational and social treatments. These additional measures have significantly reduced the number of relapses and readmissions to mental hospitals.

The Rauwolfia Alkaloids

The term "tranquilization" was first applied to an observed effect of the rauwolfia alkaloids. These drugs are not as extensively used in psychiatry as the phenothiazines which, appearing at about the same time, were both more effective and more easily controllable. The rauwolfia alkaloids are now used primarily when an individual cannot tolerate phenothiazines, or when it becomes desirable to combine an antihypertensive and a sedative effect, or when a "trial" is attempted following therapeutic failure with other drugs. The synthetic drug reserpine was the first alkaloid isolated in pure form from *Rauwolfia serpentina* (Fig. 2).

Descriptions of the use of extracts from rauwolfia plants have been found in documents of the ancient Hindu civilization. Even then they were used in the treatment of hypertension, epilepsy, insomnia and insanity, and also for snake bites. *Rauwolfia serpentina*

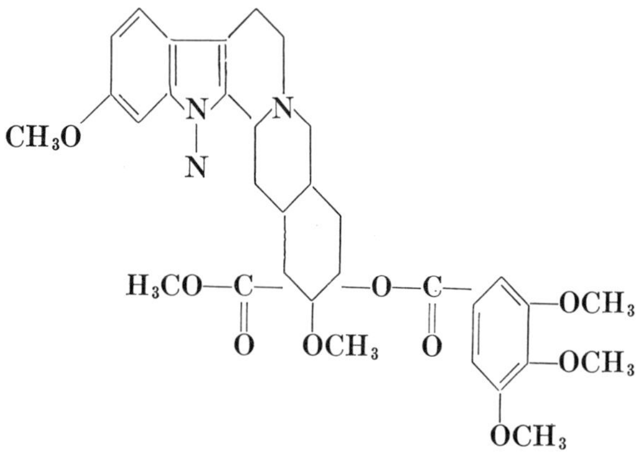

Reserpine

FIGURE 2.

is a climbing shrub indigenous to India and neighboring countries, although it is now cultivated in the United States and in Europe (Fig. 3).

Therapeutic applications for the treatment of psychoses and hypertension were first noted in an Italian medical journal in 1931. Little attention was paid to these effects until the 1950's, when several studies on the antihypertensive properties of rauwolfia were conducted. By 1954 the alkaloid reserpine had been prepared in pure form and shown to be effective in the treatment of psychotic patients exhibiting anxiety, restlessness, and hypermotility. It was also found that arousal was easy and that there was no dysequilibrium, a side effect induced by barbiturates.

The structurally complex rauwolfia alkaloids have the ability to deplete various storage sites in the body of their biogenic amines. These amines are thought to be important in various stress reactions. Major clinical effects of the rauwolfia alkaloids resemble those of the phenothiazines. The drugs induce a calming effect, an indifference to environmental stimuli, a tendency to sleep, and a quick arousability by strong or interesting stimuli.

Mental depression remains the most serious—though uncommon—adverse effect of reserpine. The depression can be quite severe and can even lead to suicide. This has largely been observed not

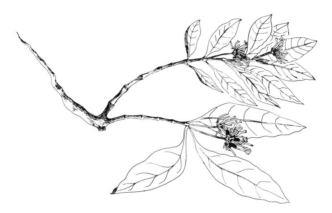

FIGURE 3. *Rauwolfia serpentina.*

in mental disorders but, strangely enough, in hypertension. Other effects are very similar to the previously discussed minor effects of chlorpromazine. Because the phenothiazines are more rapidly acting and more useful for prompt effects in emergency situations, rauwolfia compounds are not frequently used.

Drugs for Anxiety

Like the condition of anxiety itself, the calming effect of drugs cannot be adequately analyzed. This effect must be subjective and its behavioral signs and consequences are therefore variable, too difficult to pin down with precision. The mild drowsiness and relief of tension produced by these drugs are generally pleasant, similar to those produced by alcohol and the barbiturates. Meprobamate, commonly known as Equanil or Miltown, is one of the more popular drugs used in the treatment of anxiety. Its structure reveals how clearly different it is from reserpine and chlorpromazine (Fig 4). Of little value is the treatment of psychoses, the drug has a place in the less serious mental disturbances. Some would classify it as an hypnotic, but it is generally referred to as a tranquilizer.

Meprobamate was originally synthesized as a potential muscle relaxant in 1951. Four years later the first papers reporting its use in clinical psychiatry were published. The drug has since gained widespread popularity, mainly because it relieves anxiety without causing significant side effects. In the usual dosage meprobamate does not impair psychological performance as comparable doses of

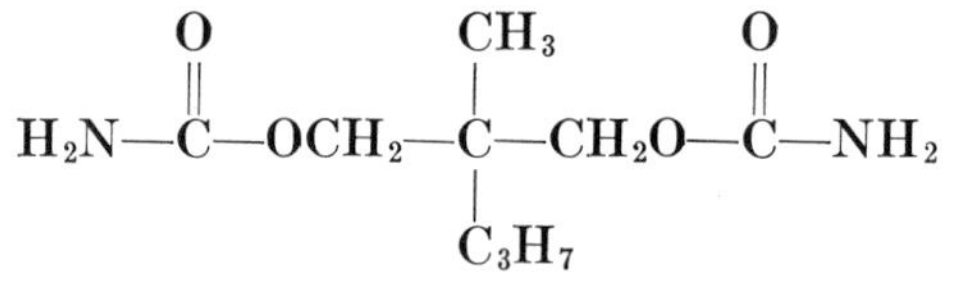

$$H_2N—\overset{\overset{\text{O}}{\|}}{C}—OCH_2—\overset{\overset{\text{CH}_3}{|}}{\underset{\underset{C_3H_7}{|}}{C}}—CH_2O—\overset{\overset{\text{O}}{\|}}{C}—NH_2$$

Meprobamate (Miltown, Equanil)

FIGURE 4.

barbiturates may. As dosage increases, however, a tendency toward a mild euphoric state has been noted. It appears to be as safe or safer than the barbiturates, although various allergic blood disorders, agranulocytosis, or high white cell counts, have occurred, though rarely. A hypotensive (lowering of blood pressure) effect is commonly seen in elderly individuals.

Compulsive and physical dependence may occur with the use of this drug. It has a potential for abusive and escapist rather than selective use—just as alcohol may be so abused. Withdrawal convulsions and/or coma may result from an abrupt discontinuance of quite prolonged high doses.

Meprobamate is used at all hours in a variety of situations involving anxiety: as a daytime sedative or as an hypnotic in the treatment of insomnia. But the drug appears to have its most pronounced effect in neurotic patients, increasing their ability to concentrate, lessening their feverish distractability. When is the drug administered? Apprehensiveness, insecurity, and insomnia are all signs of anxiety to the physician and he may prescribe the drug to alleviate these conditions. Ulcers, ulcerative colitis, and other psychosomatic diseases may be indirectly alleviated by the drug as well. Anxiety is manifest in numerous symptoms and signs, and has a varying etiology. It is highly difficult to determine precisely why these drugs are effective, since anxiety is variously caused and expressed.

Librium—chlordiazepoxide—is also used against anxiety and is specifically helpful in the treatment of delirium tremens and alcoholism. More potent than meprobamate, Librium induces perceptual misjudgments (in driving, for example), and it clearly can be abused. Sudden withdrawal of the drug after sustained high dosage leads to withdrawal symptoms. However, most physicians will not prescribe either meprobamate or chlordiazepoxide in dosages that lead to withdrawal effects.

LSD

Some people who have taken this well-publicized drug report how wonderfully it changes reality. The leaves of a petunia suddenly take fire; fantastic geometric shapes, detached from their material objects, float in air; the ring of a telephone stirs the same undertow of feelings aroused by a Brahms symphony; long-forgotten memories of childhood return with exquisite beauty. Other people, however, undergo profound depression, and attempt to do rash things. Law officials speak of addiction to LSD. But those who take it, usually a smart, well-educated set, claim that addiction applies to lower-class heroin takers. With the LSD people, the effect is an *experience*. In fact, one LSD fan who has taken this drug over a hundred times ironically claims that he is not addicted.

To the pharamacologist, of course, the term addiction refers to a dependence on drugs, the withdrawal of which produces symptoms and signs that require still more drugs (see Chapter 13). Thus morphine, heroin and codeine are addictive narcotics; alcohol can be an addictive intoxicant drug; marijuana is neither a narcotic nor an addictive drug, nor is amphetamine (pep pills), nor cocaine, though many people habitually use these latter drugs for various euphoriant or stimulating effects. And neither is LSD.

Our current laws are not based on pharmacologic or scientific knowledge, but on response to social problems and public opinion.

Accordingly, the tax bureau monitors the narcotics, opium derivatives such as morphine, and even marijuana. The Bureau of Drug Abuse Control of the Food and Drug Administration is charged with the control of traffic in amphetamines, barbiturates, and LSD. All of these drugs can be abused, i.e., used habitually in such a way that control over intake can only be dubiously exercised by the consumer. Some produce withdrawal effects, others do not. Some are associated with crime (cocaine, heroin), and some are not (marijuana, LSD). Some produce impulsiveness or lack of control (alcohol, cocaine), others tend not to (marijuana, opium); and some, like LSD, may impair judgment and threaten the individual's control—not so much of his actions, but of his mental processes.

The government now keeps LSD under tightest control, and yet it can be speedily synthesized by an organic chemist with easily procured chemicals. In short, LSD—like many drugs of abuse—is a paradox, and that makes talking about it so easy—and so difficult.

Dr. A. Hofmann accidentally discovered LSD during research on compounds derived from a black fungus called ergot, which develops parasitically on rye and some other grasses. In his now classic laboratory report Hofmann wrote:

> Last Friday afternoon, 16 April 1943, when I was working on this problem, I was seized by a peculiar sensation of vertigo and restlessness; objects as well as the shape of my associates in the laboratory appeared to undergo optical changes. I was unable to concentrate on my work. In a dreamlike state I left for home, where an irresistible urge to lie down overcame me. I drew the curtains and immediately fell into a peculiar state similar to a drunkenness, characterized by an exaggerated imagination. With my eyes closed, fantastic pictures of extraordinary plasticity and intensive color seemed to surge toward me. After two hours, this state gradually wore off.

Dr. Hofmann suspected some connection between this peculiar state and the drug with which he had been working. He decided to experiment on himself, and, using the dosage of other ergot alkaloids as a guide, he took only 0.25 milligram orally. This is now known to be 5 to 10 times the usual dose of LSD. The reaction he had to such a large dose was—so far as reported subjective experiences go—quite spectacular. Subsequently, in 1947, a co-worker, Dr. A. Stoll, reported the results of a systematic investigation of LSD in human subjects made at the psychiatric clinic of Zurich University and the original findings of Hofmann were essentially confirmed. Stoll regarded the LSD psychosis as an exogenous toxic reaction, although the confusion and clouded consciousness were lacking. One observed a mental clarity, even a looseness or fragmentation of perception and thought, which at the same time seemed intensified.

The drug has been continually used in Europe for "pharmapsychotherapy," as some refer to drug-oriented psychotherapy. European doctors give the drug to loosen old habits and viewpoints, to relax the usual restraints, and to allow a person to recognize with great intensity what he normally would reject. The ability to filter, to select, to respond to immediate and ongoing experience, is partly conditioned by what one *wants* to experience for one or another reason. LSD alters the filter or the selector; it alters responses to external stimuli, thereby allowing common experiences to appear thoroughly novel, interesting, sometimes beautiful, certainly intensified, but always elusive. The altered perceptions give rise to newer meanings, and consequently some LSD-takers refer to their experience as somehow poetic.

In America it is just this esoteric aspect of LSD that has been exploited to the full. A "psychedelic" or "mind-revealing" experience results from a massive dose. With such doses some persons may attain what is known as a conversion experience. In this state, the value of things, the whole matter of life appears, as it were, before the individual—differently. Such procedures are employed with the hope that the experience might play a role in future behavior patterns. The Psychedelic Movement derives its strength from these alleged conversions, as well as from lurid and seductive accounts of them.

Psychoanalytic therapists in Europe and America have used the drug in a more rational manner. By giving a patient a small enough dose, the psychiatrist may induce a moderate LSD experience, during which the patient will stay fully aware of the doctor and the situation. As the ability to control this "TV show in the head" becomes more difficult, the patient increasingly depends on the doctor or his surroundings for orientation. He becomes more willing to talk, even while fearing what is being talked about. Patients will then look at certain problems or express certain feelings or wishes very strongly; these become the topic for discussion in later therapy without the drug. Use of LSD is not a short-cut procedure; it is an aid to overcoming obstacles in psychotherapy.

Normally we all view the world in a particularly structured way. The mind provides constancy wherever our sense organs deal with variability. These correctional systems help keep the world in order. Just off a boat, an individual continues to act as if he were still on board. For a few minutes he cannot stop waddling. One may put on lenses that alter the world by turning it upside down; yet in a few days, the world will have righted itself in the mind and one may move about normally. Taking off the lenses will turn the world upside down again, and it takes several more days to adapt to the world as it actually is. Habits, constancies—sets— smooth out our perception and actions; they also can persist when they are not useful and this can lead to confusions and inappropriate responses.

In a sense the drug affects these sets of perceptual anticipations; it rearranges our ideas of order. When one tells a child that the people ten stories below in the street are not really "little people," one rearranges his ideas of order. LSD affects this type of rearrangement. It makes the world new and unhinges us from our constancies. With the drug one may become fascinated by his shoe, next by a little colorful design on his glasses. People may look small (micropsia) or big (macropsia) regardless of their location. A hallucinogen, LSD obviously has many profound effects on mental functions. Many illusions or hallucinations are produced by the inability to hold down or suppress a prior perception. What is currently seen and what was just seen coexist and fuse; old visual memories suddenly gain the status of a present perception.

LSD is not the only hallucinogen. Mescaline has long been used in religious rituals by certain tribes of American Indians in the Southwest. It is derived from peyote, the dried tops of a cactus found in that part of the United States. Although it produces effects similar to LSD, it is structurally quite different. Mescaline is, in fact, closely related to chemicals within the sympathetic nervous system—epinephrine and norepinephrine. LSD and, more strikingly, psilocybin (derived from certain mushrooms) are indole structures resembling tryptamine derivatives such as serotonin, which is found in the brain (Fig. 5).

When a soldier is deprived of sleep, when a religious ascetic fasts for days or weeks, when a person goes into a trance from rhythmic dancing, certain psychophysiologic states may occur, such as dreams or hallucinations. Like LSD, mescaline suppresses the ordinary responses to external stimuli, allowing bizarre phenomena to take place. And while thinking may proceed, it may take unexpected turns—both dangerous and exciting.

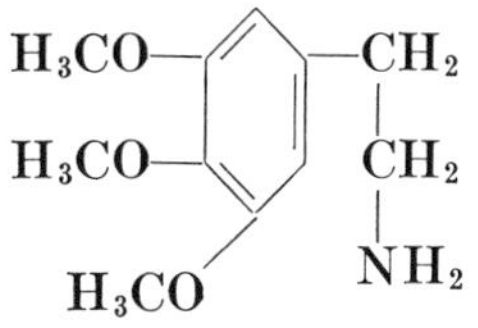

Mescaline

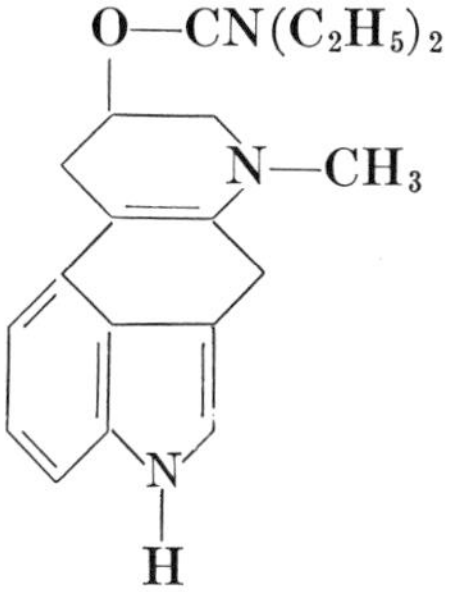

Lysergic acid
diethylamide
(LSD-25)

FIGURE 5.

LSD and mescaline have obvious value to psychiatry, but law officials question whether they should be allowed "on the market." The U.S. Food and Drug Administration has cautioned: "This drug (LSD) is considered one of the most powerful chemical agents known. It is capable of causing serious mental changes with extremely small doses. It may cause nervous breakdowns and suicidal states." There are those who would advance arguments against this stern "official" position. Shouldn't an individual be permitted to control the private life of his mind?

Of course, there are other aspects to the question. The French poet Arthur Rimbaud wished to derail his senses systematically, a terrifying thought, in order to *see*. Yet his countryman, the artist Cézanne, wished only to "portray the intensity that continually unfolds before me." For him nature was beautiful enough. And the

English Romantic poet Wordsworth remarked in his preface to *Lyrical Ballads* (1800): ". . . the human mind is capable of being excited without the application of gross and violent stimulants." Like Wordsworth, most artists attempt to find order and beauty in their own perceptions and meditations, rather than to destroy their grasp upon the natural world, the world we all have in common. Perhaps drugs actually remove one further from meaningful artistic experience, and perhaps this is why "LSD art" has not the harmony, the beauty and the richness we have come to ask of a work of art.

Many individuals have indeed used the drug without harm. Others have had "bad trips"—panic states during the period of drug action. Others are disturbed for a long time by the altered experience or the thoughts and perceptions in it. Others have recurrences—benign or frightening—of the drug experience without taking the drug, like Dr. Jekyll spontaneously metamorphosing into Mr. Hyde. Disturbances of vision in which objects are seen as larger or smaller than they actually are may be experienced, and there may be fears of loss of control. Since judgment is not enhanced during the drug, a group or "guide" is naturally sought to lend direction to the experience and to support the individual afterwards. It is not easy to put together these fragments—these waking dreams—and to draw insights from them. Groups or "religious" cults claim to bind the loosened experiences into some sanctioned or comprehensible meaning. In addition to these considerations, supplies of LSD may create problems with the law. The individual experimenter in effect takes a chance with LSD. If a person is sufficiently in command of himself, he may be able to judge the effects of the drug, if not, the drug may prove dangerous. Some experimenters frankly cannot control themselves and use LSD either to provoke society or to retreat from it; this is an inescapable feature of our current culture.

The publicity the drug has received, the manner in which it has been abused, make certain that much time must pass before we can consider it with some perspective. Thus far psychiatrists—not without some unfortunate exceptions—have been able to use the drug for therapy without recrimination by state and federal officials. Its use in the treatment of alcoholism is an important example. Whether, in an atmosphere of bureaucratic and legislative hysteria, scientists will be able or willing to use this drug to learn more about how the mind functions (as hypnosis, dreams and psychoses teach the investigator much about behavior) is not at all clear. Further, since but a billionth of a gram of LSD per gram of brain is effective, the search for its sites and mechanisms of action could lead to fundamental knowledge about the biology of altered mental states. Whether these fundamental approaches can continue in the presence of escalating, premature and self-seeking publicity is now problematical.

SUPPLEMENTAL READING

Redlich, Frederick C., and Freedman, Daniel X., Theory and Practice of Psychiatry, Chap. 11, Basic Books, Inc., New York, 1966.
Pollard, John C., Uhr, Leonard, and Stern, Elizabeth, Drugs and Phantasy: The Effects of LSD, Psylocybin, and Sernyl on College Students, Little, Brown & Co., Boston, 1965.

Chapter 13

Narcotics and Dependence on Drugs

The physicians of ancient Greece prescribed opium for everything from deafness and leprosy to the silencing of noisy children. Narcotics were practical tools of medicine for the ailing and a legitimate means of entertainment for the enjoyment of the healthy. Surprisingly little was recorded by the ancients about the addictive qualities of these drugs, but there can be little doubt that both opium and cannabis were used widely in early Greece and Rome to cure disease, relieve pain, and produce pleasure.

In our own day, these drugs are no longer used as curative agents. The medical profession has come to realize that opium and cannabis relieve only the most superficial symptoms of many organic diseases and that a mere narcotic can hardly be looked upon as a panacea. Biological scientists have also produced more refined analgesics to take the place of opium as a painkiller. Indeed, the classic narcotics have been virtually expelled from the realm of useful, everyday medical practice. Even that last ancient function of drugs—the search for pleasure—has been altered in many respects. Opium can still produce the same feeling of ease and relaxation that the earliest historians described 23 centuries ago, but attitudes concerning this artificial euphoria have changed drastically. The Greeks called it a gift from the gods. Our own society shuns the same phenomenon as the deadliest of forbidden fruits.

The Addict and the Law

The condemnation of narcotics by law appears to be so irrevocable because we have learned more of the ugly consequences that can result from their use. Frequent recourse to opiates inevitably causes drug addiction. With continued use, a form of tolerance develops to the most desirable effects of opium and its derivatives, such as morphine and heroin. A consumer of these drugs takes ever increasing quantities to achieve the same relief and sense of well-being (euphoria) he felt originally. As tolerance continues to build in the body of the consumer, a state of altered physiological excitability begins to emerge. This state of physical dependence characterizes the opiate addict. Now the motive for using opiates is not only pleasure, but also the avoidance of pain. The body cells have learned to function normally when bathed in an opiate. They will react adversely if this artificial equilibrium is not maintained. The addict finds that at this stage he must take much larger doses in order to stave off physical discomfort. As the user becomes increasingly dependent on the narcotic, the drug has proportionately less power to produce even the desired feelings of pleasure.

Unless he has an inexhaustible supply of opiates, the addict now faces a desperate and hopeless situation. The signs and symptoms of withdrawal sickness begin to appear a few hours after his access to narcotics ends. At first, he feels vaguely uncomfortable, yawns frequently, has watery eyes and a stuffy nose, and begins to sweat. He then may enter into fitful, disturbed sleep called the "sleepy yen." As the abstinence syndrome becomes more intense, the sufferer wakes and becomes restless. He perspires profusely and is bothered by goose flesh and hot and cold flashes. Forced into a fetal position by cramps, he develops back and leg pains and twitchings of various muscle groups. The term "kicking the habit" derives from this grim spectacle. Nausea, vomiting, and diarrhea soon follow. Other disorders of the autonomic nervous system (see the chapter "Nerves That Control . . .") include increases in blood pressure, respiration, and temperature.

The peak of the abstinence syndrome is reached 24 to 48 hours after the drug is withdrawn and declines fairly rapidly. The patient may continue to complain of weakness, nervousness, insomnia, and muscle pains for weeks; and it may take six months or more for basal metabolic rate, and other physiological processes, to approach a stable level.

This prolonged misery of "cold turkey" withdrawal has been a strong factor in moral and legal restrictions placed on the use of narcotics today. It helps to demonstrate that narcotic addiction is an illness—an illness that can totally engulf the personality of an addicted individual. Too often we forget this fact in our haste to blot out the evils of dope addiction. Although the American Psychiatric Association has warned that drug addiction is usually due to psychiatric illness, many of our courtrooms continue to treat drug users as if they were criminals deserving punishment instead of as sick individuals in need of care. Though there are many drug users in treatment facilities receiving medical and psychiatric care, there are many more doing time as moral degenerates.

American narcotic laws are among the harshest in our entire legal system. The Narcotic Control Act of 1956 provides for extreme and mandatory sentences, the removal of discretionary power from judges, and the abolition of probation and parole for many narcotic offenses. Under the Act, a person may be sentenced for up to twenty years on his second offense for the possession of narcotics. Moreover, an offender who knowingly does something to supply heroin to a person under eighteen years of age may be imprisoned for life or suffer death if the jury so decides. At the very least, he receives a ten-year sentence.

Under practical application of the law, a person convicted on two or more counts may receive sentences that amount to life imprisonment. In 1957, a thirty-two year old man, honorably discharged from the Army as a corporal four years previously, was given a fifty-year sentence in a California court and fined $5000 for the sale of marijuana. He had no previous arrest record but was not eligible for parole. In the same year and the same state, a young addict, suffering from epilepsy and mentally handicapped by an I.Q. of 69, was sentenced to life imprisonment on two counts. By permission of a municipal judge, a minor had been used in this case as a decoy to buy heroin from the offender. In sentencing the twenty-one year old prisoner, the judge reminded him that his offense might have been punished by death. In the severe words of the court, "the jury gave you back your life, now society should use your life to set an example for others." If the offender had been a rapist, murderer, burglar, or arsonist, he might have been eligible for parole after a few years. As a sentenced drug addict, he remains a lifer with no chance of eventual release. Addiction *per se* is not a crime and less harsh legal measures are available if the prosecutor will make use of them.

Our legal system remains convinced that drug law offenders are criminals, and a threat to civilization. Certainly a large proportion of them have prior criminal records. The medical profession, however, has shown some uncertainty as to what "addiction" embraces. Cocaine, marijuana, as well as opium and the potent analgesics are often loosely termed addictive drugs. But their properties differ so widely that they are similar only in being subject to abuse and in creating "social dangers." Indeed, it is not uncommon to see the term addiction applied to any misuse of drugs outside of medical practice that will cause serious harm to the individual and to society. Such broad usage, however, often creates unnecessary misunderstandings when abuse of drugs is discussed from different viewpoints.

A drug user resorting to heroin in large daily doses is obviously "an addict," but what of the middle-aged woman who is dependent on her four packs of mentholated cigarettes a day, or the teenager who experiences color dreams by sniffing airplane glue with his head encased in a paper bag? If he is a compulsive user, the teenager can suffer as strong a craving as the classic opium addict, and is likely to experience strong anxiety and frightening hallucinations when deprived of his drug. Clinical experience shows that cocaine and marijuana do not produce physical dependence at all. Abrupt withdrawal after prolonged use causes no abstinence syndrome. Is airplane glue a drug of addiction and cocaine and marijuana not? Some of the definitions of addiction currently offered would lead us to believe so.

The difficulties in terminology become increasingly apparent with the continuous development of new agents and changing patterns of use in others. Pep pills (amphetamines), goof balls (barbiturates), and many of the more recent sedatives have characteristics common to other addictive drugs, but with notable variations that make a single definition an impossibility. The fact that the enforced restrictions on such drugs are different discourages even a straight legal definition.

Simplicity, we are reminded, is often a virtue. Nonetheless, it is obviously not enough to say that a drug is addictive if the human body can develop a compulsive need for it. There is scarcely an agent that does not give some individuals a satisfactory or pleasurable reaction, persuading them to its continued use to the point of abuse. One can even find cases on record of people developing a compulsive craving for water. Told by both parents to take a drink whenever he felt upset, one such patient developed an insatiable craving for water whenever he felt the slightest apprehension. The World Health Organization (WHO), aware of its international responsibilities, has attempted to meet many of the problems in terminology head on. It offered comprehensive definitions of its own in 1950, 1952, and 1957. Accordingly, drug addiction was defined as a "state of periodic or chronic intoxication, detrimental to the individual and to society, produced by the repeated consumption of a drug (natural or synthetic). Its characteristics include: 1. an overpowering desire or need (compulsion) to continue taking the drug and to obtain it by any means; 2. a tendency to increase the dose; 3. a psychic (psychological) and sometimes a physical dependence on the effects of the drug." This definition received some acceptance, but much criticism even after several modifications. Its defenders suggested that it was not meant to be pharmacological, nor strictly speaking scientific, but practical—to include the diverse substances currently under international narcotics control. Unfortunately, as many have quickly demonstrated, the definition failed even in this, since it could be applied not only to drugs designated in narcotic statutes but also to many drugs which are not so specified.

Much thought has been devoted recently to these endless debates, which seem to arise mostly out of semantic confusion. Resulting discussions have focused on the possible substitution of a new term that will cover all kinds of drug abuse and avoid the popular mythology and explosive social connotations of the word addiction. The component that is common to all drug abuse appears to be dependence, whether psychic or physical or both. Hence, almost in despair, most careful consideration has been given to the term "drug dependence." In its thirteenth report, the WHO Expert Committee on Addiction-Producing Drugs has, in fact, recommended the substitution of the term drug dependence for both drug addiction and drug habituation.

Drug dependence, they said, is "a state of psychic or physical dependence, or both, on a drug, arising in a person following administration of that drug on a periodic or continuous basis." The important fact to remember is that the characteristics of such a state will vary with the agent involved and that these characteristics must always be made clear by designating the particular type of drug dependence in each specific case. Without a modifying phrase linking it to a particular drug type, the term drug dependence has little meaning. It simply is not possible to delineate or to define independently of the particular agent involved.

With this in mind, a few cautious generalizations may be added. First, individuals may become dependent upon a wide variety of chemical substances that produce central nervous system effects ranging from stimulation to depression. All of these drugs have one effect in common. They are capable of creating in certain persons a particular state of mind called "psychic dependence." The user feels strong satisfaction and develops a psychic drive that requires periodic and continuous administration of the drug to produce pleasure or to avoid discomfort. This mental state looms as the most powerful of all the factors involved in chronic intoxication with psychotropic (mind-changing) drugs. With certain drugs it may be in fact the only factor involved, even in the case of most intense craving and perpetuation of compulsive abuse.

Second, there are a very great number of variables. Psychic dependence can and does develop—especially with stimulant-type drugs—without any evidence of physical dependence and without an abstinence syndrome developing after drug withdrawal. Conversely, physical dependence can be induced by other drugs without notable psychic dependence. Intense physical disturbance is, in fact, an inevitable result of the pharmacological actions of some drugs if they are taken repeatedly and in sufficient amounts. Psychic dependence, while also related to pharmacological action, is more particularly a manifestation of each person's reaction to the effects of a specific drug. Consequently, it varies widely with the individual as well as with the drug. Many of the drugs that induce dependence, especially those that create physical dependence, also induce tolerance characterized by a diminished response to the same quantity of drug. But both drug dependence and drug abuse may occur without the development of demonstrable tolerance to the effects of the drug.

Third, drugs that are capable of inducing dependence also may be associated with psychotoxic effects that cause profound alterations in behavior. Thus, a college senior, scheduled to graduate with honors in psychology within a week, becomes capable of beating a woman and biting two policemen while under the influence of the psychotropic drug lysergic acid diethylamide (LSD). Again, it is difficult to generalize. This was but one user's reaction to LSD. Patterns of abnormal behavior are, within limits, characteristic for each drug type, but wide variations occur in individual responses. The pre-existing mental health of the person involved and the circumstances under which the drug is taken are influential here. Opium addicts have a very different reaction from the uncontrollable and violent urges that sometimes arise with LSD. The intoxicated are almost always serene, sedate, and lethargic when under the influence of heroin, morphine, or opium. Needless to say, this accurate description of mental and physical lethargy hardly corresponds to the popular myth of the dope fiend, capable of committing the most evil and sadistic acts of aggression while under the influence of heroin. The actual psychotoxic effect of this drug is one of the most misunderstood aspects of drug abuse today.

Finally, one last word of warning must be given before we outline and trace the differences between one generic type of drug dependence and another. Much of the confusion in the study of drugs stems from the fact that the significance of drug abuse or misuse may be considered from two contending points of view. One relates to the interaction between the drug and the individual, the other to the interaction between drug abuse and society. Crucial and conflicting assumptions are inevitably made, depending on which framework is emphasized. The first is concerned with drug dependence and the interplay between actions of the drug and the psychological status of the individual. Here, drug abuse is accepted and treated as an illness, like veneral disease or tuberculosis. The second viewpoint (the interaction between drug abuse and society) concentrates on the wide range of environmental, sociological, and economic origins of drug addiction. The emphasis here is usually upon the prevention and deterrence of antisocial behavior.

The World Health Organization ran into difficulty when it tried to encompass both frameworks in its definition of addiction. The Expert Committee probably caused confusion and debate instead of the consensus it sought. To avoid such confusion, an attempt will be made here to treat each viewpoint in turn—starting with drug dependence as an individual illness.

Morphine and Heroin

The generic type of opium drugs or morphine-like compounds includes many narcotics with differing chemical constitutions but similar pharmacological profiles. Morphine, as the chief alkaloid of opium, is generally used as the standard of reference. This drug, plus heroin, paregoric, Demerol and Dilaudid, is among the variations within the grouping to which addicts resort. Another drug, codeine, is used sometimes by addicts to fill their need by means of any one of a number of common cough syrups sold in drug stores. Morphine and codeine directly, heroin and Dilaudid indirectly, have their sources in opium, the dried juice of the poppy capsule (*Papaver somniferum*) grown mainly in the Mid-East and Asia. Demerol was prepared in the laboratory and developed by the chemical industry. All of these agents depress the central nervous system, relieve pain and promote sleep.

The sedative properties of morphine usually produce disinterest and a light sleep from which the patient can easily be aroused. This vacillation on the edge of consciousness is known quaintly among users as "being on the nod." The term narcotic ("to benumb") is a more archaic description of the same state. The subject may well have a general feeling of easy contentment but it should be pointed out that this "euphoria" rarely achieves the melodramatic heights assumed by the uninformed. Descriptions of rich and colorful fantasies or hallucinations are rarely obtained from patients receiving opiates. It is true, however, that patients suffering from pain, tortured fears, and anxieties do obtain a marked and welcome relief from these disturbing symptoms and emotions.

Morphine-like compounds relieve practically all forms of pain. In their analgesic (pain-relieving) action, they differ significantly from the nonnarcotic analgesics such as the salicylates, e.g. aspirin. The latter group of drugs is quite ineffective against visceral or internal pains, whereas morphine is a potent analgesic against all modalities of suffering. The reason for this difference has never been explained in a thoroughly satisfactory manner.

As an analgesic, morphine acts on two fronts—by elevating the pain threshold, and by altering the reaction of the individual to the painful experience. In addition, sleep in itself may contribute to the analgesic effect. The effect of morphine on the psychic reaction to painful experience is probably the essential feature of the analgesic action. Beyond this point, our knowledge ranges from educated guesswork to the merest conjecture. In pinpointing the effectiveness of morphine, there are differences of opinion concerning the relative importance of elevating the pain threshold and altering reactions to pain. Much of the disagreement stems from the fact that the exact site of the analgesic action of morphine has not been positively identified. A subcortical site of action has been suggested on the basis of the observation that the drug can inhibit the lip twitch following electrical stimulation of a tooth, this response being integrated subcortically. It has also been suggested that morphine may act simultaneously at many sites of transmission in the spinal cord, thalamus (base of the brain) and cortex.

One of the more interesting phenomena of morphine in the area of analgesic action is that subjective depression and maximal pain-killing action are by no means concurrent. When morphine is injected intravenously, the maximal subjective depression occurs in about five minutes. The maximal analgesia occurs some fifteen minutes later. This demonstrates that morphine is probably far more selective with regard to analgesia than could be expected from a nonspecific depression of the central nervous system. Beyond this point, however, the learned debates begin anew.

Other central nervous system effects are not shrouded in such mystery and controversy. It has been recognized for years that the respiratory center is markedly depressed by morphine—so much so that its paralysis is the major cause of death in morphine poisoning. Significantly, the respiratory system also develops a tolerance not dissimilar to the tolerance to the analgesic and euphoric actions of morphine—explaining how an addict may exhibit resistance to otherwise lethal doses of morphine. It also explains how a user can easily die if he fails to keep his drugged wits about him. If the user takes his usual dose after a period of abstinence, he may have lost the necessary respiratory tolerance to handle it. Respiratory exchange decreases, and carbon dioxide retention ensues. Eventually the addict loses consciousness, goes into a coma, and literally suffocates to death unless he is found quickly. A person in this state can be quickly identified by his pupils which are nearly the size of a period. Slowness of respiration and a bluish coloration of the skin denoting lack of oxygen are other signs.

Morphine exerts widespread effects within the rest of the organism as well. Pupillary, gastrointestinal, biliary, cardiovascular, bronchial, and metabolic mechanisms are seriously affected. In fact, an opiate is one of the time-honored remedies in the management of both diarrhea and whooping cough.

The other opiates produce similar nervous system effects but with varying intensity. Codeine, or methylmorphine, is a very important drug for relieving pain and subduing a cough. In therapeutic doses, it is less sedative and analgesic than morphine, but the tolerance to the drug also develops more slowly and codeine is less addictive than morphine. It has a correspondingly weaker effect on the gastrointestinal and urinary tracts and on the pupils than morphine. Codeine phosphate is widely used by mouth in doses of 15 to 64 milligrams for moderately severe pain when the nonnarcotic analgesics prove to be ineffective. When consumed, the drug is partly changed to morphine by the body. On the other side of the spectrum, Dilaudid is up to four to five times as potent an analgesic as morphine. Its respiratory depressant effect is also greater although the drug may be less nauseating and constipating.

Heroin (diacetylmorphine) is dose-wise more powerful than morphine and qualifies as one of the highly euphoric and analgesic members of the opiate family. In fact, "horse", or just "big H", remains the drug that addicts abuse most in our society. One in every 3500 United States citizens is addicted to "hard" narcotics. Ninety-two percent of these are heroin users.

Certain peculiar characteristics of heroin experienced by the drug addict go a long way toward explaining this preference. Although it is known that heroin is converted in part to morphine in the body, addicts can readily differentiate between the two agents when they are given intravenously. When morphine is injected, a flush is produced and the patient experiences a transient dizziness, lightheadedness, and a "pins and needles" sensation. These effects are only rarely observed when heroin is administered intravenously. Moreover, heroin has a more rapid onset of action than morphine.

Many addicts have compared the sensation to that of sexual orgasm except that it is located in the abdomen rather than in the genitals. Needless to say, heroin has a high addiction potential as well as being the most generally preferred of the morphine-like compounds. The drug may not be legally manufactured in or imported into the United States and is banned from medical use in most countries of the world.

All of the classic characteristics of drug dependence—psychic and physical dependence as well as tolerance—arise from the abuse of morphine-like compounds. The unique element is that these characteristics can be initiated by the repeated administration of small doses and will increase in intensity as the dosage is increased. It follows that dependence on drugs of this generic type may be created within the dosage range generally used for therapeutic purposes and that its mechanism appears to be set in motion by the first dose administered.

Of the primary characteristics, tolerance is perhaps the least understood in morphine dependence. Scientists believe the phenomenon must be one of true cellular adaptation of some neural structures, including the respiratory center. It is clear that alterations in absorption, metabolism, or excretion to explain it have not been demonstrated.

An abstinence syndrome appears in the opium user within a few hours of the last dose. It reaches peak intensity in 24 to 48 hours and subsides spontaneously. Intensity and duration vary with the degree of dependence. The extraordinary feature that distinguishes the morphine abstinence syndrome is that it manufactures changes in all major areas of nervous activity including alteration in behavior and dysfunction of the autonomic nervous system. The complex of signs and symptoms already described includes anxiety, restlessness, insomnia, yawning, tearing, perspiration; also hot flushes, nausea, diarrhea, elevation of body temperature, blood pressure and respiratory rate, and muscle cramps.

Morphine-like compounds vary in potency from substances with low activity to others that are several thousand times as potent as morphine. They are alike in that they all produce and maintain some degree of physical dependence, tolerance, and psychic dependence. Their use will also always prevent the appearance of the abstinence phenomena of any one of the others. Morphine and similar compounds are mutually interchangeable by substitution, although obviously not on a milligram for milligram basis. The time from the beginning of administration to the appearance of demonstrable physical dependence also varies with the agent. With morphine, the interval may be less than three weeks. It is shorter for ketobemidone and definitely longer for the weaker codeine. All of these last characteristics are of crucial importance in chemopharmacological approaches to addiction problems and they will be discussed in this context later.

Dependence on Cocaine

For centuries, a large percentage of the Indian population in the high Andes of South America have chewed a mixture of coca leaves (*Erythroxylon coca*) mixed with lime to reduce sensations of cold, fatigue, and hunger. The lime releases a substance from the plant known to the world as cocaine. This alkaloid is the prototype of the psychotropic stimulants that are capable of inducing euphoric excitement and hallucinatory experiences.

As a stimulant, cocaine is not pharmacologically a narcotic at all since only those drugs that literally "benumb" and produce stupor technically qualify. Still the drug ranks high in the esteem of experienced drug users and leads to the highest degree of psychic dependence. It is included in most of the narcotic control laws. Moreover, its characteristic effects are much more in line with the vague notions most people have regarding "dope addiction" than are those of the opiates.

Cocaine produces intense excitation and a corresponding release of normal inhibitions that can result in aggressive and criminal behavior. An induced feeling of great muscular and mental strength often leads the individual user to overestimate his own capabilities disastrously. Visual and auditory hallucinations follow with paranoid delusions frequently occurring. In addition, psychopathic tendencies are often unmasked (but *not* induced) by the drug.

An advanced user can inject cocaine intravenously at intervals as short as ten minutes and can reach levels of consumption as high as ten grams a day. Strong psychic dependence always develops from the ecstatic thrills produced. The cocaine user also pays for his habit with digestive disorders, nausea, loss of appetite, emaciation, sleeplessness and occasional convulsions. Continued, excessive dosage also increases paranoia to the point where the user becomes fearful and suspicious of everyone. An addict in this state is incapable of planning a deliberate crime. But he may commit crimes of violence out of an imaginary fear of imminent dangers, or apprehension. One cocaine user has been reported to have used a hatchet in order to attack a laundry bag in his bathroom, convinced that it concealed a policeman. The incident is bizarre but not atypical.

Continuous abuse, however, is rare. The user reaches such a state of excitement that he voluntarily seeks sedation to counteract frightening hallucinations and delusions. A current practice is to antagonize the exciting effects by administering morphine and cocaine alternately. The "speedball" is also extremely popular among users today; the mixture consists of cocaine and heroin.

Cocaine, a stimulant, could hardly be more antithetical to the opiates, which are depressants. Cocaine produces no physical dependence and there is no characteristic abstinence syndrome on abrupt withdrawal. Again, unlike the opiates, cocaine never causes tolerance in the body of a user. No diminution of the drug's subjective or objective effects occurs with repeated use. Indeed, these effects become enhanced, creating the sensitization phenomenon that leads to the cocaine abusers' search for sedation.

Significantly, cocaine presents other and, in a certain sense, more profound dangers to the drug user. Strong psychic dependence on the euphoria produced by the drug brings a craving every bit as strong as the opium user's combined psychic and physical desire. In addition, according to the White House *ad hoc* Panel on Drug Abuse, long continued abuse of cocaine can lead to serious mental deterioration. At the very least, severe depression will occur when cocaine is withdrawn, complicating any existent mental imbalance. The user may also suffer from continuing delusions after forsaking the drug, regardless of the state of his health. Cocaine, in short, is probably the best example of a substance to which neither tolerance nor physical dependence develops, but through which psychic dependence can lead to a profound and dangerous type of drug abuse.

Fortunately, cocaine abuse is on the wane. The drug has lost popularity among addicts in the United States today because of its high cost and scarcity. Advances in medical knowledge have undoubtedly played a part. Cocaine has been replaced as a local anesthetic by synthetic drugs that do not produce comparable psychological effects (see the chapter "Localized Pain Control"). Hence, a large legal supply of cocaine is not available and illicit traffickers have concentrated mainly on heroin.

Cannabis (Marijuana)

Marijuana, ganja, bhang, "pot," and hashish are all synonyms for preparations containing a resin from the flowering tops of the cannabis plant. Abuse of this narcotic has been more widespread than that of any other single drug in the world. Its uses have been manifold. Societies of hired killers are alleged to have taken the drug in search of the artificial courage needed to ply their trade. The French word "assassin" comes from hashish, as it were, in honor of this practice. Other areas of the world have different outlooks. In many countries, smoking, chewing and even eating cannabis or marijuana are as socially acceptable as drinking in our own land (Fig. 1).

One should remember, in this context, that indulgence in cannabis is essentially a gregarious habit. The isolated user of cannabis is practically unknown, in striking contrast to the solitary morphine addict. Marijuana and company seem to go together; thus, the term "pot party."

The principal characteristics of marijuana often fit in well with such occasions. Some of the prominent subjective effects of the drug are: hilarity, often without apparent motivation; carelessness; loquacious euphoria; and distortion of one's sense of time and space. A lowering of the sensory threshold—especially for optical and acoustical stimuli—often brings an intensified feeling of appreciation for music, paintings, and other works of art. Repeated administration, however, will cause hallucinations, confusion, illusions, anxiety, and deep depression.

Drug dependence of the cannabis type causes moderate psychic dependence but no physical dependence or abstinence syndrome.

There is no evidence of tolerance either. Generally, marijuana is relatively mild in all respects. It is dangerous mostly because of its associations. The reefer smoker easily becomes involved with social groups and subcultures using more dangerous drugs. The psy-

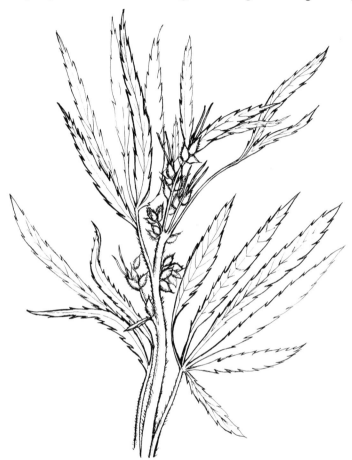

Cannabis sativa (*marijuana*)
FIGURE 1.

chological dependence created by marijuana often provides an excuse and incentive to try the stronger, and readily available narcotics. Not surprisingly, many youthful drug abusers begin their habits by lighting a stick of marijuana. It is neither difficult to obtain nor expensive in spite of legal attitudes and vigorous control measures.

Barbiturates

Patterns of drug abuse in the United States have undergone significant changes in recent years. A prominent feature has been a shift from the narcotics to the barbiturates, amphetamies, alcohol, or more often a combination of these. Vigor of control measures may have been partially responsible for this phenomenon by reducing the supply of cocaine, heroin, and morphine on the illicit market, but ready availability of the other agents and experimenting have played an important part. Drug abusers have tended to resort more and more to the easily available and less expensive agents. On account of this expansion, barbiturates and amphetamines are coming more and more to public attention.

Abusers may gobble as many as 20 to 40 barbiturate pills or "goof balls" a day. They get a relaxed feeling from the sedative which depresses the central nervous system. Mental confusion and muscle incoordination are among the more annoying side effects that follow. Barbiturate abusers also have to put up with all three characteristics of true drug addiction—tolerance, and both physical and psychic dependence.

These similarities to dependence on drugs of the morphine type are often stressed, but there are notable differences during the course of barbiturate intoxication and withdrawal. Physical dependence on barbiturates appears to require for its inception and maintenance continuous administration at a level significantly above therapeutic levels. Psychic dependence at least can certainly develop with regular administration of ordinary doses and is likely to incite to the taking of larger amounts particularly if tolerance develops.

When the daily dose is increased appreciably, tolerance as well as dependence will occur, but with marked variation. In contrast with tolerance to morphine, tolerance to barbiturates will not develop indefinitely. There is a definite limit. This limit is a characteristic of the individual patient and varies widely. Tolerance is also lost rapidly when barbiturates are withdrawn. Thereafter, experimental evidence indicates increased sensitivity to the drug, greater than that prior to chronic intoxication.

The abstinence syndrome is perhaps the most characteristic and distinguishing feature of drug dependence of the barbiturate type. It begins to appear only about 24 hours following withdrawal of the drug, and reaches peak intensity in two or three days, then subsides very slowly. The complex of signs and symptoms in approximate order of appearance includes: anxiety, involuntary twitching of muscles, tremor of hands, weakness, dizziness, distortion in visual perception, nausea, convulsions, and eventually a delirium resembling alcoholic delirium tremens. In other words, the barbiturate syndrome combines the worst features of heroin and cocaine withdrawal.

Large doses of barbiturates can have seriously detrimental effects in other ways. Loss of coordination and emotional control make a user extremely accident prone and unreliable in judgment. Heavy use can even produce a major psychotic episode. Most serious of all, the unique characteristics of barbiturates can easily cause involuntary suicide. This last danger is caused by three factors. First, barbiturate intoxication at a given level causes perceptual time distortion. Second, the body absorbs barbiturates somewhat slowly, and the presence of a large quantity of the drug in the stomach diminishes gastric and intestinal functioning, further delaying absorption. Finally, as already noted, tolerance develops to barbiturates, but it is not sufficiently great to increase significantly the size of a lethal dose. Too often, the combination brings untimely death.

The barbiturate user often fails to obtain the desired effect from a prescribed dose within what seems to him to be a long period of time. Frequently, he will ingest tablet after tablet in search of the "kick" that is already on its way. In this manner, slow absorption makes it possible for him to take a lethal dose before he becomes unconscious. More than 3,500 Americans died this way just last year.

Many of these unnecessary tragedies could easily be averted if all physicians refused to write, and druggists refused to fill, prescriptions for large quantities of barbiturates, and even if small prescriptions were non re-fillable. The barbiturate abuser cannot become physically dependent without the continuous ingestion of his drug usually in large doses over a prolonged period.

Amphetamines

The amphetamines are known intimately by two widely divergent elements in our society—students and truck drivers. Both use these drugs under their more familiar names of Benzedrine or "bennies" and Dexedrine to stave off sleep and remain alert for long hours. Hardened drug abusers use amphetamines to obtain cocaine-like effects or to eke out their drug need when their demand for heroin is unsatisfied. Like cocaine, the amphetamines are stimulants and they produce somewhat similar psychological effects. Their abuse originates and is perpetuated by a psychic drive to maintain maximum stimulation and euphoria or the psychological thrill which the drug engenders. No overt physical dependence is created.

A unique feature of the amphetamines is their capacity to induce tolerance . . . a quality possessed by very few central nervous system stimulants. Although tolerance develops slowly, a progressive increase in dosage permits the eventual consumption of amounts that are several hundredfold greater than the original therapeutic dose. A user may take up to 150 "pep pills" daily trying to attain the original floating feeling created by just one tablet. The amphetamine abuser too is accident prone because the stimulation and alerting effect may fail him at a crucial moment.

Although an individual may survive the oral administration of very large quantities, he may still pay for his folly. Such ingestion may produce profound behavioral changes that are often of a psychotic nature, including hallucinations, delusions, etc. Intravenous injections are even more severe. They are taken for the express purpose of obtaining bizarre mental effects. Sexual fantasies resulting in orgasm are not uncommon. This type of abuse has been increasingly frequent in recent years with changing patterns of drug abuse.

Approaches to the Problem

Great strides have been made in the various aspects of drug dependence. Working categories have been set up; psychological and physical effects have been carefully tabulated; and the molecular structures of the various drugs involved have been exhaustively probed. Subsequent explanations of the pharmacological mechanisms of drug action in the human body have become increasingly accurate and precise. Unfortunately all has been less promising than hoped for. In spite of our knowledge, attempts to solve the drug addiction problem have met with little success. Clinical expertise, social ostracism, the harshest of legal penalties and even the horrors of "cold turkey" withdrawal seem to have had little effect on the junkies of this world. Out of every hundred drug abusers receiving treatment today, only a few will remain free of drugs; for the others, treatment and punishment amount to little more than an enforced pause. But any remission in drug consumption is an improvement and there are other worthwhile criteria on which to judge the effects of treatment. The approaches to the problem are varied and some attention should be given to each of them.

The Chemopharmacological Approach

At the turn of the century, cocaine abuse had reached what one physician called "epidemic proportions." The abuse waned following the synthesis and introduction of Novocain, which lacked the capacity to produce some of the central effects of cocaine, but could be used in place of the latter, as a powerful local anesthetic. Cocaine abuse subsequently lapsed in part at least because of the drug's decreased availability and certainly in part because of changes in medical practice. Fewer persons were exposed to its effects. Not surprisingly, Novocain seemed to constitute a shining example for organic chemists in their attempts to separate the dependence producing qualities and the analgesic action of morphine through chemical modifications. If cocaine abuse could be eliminated by chemical success, why not morphine dependence as well? The hypothesis was a useful stimulus to activity in this field but erroneous really because of lack of appreciation of the differences between dependence on cocaine and dependence on morphine. The molecule of morphine— identified as the most active element in opium—has received the closest examination for almost half a century.

Over the years, each of the parts of the morphine molecule has been altered, rearranged, and some have been eliminated. Hundreds of morphine modifications have been made and a few have become useful therapeutic agents. Many hundreds of other derivatives have resulted from the ingenuity of the organic chemist, sometimes incidental, sometimes by design, always with the separation of analgesia and physical dependence the objective. Now and again in this parade a "miracle drug" has been hailed only to prove a disappointing false alarm. Heroin was the first of these, obviously a potent agent, thought to be nonaddictive because it was not understood that satisfactory substitution for morphine in an addicted person was evidence of its own addiction liability. This kind of mistake has become increasingly unlikely as our knowledge of drugs has grown, but the miracle drug in which analgesia and physical dependence are separated (a practical analgesic with little or no abuse liability) has continued to elude us. No substance has been found which will significantly suppress morphine abstinence phenomena that will not itself produce physical dependence.

Only very recently has the clue to success in this search emerged. Some of the specific opiate antagonists relieve pain in man; because of this fact, antagonistic action may be practical clinically without the liability of dependence.

Of the synthetic series of drugs that have emerged from laboratories in the past 25 years, methadone is one of the most useful. This substance duplicates the effects of morphine in nearly every respect except time. The time course of the abstinence syndrome which follows abrupt withdrawal of methadone differs radically from that of morphine. The abstinence symptoms of the former are not apparent until about 48 hours after the last dose of the drug. More important, they never reach more than low intensity and are prolonged for about two weeks.

By substituting methadone for other narcotics, there has finally been discovered a satisfactory management of the withdrawal phase of the narcotic-dependent person. Such addicts need no longer "kick" the habit through "cold turkey" illness. It is a measure of the controversy surrounding the whole subject of narcotics that some law enforcement agencies are reluctant to adopt this practice. Many feel that the "dope fiend" is not getting his due if he avoids the more unpleasant aspects of his illness.

Other drugs have been similarly useful, but none presently available has achieved the ultimate goal. Assuming, however, that some substance eventually proves to be a sufficiently powerful analgesic without causing dependence and undue side effects, it will not solve the drug abuse problem overnight. There will still be countries economically dependent on opium that will oppose any attempt to stop poppy cultivation. The established machinery for illicit production and distribution of heroin will remain. More recently discovered addictive agents will still be on the market. Most important, we shall still have the social and psychological forces that encourage potential addicts to hide from their problems in a dream world of drugs. A potent analgesic lacking dependence-producing qualities will supply a sound basis for a strengthening control over the current morphine-like agents. But this day of discovery has not come. When it does, a contribution and not a solution will have been made.

The Sociolegal Approach to Drug Abuse

Clearly, the solution to drug abuse depends upon a sound system of preventative measures and a program of rehabilitation techniques. Drug dependence is a symptom of mental imbalance. There is nothing in its make-up to justify, for that reason alone, the treatment of those who suffer from it as criminals and moral degenerates bent on perversity. The problem is essentially one of mental health. Federal and state laws calling for long terms of imprisonment for all narcotic offenders and cumulative penalties for a single drug offense have lost sight of this fact. The primary problem is the dependence and the drive of the person to maintain his drug supply. What is more, repressive measures have too often proved ineffective, as the high recidivism of drug abusers amply demonstrates.

Narcotics are the crutch that an unbalanced person uses to hide his real or imagined inadequacies and anxieties. Long prison sentences and rehabilitative efforts without an understanding of the problems merely underline these feelings and reinforce the user's need for his medicine. Only an integrated program of treatment, follow-up, and social rehabilitation can really answer such problems. Meaningful solutions must attempt to help, not insist on punishment only.

Current repressive measures do little but disguise this one simple fact. At the moment, only a few general hospitals even bother to admit drug addicts and private hospitals accepting addicts are as rare as they are expensive. Laws that place drug abusers in the hands of skilled professionals capable of giving meaningful treatment are just as scarce. Obviously, there is much to be done before the drug abusers in our society receive proper care and psychiatric aid in proper hospitals, halfway houses, and aftercare centers and to this end the fullest cooperation of all elements of the community is essential.

Effective legal measures for the prevention of drug dependence must focus on the production and distribution of drugs and the source materials from which these drugs are derived. In this area our national laws and international conventions have been undergoing revision. In 1960 our newest Narcotics Manufacturing Act became effective, establishing classes of drugs and yearly quotas, making possible change in the scope of control of a drug in either direction and establishment of exempt status for preparation of synthetic analgesics, for example, for which no such provision existed in previous laws. Also it has become apparent that stricter control over nonnarcotic drugs of abuse, the barbiturates, amphetamines, LSD, etc., is essential and Congress has recently enacted the Drug Abuse Amendments, making such added control possible. At the international level, the Single Convention on Narcotic Drugs was drafted in 1961 and came into force in December 1965. In addition, consideration is now being given to international control of the nonnarcotic drugs of abuse.

Perhaps the ugliness itself will never be completely erased, mostly because there will always be some people who find beauty within it. Thomas DeQuincey (1785–1859) was a life-long addict and knew full well the price he had to pay for his habit. In *Confessions of An English Opium Eater* he tells us, "Oh just, subtle, and mighty opium, thou hast the keys to Paradise." More than a hundred years later, today's junkie might easily agree with these sentiments and there will always be others trying to find out for themselves. We may carefully control those who insist on living this way, if the proper methods are used, but there always will be a few who will insist. The attitudes that we ultimately adopt toward this last element may well depend on how hastily we make them.

Chapter 14

Penicillin

While bombs were falling outside, research proceeded in a London laboratory—1940. A team of scientists led by Howard Florey inoculated a group of mice with deadly bacteria. Some of these they also inoculated with a promising new bactericidal substance, penicillin. A day later all mice that had received both the bacteria and the penicillin were alive, and all those not treated with the new drug were dead.

When this test was conducted, England was bearing the full weight of World War II. The country was unable to expend the effort needed to develop techniques to mass-produce the drug. But the success of Florey's tests inspired a massive developmental program in America, and in 1943 the drug became clinically available. Since then, public and private expenditures on antibiotics have continued to grow. In 1962 the United States alone produced over 6.3 million pounds of antibiotics.

The impact of antibiotics is incalculable. Typhus has practically disappeared from most areas of the world. Tuberculosis, rheumatic fever, pneumonia, scarlet fever, bubonic and pneumonic plagues, and many other diseases which used to cripple or kill, now take only a minor toll. A longer life-span has resulted from the application of antibiotics; we are less conscious of infectious disease. Antibiotics can thus be said to have altered all of human society.

The achievement of 1940 had been long in preparation. In 1877 Louis Pasteur, who had proved that microbes cause infections, observed two different types of microbes forced to live together in close quarters. He found that neither species could grow, even when plenty of food was available. Apparently, each species could prevent the other from growing. Pasteur summed up his observation in a famous dictum: "Life hinders life." Other scientists confirmed Pasteur's work, using a large number of species; the results were always the same. It became evident that even at the tiny level of microbes and cells, a continuous struggle for life is waged, each species trying to multiply at the expense of the others. Multiplication, in fact, is a definition of their life.

The hindrance of one species' growth by another species is the result of a specific substance secreted by the microbe into its environment. The word "antibiotic," meaning "against life," was applied to the active substance.

Several years after Pasteur's observation, a group of scientists noticed that a certain fungus, a *Penicillium,* could kill the bacteria with which it came into contact. One of these men, Ernest Duchesne, in 1897, actually went so far as to inoculate mice both with bacteria and with a broth on which *Penicillium glaucum* had grown. All the mice that received the broth lived, and all that did not receive the broth died. The experiment was just as successful as that which Florey was to carry out more than forty years later, but it was ignored and soon forgotten.

Alexander Fleming finally realized the clinical importance of antibiosis. A mold had accidentally fallen into one of his staphylococcal cultures and he found that it had inhibited the growth of colonies of this dangerous bacterium. Fleming recognized the mold as a member of the *Penicillium* family, and named the antibiotic substance which it produced, penicillin. He argued that this substance, penicillin, was solely responsible for the ability of *Penicillium* extracts to kill bacteria. Furthermore, he proposed that it be used to cure disease in man. But Fleming was unable to purify penicillin sufficiently. He was afraid it would be very toxic, and he gave up. Ten years later, after penicillin had been successfully purified and extensive toxicity tests had been made, Florey's experiments gave the wonder drug to the world.

Meanwhile, another man was making a great contribution to the search for antibiotics. René J. Dubos was puzzled by the fact that dangerous bacteria are not found in the soil, even though animals are continually dying of infectious diseases and discharging the bacteria into the soil. Could it be that organisms living in the soil are killing the bacteria? If so, perhaps soil organisms could produce antibiotics which might be useful to man. In 1937 Dubos began his full-time hunt for an antibiotic from the soil. Among the many soil samples tested, he found one that could kill the pneumococcus, the agent of pneumonia. The short bacteria isolated from the sample he named *Bacillus brevis*. The substance, tyrothricin, produced by *Bacillus brevis,* proved to be very active in killing most bacteria. However it proved to be fatally toxic to animals if given internally. Still, the success of Dubos's systematic search for antibiotics among the soil microbes served as a prototype for the series of investigations which have given us most of the important antibiotics.

The Agents of Disease

The infectious diseases which can be treated with antibiotics are caused by bacteria, fungi, rickettsiae (infectious agents smaller than bacteria but larger than viruses), and a few viruses. Protozoa, or one-celled animals, are responsible for amebiasis, malaria, and sleeping sickness, but only the ameba, which causes amebic dysentery, is affected by antibiotics.

The bacteria are primitive single-celled organisms which differ from animal cells in several important ways.

1. Bacteria lack a normal nuclear membrane (see Fig. 1). The genetic material is not, as in higher plants and animals, packed into chromosomes and protected by the nuclear envelope, a membrane which surrounds the nucleus of higher forms of life. In fact, bacteria have one or several "nuclei" in a cell,—(not recognized as discrete structures). Staining indicates, however, that these nuclei, like regular nuclei in cells of man, do contain DNA and RNA (see Chapter 18).

2. Like plants, bacteria have a cell wall, a rigid sheath enclosing the entire bacterium, exterior to the cell membrane. If, for some reason, this cell wall becomes damaged, the cell membrane itself is not strong enough to maintain the shape and integrity of the bacterium, and the bacterium disintegrates. Since the cells of the host animal do not possess cell walls, agents which attack the cell wall will kill bacteria without necessarily harming the host animal. The cell wall contains many substances which are radically different from any substance found in ani-

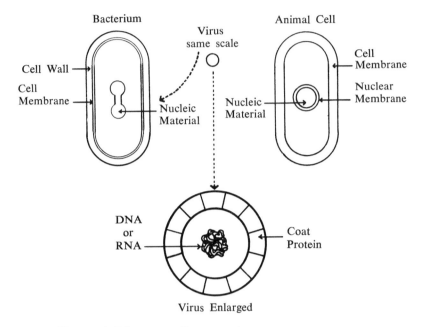

FIGURE 1. *Diagram to illustrate relative sizes and structures*

mals. Penicillin acts by preventing proper construction
of the bacterial cell wall, but leaves host animal cells
unaffected.

3. Metabolism is a system of chemical reactions essential
to life. In a bacterium these reactions are different from
those in animal cells. Some differences are subtle, some
radical.

All living things rely on the same basic chemical system.
This system is described elsewhere but we should review briefly its
important features. A chemical substance called deoxyribonucleic
acid (DNA) is the carrier of the genetic information. In an active
cell, this genetic information is continually copied onto ribonucleic
acid, RNA. RNA serves as a messenger. It carries the genetic information to small structures called ribosomes. The ribosomes serve
as factories where proteins are manufactured out of small molecules

called amino acids. The proteins made in this way are responsible for the structure of the cell, and for controlling all the metabolic activities of the cell, including the synthesis of more DNA, RNA, ribosomes, and cell wall. It is these activities, and the proteins which carry them out, which vary so greatly from species to species, and even from individual to individual.

Obviously, if a chemical is found which somehow interferes with protein synthesis, it will have a devastating effect on an organism. For use as an antibiotic, the chemical would have to have the additional property of specificity. It should be able to ruin the bacterial protein factory, but not that of man, and the astounding fact is that the protein factory of a bacterium is very similar to ours. The biochemist can add RNA from a virus or a bacterium to a test tube containing a mixture of ribosomes from a rabbit, let us say, with several other enzymes and metabolites from some other type of organism. Then all the parts of the factory will function together as though they came from the same organism, the bacterial RNA will be copied, and bacterial protein will be made.

Because all living things make proteins with nearly identical machinery, chemicals which ruin one protein factory are likely to ruin them all. That is, if an antibiotic kills bacteria by preventing protein synthesis, it is likely to kill man by doing the same thing to him. After this pessimistic introduction, it is necessary to admit the surprising fact that some substances have been found which do interfere with protein synthesis by certain bacteria but not that by human beings. Among these substances are the very important antibiotics streptomycin and the tetracyclines. The existence of such drugs merely emphasizes the importance of the infinitely subtle variations among nature's creations.

Bacteria can be grouped into two categories, Gram-positive and Gram-negative. One group can, and the other cannot, be stained by a certain process discovered by a man named Gram. The species in each group are fairly similar to each other in the way in which they respond to the various antibiotics.

Viruses are, in general, much smaller than bacteria. The smallest viruses are extremely simple organisms. They consist of a DNA or RNA molecule, carrying all the genetic information of the virus, coiled up inside a simple box-like container or "coat." This coat is made up of a single layer of protein molecules. The virus has no system for protein synthesis and lacks the enzymes and small molecules necessary for metabolism. The virus would seem, then, to be a completely dead thing. But when it comes into contact with the right kind of cell, all this is changed. The DNA or RNA inside the virus is propelled into the host's cell, where it unwinds and somehow takes control of the cell's synthetic apparatus. The cell is no longer allowed to turn out its own RNA and protein, but instead manufactures copies of the viral RNA or DNA, and viral protein. The new viral RNA or DNA and viral protein molecules participate spontaneously in the formation of new viruses identical to the original one. They are released when the cell, now dead, deteriorates. A more destructive and completely parasitic life-cycle cannot be imagined.

A chemical which will act selectively on viruses will be hard to find, since a virus does nothing and requires nothing until it enters the host's cell. Once a virus has entered a cell, killing the virus would seem to require killing the infected cell without killing uninfected cells. This has not yet been accomplished. Antibiotics are futile against true viruses. A viral infection must be fought with a serum which builds up the body's defenses, the antibodies, against the virus.

However, some of the more complex viruses, if they may be called viruses, do show some sensitivity to a few of the antibiotics. Also, fortunately, some true virus infections, such as the common cold, subside by themselves after a short time. Antibiotics have no effect on measles, chickenpox, and smallpox, which are all caused by viruses. Viruses as agents of cancer are discussed in Chapters 16 and 17.

The rickettsiae are very small, primitive organisms which may be intermediate between viruses and bacteria. Unlike some bacteria, the rickettsiae do not readily acquire resistance to antibiotics, but are often less susceptible to antibiotics in the first place. Rickettsiae are responsible for such diseases as Rocky Mountain spotted fever, Q fever, spotted fever, and typhus.

Fungi are a few steps up the scale of complexity from bacteria to higher plants. The cells have nuclei and cell walls, and the fungi have varying amounts of multicellular organization. The antibiotics which affect fungi are entirely different from those which affect bacteria.

Curing an Infection

Upon first inspection, the way an antibiotic cures an illness may seem simple: it gets rid of the germs. But this process is complicated. A "cure" depends ultimately upon the natural defense mechanisms of the body. Usually, the antibiotic merely holds the germs in check until the body can rally and destroy them. Improper application of an antibiotic may do more harm than the disease it was meant to cure.

When a sufficiently large amount of a foreign substance enters the blood stream, certain cells in the plasma are stimulated and begin to produce antibodies, which form a complex with the foreign substance, causing it to precipitate. If the intruder is a bacterium, formation of the complex will render the bacterium helpless against such cells as the white blood cells which, ameba-like, engulf the bacterium, swallow it whole, and digest it. The site of a virulent attack becomes a chaotic battleground for the fight between the bacteria and the protectors of the body. It is at this crucial point that an antibiotic can turn the tide and become the difference between life and death. The antibiotic may kill many of the bacteria outright, thus leaving the body defenses a "mop-up" job. More commonly, however, the antibiotic merely makes the bacteria sick enough so that they stop growing and multiplying. The blood cells then slowly kill off the bacteria. And since there are no new bacteria to replace the dead, the bacterial population dwindles and finally succumbs.

An antibody is a substance made by a type of plasma cell called the lymphocyte. Each antibody reacts only with a very specific type of chemical compound. Research has shown further that each antibody attacks only a specific small site or area on a large molecule. Small molecules do not cause antibody formation, unless they become attached to large molecules. These defensive mechanisms perform an indispensable part in almost all cures. When a patient is so weak that his defenses are not functioning properly, the doctor must try to sustain him with antibiotics and agents which will relieve the symptoms of the disease until the patient's defenders have recovered and become capable of doing their part.

Dangers of Antibiotics

When the "miracle drugs" first appeared, the public, as usual, tended to assume that intensive research would quickly develop drugs which were both infallible and completely safe. But as more experience was gained with the known antibiotics, setbacks occurred which clouded early visions. Rarely, but often enough to cause great anxiety, a patient under penicillin therapy would be recovering admirably, then suddenly, for no apparent reason, would suffer a relapse and die in a matter of hours. Some patients experienced mild, others severe reactions immediately upon application of an antibiotic. Very severe reactions have even resulted from a physician's administering a very tiny amount of a drug only to determine whether the patient were allergic. Yet most people would be unaffected by doses thousands of times as large as these "test" doses. Why?

The reactions described above are distinctly different from those caused by toxic, or poisonous, effects of a drug. Poisonous effects are greatly decreased when the dosage is lowered. Yet a few patients are still seriously affected by absolutely minute amounts of antibiotics. This phenomenon is an allergic reaction, called hypersensitivity. Although it is now understood fairly well, hypersensitivity is still quite unpredictable. The villains of the tragedies are the body defenses, the antibodies, themselves. In a very small minority of people, the presence of a certain drug or its breakdown products in the blood stream can cause an abnormal and disastrous antibody reaction.

Most antibiotics are small molecules, but some of them become bound to large molecules, proteins. It is the complex of the small molecules with the large molecules which incites the catastrophic attack of the antibodies. The reaction may be delayed until a week or more after the application of the drug. Immediate reactions usually occur only in people who have been exposed to the drug before. They have had time to build up antibodies against the drug as a result of the previous contact.

Sometimes, breakdown products of the antibiotic are what produce the reaction. If this is true, careful modification of the techniques of handling it may lower its tendency to cause allergic reactions. Ointments applied to the surface of the body are especially likely to induce allergic reactions. Penicillin, streptomycin, and the tetracyclines are very dangerous when applied to the skin. Hence, they are rarely used in this way.

The possibility of severe hypersensitivity reactions to an antibiotic means that it must not be used indiscriminately, especially on a person who has previously shown a tendency to react to the drug. However, the side effects of some antibiotics are routine and relatively harmless. Only an experienced physician is in a position to evaluate a reaction to an antibiotic.

Bacterial Populations and Antibiotics

One of the dangers of using an antibiotic is that it may drastically reduce and alter the normal bacterial population in the digestive tract. In a normal person there are millions upon millions of these bacteria in every cubic inch of the lumen or inner cavity of the intestines; yet the person suffers no ill effects. In fact, these bacteria are capable of producing many substances that man can not, among them certain vitamins. When certain drugs are taken orally, most of these bacteria may be killed off, resulting in nausea and diarrhea. If the bacteria are destroyed and the diet is inadequate, a possible side effect is harmful vitamin deficiency. This can be corrected by simply giving vitamins with the antibiotic.

Unfortunately, other side effects which result from killing the intestinal bacteria are not as innocent. When the normal bacteria are killed, their place may be taken by much more dangerous microbes. Extended treatment with an antibiotic may result in an overgrowth of fungi, which may completely cover the lumenal surface of the small intestine. It must be realized in this connection that the "inside of the intestine" is technically external to the body. Cells on the inner surface of the intestine belong to the same class of cells as skin cells. A substance not absorbed through the intestinal wall will pass through the digestive tract without actually going "inside" the body, without ever coming into contact with the blood stream. A drug taken orally may build up to a very high concentration in the lumen of the intestine if it is not rapidly absorbed into the blood stream. This is helpful, since it means that a drug which is toxic if injected into a vein may be taken orally without ill effects, assuming the drug is not absorbed through the intestinal wall. Of course, such an antibiotic is only effective against intestinal infections.

When virulent, pathological microbes replace the beneficial or harmless bacteria, the new infection is called a "superinfection." The intestinal superinfection caused by oral use of an antibiotic may be more serious than the illness for which the antibiotic was given. It may be very difficult to distinguish between normal digestive disturbances and the early stages of a serious superinfection. If the physician does suspect a superinfection, he examines a sample of the bacteria in the feces of the ailing patient, where dangerous strains of bacteria abound. If this confirms the superinfection, the physician may stop the antibiotic treatment of the original disease immediately and switch to an antibiotic which will destroy the new intruder.

The dangers of hypersensitivity reactions and superinfections must be taken into account every time an infectious disease is treated with an antibiotic. The dangers of the infection, if left untreated, must be weighed against the possible dangers of treatment. If the disease is a relatively mild one, running its course quickly without aftereffects, it may be wisest to use no antibiotic at all. On the other hand, many diseases have such dangerous possible effects that even the great risk associated with use of a toxic drug may be acceptable in the hope of a cure.

The antibiotics seemed at first to be a complete answer to the threat of certain diseases. Some diseases which had never before responded to therapy, such as staphylococcal infections, succumbed quickly and consistently to the proper antibiotic. Then one day, after years of astounding success against a particular infection, a physican would find a patient with the same disease who failed to respond to the antibiotic. Days or months later, another such case would be reported, and eventually such "resistant" infection would be reported everywhere, with increasing frequency.

This is what had happened: out of the large number of bacteria in an infection, a very small number of them were either originally unsusceptible to the antibiotic or had become resistant to it by a random mutation. This small colony would live on and multiply while the other bacteria would succumb to the antibiotic. Resistance to the antibiotic would arise by the process of natural selection of resistant individual bacteria in a large population under the killing pressure of the antibiotic. In a hospital, where antibiotics are in constant use, the development of resistant strains is particularly rapid. Antibiotic-resistant bacteria are carried by the doctors and nurses and are present everywhere in the hospital, but, fortunately, superior sterilizing techniques and hygiene keep the total bacterial population down.

Scientists have collected all the strains of staphylococci they could find, both inside and outside hospitals. The results are startling. While only 5 to 15 percent of staphylococcal strains found away from hospitals are resistant to penicillin, fully 90 to 95 percent of the staphylococcal strains inside hospitals are resistant. Therefore, if a patient in a hospital becomes infected with a staphylococcus while there, it is most likely that his infection will have the added danger of being unaffected by the usually safer and more reliable drugs which are normally used. A less desirable drug may have to be substituted.

Staphylococci are especially prone to develop resistance to drugs. Resistant strains can be produced in a matter of hours in the laboratory. First, the bacteria are cultured in the presence of a low enough concentration of the antibiotic so that some of the bacteria, the most resistant ones, will survive and multiply. The resulting colonies of more resistant bacteria are removed and cultured in a higher concentration of the antibiotic, and the same process is repeated until the concentration of antibiotic has become more than one thousand times as great as the original one. The antibiotic itself does not cause the changes in the bacteria. These changes are the result of mutations, which are so infrequent that they usually would go unnoticed. By killing the unmutated bacteria, the antibiotic eliminates the resistant bacterium's competitors, allowing it to multiply quickly. In hours the resistant strain has countless descendants, all unsusceptible to the lethal effects of the antibiotic.

The antibiotics differ in both the manner and the likelihood of giving rise to resistant strains. In those cases where resistance does not arise, perhaps the antibiotic attacks such a vital function in the bacterial cell, that a single mutation is unable to give rise to resistance without killing the bacterium.

A startling revelation of the last few years is the discovery that sensitive bacteria can "catch" resistance to a whole group of antibiotics from resistant bacteria, as a healthy man can catch a cold from his neighbor. The basis for the spread (in such contagious fashion) of resistance to antibiotics is that bacterial genes control resistance and sensitivity. The reasons why these genes may be transferred are not clearly understood, but one carrier of the genes is understood: the virus.

In the discussion of cancer it is mentioned that a virus may alter or scramble the genetic material of the infected cell. Viruses called bacteriophages ("bacteria-eaters") infect bacteria and occasionally and inadvertently carry genetic material of the bacterium instead of genetic material of their own. A virus which first infects a resistant bacterium and then a sensitive one, may carry the genes for resistance from the first to the second. The complex forces of natural selection seem to have induced the bacterium to arrange several of its antibiotic-resistance genes in one small area of its chromosome, for the sole purpose of making resistance to the antibiotics quickly transferable. So the virus which normally would carry death to the bacterium is also part of the mechanism which enables the bacterium to adapt quickly to new dangers.

Because of the infectiousness of antibiotic resistance, the physician often must, for each new patient, test the infecting strain of bacteria for sensitivity to a large number of drugs, especially if the patient became infected in a hospital. Bacterial resistance, patient hypersensitivity, and the possibility of superinfections are all factors whose dangers are reduced only by accurate diagnosis and careful treatment. The dangers must be weighed each time the use of an antibiotic seems to be required. The person who becomes ill and takes old "leftover" antibiotics without consulting a physician may be unkowingly endangering his own life. Properly used the antibiotics are safe and effective and should not cause apprehension.

Penicillin

This chapter started with the story of the development of penicillin: Fleming's discovery of the antibiotic substance manufactured by the mold *Penicillium notatum,* and Florey's conclusive demonstration of penicillin's life-saving ability. Because of the war shortages, Florey was forced to grow the mold in bedpans, the only available vessels. By the beginning of 1941, Fleming had enough impure penicillin to try to save the life of a human being. The patient, a policeman with a mixed streptococcal and staphylococcal infection which at that time could have only been fatal, was injected over a period of days with practically the entire world's supply of penicillin. The policeman immediately started a recovery which shook the medical world. Because penicillin was so scarce in those early days, the urine of patients receiving penicillin was collected, and the penicillin refined, and used again. This situation existed until the mass-producing capabilities of America began to supply the antibiotic in huge quantities in 1943.

Some of the people working with penicillin found it was much weaker than early reports claimed. The mystery was solved when it was found that these people were using a different strain of *Penicillium,* which produced a slightly different penicillin. The more potent penicillin was given the name penicillin G, and several other natural penicillins, all differing only slightly, have been found. Other penicillins have been produced by adding certain chemicals to the broth in which the mold grows. These chemicals are designed to resemble the compounds which the mold normally makes into penicillin. The mold incorporates the synthetic chemicals into the penicillin it is making. The results of these processes are called the semi-synthetic penicillins, some of which differ from natural penicillins in ways which are very important improvements over the original. These improved penicillins will be discussed later.

Penicillin is produced commercially in enormous vats, a method called deep fermentation. The penicillin-producing mold is grown in a liquid broth, usually corn-steep liquor. When the nutrients in the liquid have been exhausted, the liquid is collected and a series of processes purify and separate the penicillin from the liquid. Some penicillin strains produce penicillin G more efficiently than others.

The most efficient strain, which is used now, was isolated from a moldy cantaloupe stem and mutated by X-rays. After the tiny laboratory beginnings, the bedpans were finally forgotten, and by 1949 annual production of penicillin had risen to ten trillion units, roughly 12 million doses.

Penicillin is a small molecule bearing some resemblance to several molecules which are important to cell processes, but small changes in the penicillin molecule render it useless. Penicillin apparently kills bacteria by interfering with synthesis of the cell wall, which is necessary to the life of a bacterium. Under the influence of penicillin, the bacterium is still able to manufacture the building blocks of the cell wall, but cannot put them together to form the wall. The little pieces go floating off into solution instead of being bound together chemically into a tough shield. This accounts for the known fact that penicillin will only kill actively growing bacteria. Bacteria which are not multiplying do not need to form additional cell wall substances. A multiplying bacterial culture, however, must continually produce such material for newly-formed cells. In the presence of penicillin, this substance is not formed. Hence, the new cells are left without a protective cell wall. Thus, they are more or less at the mercy of their environment and more susceptible to the defense mechanisms of the body.

Because penicillin acts on the cell wall, its killing action works only on a class of bacteria that has a particular cell-wall structure. Gram's stain is used to stain the cell wall, and penicillin works best on the bacteria which are stained blue by this method. That is, penicillin is effective on Gram-positive bacteria, with some exceptions.

The spectrum or the group of microbes susceptible to penicillin includes the following Gram-positive bacteria and diseases: Staphylococci (responsible for a wide variety of infections, usually pus-forming), streptococci (scarlet fever, pneumonia, meningitis, "strep throat," peritonitis, rheumatic fever), *Bacillus anthracis* (anthrax), *Treponema pallidum* (syphilis), pneumococcus (pneumonia, arthritis, meningitis), *Listeria* (meningitis), and *Actinomyces bovis* (actinomycosis). Penicillin also attacks *Neisseria,* Gram-negative bacteria which cause gonorrhea and meningitis; and clostridia, which cause tetanus and gangrene; but these last diseases are more resistant, and penicillin is totally without effect on the toxins (poisons) which are the source of danger in these infections. Note that words like "pneumonia" refer to the locus of the disease and its symptoms, and that several different agents may be the source of one type of disease. Meningitis, an inflammation of the membranes surrounding the brain and spinal cord, may be caused by tuberculosis germs, by pneumococci, by streptococci, or by meningococci, and others. The disease may require a different treatment in each case.

Some of the infectious diseases which cannot be treated with penicillin include tuberculosis, typhoid, typhus, plague, granuloma inguinale, urinary tract infections.

Penicillin G (benzylpenicillin), the most common natural penicillin, has several disadvantages and limitations. It causes a relatively large number of hypersensitivity reactions. It is partly broken down in the stomach, so that oral administration requires larger doses; oral administration is not used in serious infections. Penicillin G is excreted so rapidly through the kidneys (80 percent of the original dose is expelled into the urine within four hours) that it is hard to maintain effectively high levels of penicillin in the blood. Finally, most Gram-negative bacteria and some Gram-positive bacteria are unaffected by penicillin G.

The synthetic penicillins were developed in an attempt to overcome some of these limitations of penicillin G. Oxacillin (Prostaphlin) and methicillin (Staphcillin) are two very important synthetic penicillins. Penicillin G is destroyed by the enzyme penicillinase, which inactivates the antibiotic. Most of the penicillin-resistant staphylococci are penicillinase producers, and are, therefore, resistant to treatment with this drug. Since penicillin G has had no effect on penicillinase-producing strains, it has not been possible to eradicate these strains. But the chemical modifications present in such semi-synthetic penicillins as methicillin and oxacillin allow them to resist destruction by penicillinase and to kill the staphylococcus. Since these new penicillins do not seem to kill most other bacteria as effectively as penicillin G and are more expensive, their use is restricted to treatment of diseases caused by penicillinase-producing strains of staphylococcus.

Ampicillin (Penbritin), too, is destroyed by penicillinase, but has a broader spectrum of effectiveness than penicillin G. It is effective against many Gram-negative bacteria which are unaffected by penicillin G. But it is very costly, so that penicillin G is still used against Gram-positive bacteria, against which it is more effective than ampicillin in the first place.

Phenethicillin and penicillin V are resistant to inactivation by gastric acid and so may be taken orally; but it seems to be as effective to give larger doses of penicillin orally.

No method has been found of overcoming the high tendency of penicillin to cause hypersensitivity reactions. Procaine penicillin G, which is used to provide a long-lasting depot in muscles from which the penicillin slowly diffuses into the blood stream, has a reaction incidence of 5 percent. Aqueous penicillin G causes allergic reactions about 2 percent of the time if administered through a vein, and only 0.3 percent if given orally. Methicillin may be more apt to cause reactions. The possibility of causing the patient to become dangerously hypersensitive to penicillin means that it should not be used in diseases which are not really serious. Too often, a sick person will foolishly attempt to pressure the physician into giving him penicillin when it would be wiser to do without it.

Although it occasionally induces allergic reactions, penicillin G seems to be almost devoid of toxicity in man. Doses thousands of times larger than those necessary to cure most diseases are without ill effect on the great majority of patients. It is apparently impossible to give amounts of penicillin G capable of producing toxic effects. Only the staphylococcus has gained significant resistance to the drug. For these reasons, after more than two decades penicillin remains the drug of choice against many diseases. It is effective even in cases where the patient's natural defenses are weakened, because it actively kills bacteria, rather than just slowing their growth.

SUPPLEMENTAL READING

Stewart, Gordon T., The Penicillin Group of Drugs, Elsevier Publishing Co., 1965.

Chapter 15

Newer Antibiotics

Streptomyces *griseus* is a mold-like organism found in the soil. As an undergraduate in 1915, Selman A. Waksman had discovered this organism and he became interested in the strange effects of the microbial life of the soil on bacteria. In the 1920's he collaborated with René Dubos on a series of investigations on soil organisms. Encouraged by the discovery of tryothricin by Dubos in 1937, Waksman studied his "own" soil organism, *S. griseus,* and found that it produced a rather weak antibiotic. A widespread search for better strains of *S. griseus* was launched—final success coming in the form of a strain isolated from the neck of a sick chicken. This strain produced in large amounts a potent antibiotic which was named streptomycin.

Universities and industry banded together at tremendous expense to develop and test the new wonder drug exhaustively. Streptomycin was finally released for general use in 1947. It is currently mass-produced by methods similar to those used to produce penicillin.

Streptomycin

Streptomycin has a wider spectrum of antibacterial activity than penicillin. Penicillin does not affect most Gram-negative bacteria. Several very well-known diseases are produced by Gram-negative organisms. Tuberculosis, influenzal meningitis, bubonic and pneumonic plague, and tularemia are among the most severe. Streptomycin destroys Gram-negative bacteria (by interfering with protein synthesis) and effectively controls these and certain other diseases caused by Gram-negative organisms.

Prolonged use of streptomycin has raised special problems. A large number of patients using the drug began to experience trouble with their sense of balance. They could retain their balance if they kept their eyes open but even then only with difficulty. This vertigo, or dizziness, was soon shown to be the result of a

243

direct toxic effect of streptomycin on the auditory nerve. The poison-ous effect, dependent upon the duration and the size of the dose, was temporary or permanent, and could cause anything from slight loss of ability to hear very high-pitched ringing sounds, to complete deafness. In some cases large doses caused kidney and liver damage. Furthermore, streptomycin is not absorbed from the intestines, and is only effective against bacteria in the intestine itself when it is taken orally. For treatment of systemic infections it must be given by injection, which of course is a less desirable form of therapy for both doctor and patient.

Scientists decided to try to develop a chemically-modified streptomycin without streptomycin's hazards. Among the many such molecules they produced, they found one, dihydrostreptomycin, which was an effective but no less toxic drug. The use of dihydrostreptomycin which had an early period of popularity has now been discontinued.

Streptomycin presents another problem. Many types of bacteria become resistant to it very quickly. Because streptomycin affects the universal and basic process of protein synthesis, its action has been studied closely. It is suggested by scientists from the available evidence that streptomycin acts by interfering with both the synthesis of intracellular proteins and the permeability of the bacterial cell membrane.

Streptomycin kills bacteria by binding to some specific site on the ribosomes, the factories of protein synthesis. As the ribosomes try to make more proteins, the streptomycin molecule takes up space, getting in the way of the moving parts of the machinery—the en-zymes and other chemicals necessary to the process. The mismatching of the machinery causes a large number of mistakes in the making of the proteins, like a machine which goes wrong and becomes entan-gled in its own defective products. The bacterium is deprived of substances necessary to its life processes, stops growing, and finally dies.

A single bacterial gene appears to be responsible for the region of the ribosome which is affected by streptomycin. This gene can mutate in such a way that the chemical nature of the ribosome is changed and the ribosome no longer binds the streptomycin mole-cule. When this happens the streptomycin can no longer bottle up the protein-making factory, and the mutant bacterium is thus resistant to the drug. Such mutations therefore are responsible for the rapid appearance of streptomycin-resistant strains of bacteria. Different cells, one might add, are resistant to different concentrations of streptomycin.

There is another interesting laboratory observation. The gene may mutate so that the bacterium becomes dependent on streptomycin for life. This mutant is killed if streptomycin is removed. In this case, the gene mutation results in the opening of a little nook in the ribosome where streptomycin becomes bound. When streptomycin binds here, the normal contours of the ribosomes are restored, and the machinery fits well and runs smoothly. When streptomycin is not present, a gap opens in the ribosome, the machinery breaks down, mistakes are made, and death of the mutant results. Streptomycin-dependent strains are most easily destroyed: simply discontinue use of the drug and the bacteria will die. However, development of such streptomycin-dependent strains has not been observed in man.

The Tetracyclines

In 1945, B. M. Duggar began an extensive search for new antibiotic-producing microbes. Thousands of soil samples were collected from all over the world and were tested for the presence of antibiotic-producing microbes. The most powerful antibiotic observed in this survey was produced by an unusually bright yellow fungus which Duggar named *Streptomyces aureofaciens,* or the gold-forming fungus. He named the antibiotic Aureomycin. Preliminary tests showed that Aureomycin had a very wide spectrum of antibiotic power. Late in 1947, not long after its discovery, Aureomycin was tested in a human being with complete success. The drug cured a man of granuloma inguinale, a venereal disease which had resisted all other forms of treatment.

The success of the organized searches which had already given the world streptomycin and Aureomycin encouraged others to try their luck. For example, the Pfizer laboratories collected and tested over 116,000 soil samples. They rediscovered Aureomycin several times, but went on with the search. Finally, in 1950, Pfizer found a new antibiotic, which they named Terramycin, produced by *Streptomyces rimosus.*

It soon became evident that Aureomycin (chlortetracycline) and Terramycin (oxytetracycline) had very similar ranges of activity. Further, whenever a bacterial strain became resistant to one of the drugs, it was found to have become resistant to the other as well. In other words, the cross-resistance between the two drugs is complete. They are both slight modifications of the molecule tetracycline. And when tetracycline was synthesized in the laboratory, it was found to be just as effective against bacteria as Aureomycin and Terramycin. In fact, all the tetracyclines are antibiotics that are generally similar chemically, but differ from one another by the addition or deletion of chemical groups.

Another altered tetracycline, demethylchlortetracycline, has been synthesized in the laboratory. Demethylchlortetracycline has the advantage of increased stability. It remains at high levels in the blood longer than the other tetracyclines, and does not have to be administered as often.

Since the tetracyclines all have nearly identical antibiotic properties, they may be discussed as a group. They are effective against most diseases that penicillin affects, and are a second choice drug in those diseases. Since they are also effective in many diseases that penicillin does not affect, they are called "broad-spectrum antibiotics." They are used if the patient is sensitive to penicillin or if the bacterial strain has become resistant to penicillin. The tetracyclines are first choice for treatment of many diseases caused by Gram-negative bacteria, rickettsiae, and some "viruses." Among these diseases are trachoma, actinomycosis, amebiasis (e.g., amebic dysentery), bacillary dysentery, lymphogranuloma venereum, certain types of meningitis, brucellosis, tularemia and psittacosis.

How the tetracyclines kill bacteria is not clearly understood. The tetracyclines are bacteriostatic rather than bactericidal: they do not kill bacteria, they just keep them from multiplying. Since they cannot actually kill bacteria, the tetracyclines do not eradicate infections unless the body's defenses are functioning properly; the body itself must do the killing. A patient whose defenses are damaged by his disease must be given a bactericidal drug instead of one of the tetracyclines. Also, even if the defense mechanisms are functioning, the tetracyclines give the bacteria a longer time to develop resistance, in which case superinfection by the resistant bacteria may occur.

All tetracyclines may be taken orally, but with prolonged use the occurrence of side effects, particularly diarrhea, are common. These digestive disorders occur because the tetracyclines are broad-spectrum drugs, and drastically reduce the number of the Gram-negative bacteria in the intestines. If these harmless bacteria are replaced by a normally suppressed bacterial flora, a superinfection may arise which is potentially fatal. The physician is always on the watch for the first signs of superinfection, and must not confuse these with temporary side effects. The chance of superinfection with the tetracyclines is higher than with penicillin and streptomycin. Also the tetracyclines have a slight toxic effect on the body's defense mechanisms.

The tetracyclines produce a wide variety of toxic effects; liver damage, and discoloring of teeth in infants are among the more common ones. Sensitivity of the skin to certain frequencies of ultraviolet light results from demethylchlortetracycline. The tetracyclines do seem to affect bone growth of a fetus, and are given with caution to pregnant women. The danger of allergic reactions is great only if the antibiotic is applied to the skin, so it is not used in ointments. But, in general, the tetracyclines are relatively safe drugs with only slight dangers.

Bacteria acquire resistance to the tetracyclines more slowly than to penicillin. Curiously, Gram-positive bacteria do not acquire resistance to both chloramphenicol (see next section) and tetracycline, but many Gram-negative bacteria do. Moreover, the tetracyclines seem to be less toxic than Aureomycin and Terramycin. They are currently replacing these drugs in the treatment of a number of diseases. But which one is best in a given instance depends on many subtle factors. These must be weighed in every case.

Chloramphenicol

Chloramphenicol (Chloromycetin) was discovered in 1947 by Burkholder as a product of a Venezuelan soil organism called *Streptomyces venezuelae*. It is now produced synthetically. Chloramphenicol is bacteriostatic for a large variety of bacteria, both Gram-positive and Gram-negative. It kills rickettsiae and some Gram-negative bacteria outright, so it is particularly useful in treatment of rickettsial diseases like Rocky Mountain spotted fever, Q fever and typhus. It is the best drug against typhoid fever which is caused by Gram-negative bacteria. Chloramphenicol is effective in most diseases treatable with the tetracyclines.

Chloramphenicol acts on bacteria by stopping protein synthesis, and bacteria cannot build resistance to the drug with a single mutation as they do in the case of streptomycin. Rickettsial infections and typhoid fever have not yet shown any tendency toward development of resistance to it, which fact, of course, increases the value of chloramphenicol greatly. If bacteria do develop resistance to chloramphenicol, they seem to do it by making their cell walls impermeable to the drug. The drug is unable to enter the bacterium and poison it. In essence the organism is protected from chloramphenicol by an effective shield.

Chloramphenicol can be taken by mouth, since it is rapidly absorbed into the bloodstream from the intestine. In the body the drug is chemically degraded, and its fragments pass out of the body in the urine. As with all wide-spectrum antibiotics, gastric disturbances occur commonly when it is taken orally. And there again is the danger of superinfection by resistant staphylococci and fungi. It was thought at first that chloramphenicol was nontoxic; but in some instances very serious side effects can occur. It attacks the sites of blood cell development, the bone marrow; and the aplasia and anemia which occur are fatal if not detected in time. Because of this danger, chloramphenicol is regarded as a risk drug, and is used only in serious or life-threatening diseases. When using it, a physician must check the blood frequently for anemia. The drug seems to be very poisonous to a fetus, but can be given to a pregnant woman safely because there is a partial barrier to its passage across the placenta from the mother to the fetus. It is safe enough for use with proper caution in children who are seriously ill, but its use is usually not prescribed in infants; they lack the glucuronide-forming enzymes in the liver that detoxify the chloramphenicol.

The Macrolides: Erythromycin and Oleandomycin

Erythromycin and oleandomycin are similar chemically, and cross-resistance between the two has been observed. Erythromycin seems to be slightly more potent, and both drugs have a similar, rather narrow spectrum of activity similar to penicillin. The main use for these drugs is the treatment of infections that are resistant to penicillin or in the treatment of patients sensitive to penicillin and other drugs. One disadvantage is that about 50 percent of all staphylococcal strains in hospitals have already developed resistance to them. Oleandomycin can be taken orally, as can a preparation of erythromycin.

Because the narrow spectrum of the drugs does not include the normal bacterial populations of the intestines, digestive disorders and superinfections occur less frequently than when streptomycin or the tetracyclines are used. The macrolides do not possess notable toxicity, although it is possible that the liver may be adversely affected (jaundice), especially in treatment of younger people.

The Peptidyl Antibiotics

The peptidyl antibiotics are relatively large molecules which do not diffuse through the skin, but are very toxic if they get into the blood stream. Because they do not pass through the skin, they do not cause allergic reactions, and therefore possess unique value when used in ointments.

Tyrothricin was one of the first antibiotics. It contains two very poisonous active substances, gramicidin and tyrocidine. It is so toxic that it is only used in ointments. Bacitracin can also be used in ointments and has a spectrum similar to that of penicillin, but its danger to the kidneys limits the scope of its application and its value.

Polymixin B has a detergent-like structure and acts on the membrane of the bacterial cell. Its main clinical value lies in its ability to kill certain types of bacteria that are not easily eliminated by other antibiotics. More toxic than penicillin, it is somewhat less toxic than the other peptidyl antibiotics. The antibiotic colistin is similar to polymixin B and particularly effective against pseudomonal infections. Indeed the drug should be reserved for use only in such infections. Because these drugs are not absorbed into the blood when taken orally, they can be used to treat infections in the digestive tract. Parenteral preparations are also available, however. Neomycin, a potent and broad-spectrum antibiotic is useful topically and by the oral route. Its toxicity has limited its usefulness.

In general, the peptidyl antibiotics are valuable therapeutic adjuncts. They frequently prove effective against certain Gram-negative bacteria which are not affected by the more generally useful drugs, and they are the only antibiotics that do not cause dangerous allergic reactions when applied as ointments. Peptidyls widen the doctor's choice of antibiotics, raising the chances for success in certain limited areas of infectious disease.

The Newest Antibiotics

Newer antibiotics are being synthesized all the time. Many drugs have been found in the search for agents which are able to cope with organisms resistant to penicillin, particularly the staphylococcus. A narrow-spectrum antibiotic, lincomycin, may be useful against penicillin and erythromycin resistant organisms. It is known to interfere with protein synthesis. Cross resistance between lincomycin and other antibacterial agents has not yet been reported clinically. Novobiocin (Albamycin, Cathomycin) and vancomycin (Vancocin) are both products of strains of *Streptomyces*. They are effective against Gram-positive bacteria which are normally sensitive to penicillin. The drugs are rather dangerous, but can be life saving in cases where serious infections are caused by penicillin-resistant staphylococcus strains.

Antifungal Antibiotics

The fungi are nearly unaffected by the antibacterial antibiotics. Organic acids like undecylenic acid have been used successfully on the skin. The antibiotics which have been found to be active against fungi are not active against bacteria.

Griseofulvin was discovered in 1939. Since it was only tested against bacteria, the antibiotic was thought to be useless at first. However, griseofulvin has proved very effective against fungal skin infections. Furthermore, it is not particularly toxic, and allergic reactions are rare. Its great advantage is that it is very effective when taken orally. Griseofulvin is used for the treatment of ringworm and athlete's foot.

Chemically, nystatin is a large molecule which is amphoteric, that is, containing both positively-charged and negatively-charged ionic groups. It does not affect bacteria, but kills the fungi which often proliferate in the intestine when the normal bacteria are killed during use of antibacterial agents such as tetracycline. These fungi are very resistant to other agents, and may cause very serious infections.

Amphotericin B resembles nystatin. Administered intravenously, it has many potentially dangerous side effects, especially to the kidneys, so close supervision by a doctor is required during treatment. It is active against many fungi that are susceptible to no other drug.

What Next?

Written accounts of man's attempts to use natural products against disease date back to the very earliest periods of recorded history. Certain soils were thought to have magical powers of healing, and were applied directly to the infected areas. Today, having isolated all our major antibiotics from soil microbes, we understand the source of whatever real healing power these preparations may have had. Antibiotics have been found in many of the herbs used in ancient and medieval medicine. But the antibiotics found in higher plants so far seem to be much weaker than the microbial antibiotics now available. Whether they really had any beneficial effect on the medieval patient is doubtful. Until this century, man was fumbling in the dark, against forces he did not understand, and with medicines whose actions were even more mysterious. Now we can isolate, purify, and identify the agents effective in the treatment of infection. What are the obstacles to further research?

Two great problems loom in the field of antibiotics. First, how can we expand the number of diseases treatable with antibiotics? Second, how can we continue using the drugs we already have in order to prevent a decrease in their effectiveness? In particular, what can we do about the ability of bacteria to acquire resistance to a drug after continued exposure to it?

Among the more important diseases which cannot yet be cured with antibiotics are the viral diseases and cancer. The problem of specificity, brought up earlier in this chapter, is relevant here. Scientists question whether there are significant differences between a virus or a cancer cell and the normal human cells which will make it possible for an antibiotic to kill the invader, but not the host. Extensive research has not yet provided a satisfactory answer.

Serious questions can be raised concerning current uses of antibiotics. As we have seen, certain types of bacteria are adept at becoming resistant to drugs after being exposed to them over an extended period. Lethal infections that formerly responded to penicillin or streptomycin, now are unaffected. New antibiotics are continually being introduced, keeping us a few jumps ahead of the resistant microbes. These work until the bacteria have had a chance to grow resistant to them. Erythromycin, introduced to kill penicillin-resistant strains, has already induced many resistant strains of its own. It is about to fall by the way. The future history of antibiotics might turn out to be a struggle between the antibiotic researcher and the bacterial resistors. Fortunately, some types of bacteria have not shown any tendency to become resistant—even after extensive exposure to some of the drugs. Proper use of drugs may slow the growth of resistance in several ways:

1. The less a bacterial strain is exposed to a drug, the less likely it is to grow resistant to that drug. Therefore, drugs necessary to combat dangerous diseases must be avoided for trivial uses where the dangerous bacteria may be exposed to the drug and attain resistance. Also, the identity of the organism and the drug sensitivity of the infecting strain of the organism should always be determined. In this way, the most effective drug will be used first, and the use of more than one drug can be avoided. Besides, taking the wrong antibiotic may actually increase the hazard of the infection. This proposition may be unreasonable only when withholding therapy may be considered unwise because of the urgency of the situation. Only in such cases should antibiotics be given before laboratory results are known.

2. If an effective antibiotic is not used in optimum concentrations, a sufficient number of bacteria may survive long enough to give rise to a resistant strain. Therefore the amount of drug given and the duration of treatment are very important.
3. Bacteria quickly become resistant to streptomycin, so the drug should not be used when another agent is just as good.

People occasionally become allergic to drugs by repeated contact with them. This is another reason that antibiotics should never be used where they are not necessary. If an allergy is built up, like a child crying wolf, that person will not be able to use that antibiotic when it is really needed.

Not long after the antibiotics were introduced, someone thought of putting antibiotics in food to keep it from spoiling. The idea worked nicely. Even ground beef, which becomes unpleasant in only a few hours at room temperature, stays relatively fresh for days when treated with Aureomycin or Terramycin. This was a valuable discovery, reducing greatly the waste and expense of shipping and selling meat and poultry.

The cost of animal products was decreased still further by the addition of small amounts of antibiotic to the feed given to the animals. Supplying the animal constantly with antibiotic seems to protect it from bothersome infections and to allow the full metabolic system of the animal to be directed to its growth and nourishment. At any rate, animals fed on antibiotics grow larger and produce more meat, eggs, and milk; there is more product for the amount of food consumed than there is from animals which are not so fed.

Both of these applications of antibiotics, as a food preserver and as an additive to animal feed, reduced the cost and therefore the price of food, increasing the nation's food supply. But such use of antibiotics may be hazardous. If the antibiotic is also used against human disease, then its widespread presence at low concentrations in food may greatly increase the rate of development of bacterial resistance to the drug, just as the use of the antibiotic in hospitals induces bacterial resistance there. Secondly, the presence of even small amounts of an antibiotic in food when it is being eaten may be enough to trigger a hypersensitivity or allergic reaction in the person who eats it. As yet, sufficient data are not available to tell what levels of antibiotic may safely be present in food. Animals grown on a diet that includes antibiotics are not given any antibiotic the last few days before slaughter, but in some cases it is not certain that all the antibiotic has left the tissues.

In the summer of 1966, a U.S. government committee released a report on agricultural use of antibiotics. The report stated that in order for an antibiotic to be used in food preservation it should not be used in medicine, should not give rise to resistant strains, or cross-resistance, and should not antagonize the effects of antibiotics in medical use. The committee advised that antibiotics given to food-producing animals should be tested to determine how much time is required for the antibiotic to leave the animals' tissues, and if this time is not known, the drug must be abandoned: the presence of penicillin in such foods is considered a serious public health hazard. Chloramphenicol was specifically forbidden from use in food-producing animals because the lag time is unknown. As always in the field of therapeutics, a proper balance must be maintained between use of relatively untested drugs on the one hand, and the need for progress on the other.

The use of antibiotics for economic reasons seems inevitably to carry some health risk; but medical use also involves the necessary risk of bacterial resistance and allergic reactions. The optimist assures us that man's ingenuity will continue to discover new drugs at a fast enough rate. He claims a cure will always be one step ahead of the disease, in this case, resistance. Let us hope he is right.

SUPPLEMENTAL READING

New Drugs, American Medical Association, Chicago, 1966.
Third International Congress of Chemotherapy, *I & II*, Hefner Publishing Co., New York, 1964.
The Medical Letter, Drug & Therapeutic Information, Inc., New York.

Chapter 16

Chemical Warfare Against Cancer

Part I

To Americans, cancer means more than a disease; the word elicits as much terror as any other in our language. When we look at the sinister side of our nation's life, nothing may be as fearful as the rising crime rate, except if we choose to call it the cancer of the rising crime rate. Neither can we forget the cancer of war, or the cancer of communism, of inflation, or of urban decay. The physician after diagnosing an ailment can say almost any word but the one word—"cancer."

Several factors nourish the terror. One is cancer's reputation for insidious surprise. Another is the protracted suffering the disease can cause. Moreover, no one seems safe. Those who exercise, avoid tobacco and alcohol, and otherwise lead exemplary lives can still fall victim to the disease. The account of a child dead of leukemia is common enough to constitute a minor genre in the newspaper industry. Finally, we fear cancer's seeming omnipresence. Among the people who have succumbed to it include the little known man down the street, as well as T. S. Eliot, the poet; Robert Taft, the U.S. Senator; Edward R. Murrow, the TV commentator; Ernie Davis, the football star; and Nat King Cole, the entertainer. The development of the disease, as it afflicted these people, is understood; its basic cause or causes are not.

Cancer—What It Is and What It Does

Essentially, a cancer cell is a normal cell that has lost its responsiveness to the normal control mechanisms of the body and the cell. The common conception is that cancer cells grow and divide much more rapidly than normal cells; in fact, however, many normal body tissues, such as the mucosa (mucous membranes) lining the gastrointestinal (G.I.) tract, the mucous membranes of the mouth, the hair follicles, and the cells constituting the bone marrow may divide and reproduce themselves faster than cancerous cells. So also

257

do cells in the new growth of incompletely organized bony structure, called the callus, around a bone fracture. The G.I. tract completely re-lines itself about every three days, and the uterine endometrium (mucous membrane lining the uterus) also replaces itself with startling rapidity after each menstruation.

The normal, rapidly reproducing cells present some serious obstacles to cancer chemotherapy. The cancer cell may develop into an abnormal shape or size; it may not die at the end of what would be a normal life span for a cell of its tissue-type. As normal cells divide and new cells are, in effect, born, they differentiate and adapt their structures and functions to serve differing purposes necessary for the well-being of the whole organism. Cancer cells, however, cease to differentiate themselves and fail to fall into step with the normal processes of their so-called "host" organism. Although cancer cells are not parasites introduced from outside, the organism that has produced them actually does play "host" to a parasitic growth once they have established themselves. The cancer cells, even if they appear and function in many aspects like normal cells, do not contribute to the well-being of the host, but continue to reproduce and to draw nourishment, often to the detriment of the neighboring normal cells, and finally with malign consequences for the organism itself. The cancerous cells in most tissue form a growth, a tumor or neoplasm (from the Greek for "new growth"). The tumor itself may cause the death of the organism by simple mechanical means. For example, it may restrict circulation of blood to vital organs; it may interfere with normal cell growth and reproduction and take over and force out essential, functioning cells. It certainly drains off necessary nutriments to feed its own uncontrolled growth. Not all neoplasms are cancerous, however. Many kinds of moles, warts, and cysts, for example, and various kinds of polyps which grow internally, are not in themselves malignant.

Cancer spreads. This characteristic is one of the chief medical problems in treating the disease. The technical word is *metastasis;* cancer metastasizes, quite rapidly in some varieties, more slowly in others. Cancers of the skin or bladder, for example, metastasize relatively slowly and are called *invasive* tumors: they spread by invading surrounding contiguous tissues. Other kinds jump from one site to another. Cancer of the colon has a noted preference for the liver as a secondary site, while some types of cancer in the blood move into the central nervous system and settle in the brain. The avenues for expansion are the body's superhighways, the circulatory and lymphatic systems. Because the primary tumor, the cancerous growth in its original site, is often not well organized, pieces of it, little groups of cells, break off and circulate through the blood stream to lodge in other, often remote, portions of the body.

Various types of cancer seem to have special preferences in their choice of secondary sites, but not all environments in the body appear to be equally suited to receive the insidious immigrants. The most common secondary sites, the most receptive hosts, are the lungs, the liver, the brain, and to a lesser extent, the bones. A variation on this circulatory system route is found in some cases in which a cancer has invaded a neighboring blood vessel and then grown out into a long string of cancer cells, rather like a tapeworm, so that long threads of cancer cells can sometimes be found running through the body's blood vessels. The lymphatic system can open the way to a less dramatic spread of cancer from its primary site. For example, cancer of the breast eventually will involve lymph nodes or glands in the area and spread through the lymphoid tissues to the major lymphatic centers about the armpit. Not all cancers succeed in establishing secondary lesions, however. This is indeed fortunate, since the more widespread the disease, the less the chances for survival. Sometimes cancers with an observed predilection for some particular site unaccountably fail to establish a "colony" there despite metastatic spread to other tissues. If a way could be found to limit all cancers to their primary sites, medicine could make considerable progress in its fight against the disease; cancer *in situ* is relatively easy to remove by surgical excision.

The cancer cell, undifferentiated as to function, rapidly growing and dividing, is a kind of primitive throwback bearing many resemblances to embryonic cells. They may be considered to represent a regressive change in cell organization. From different species throughout the plant and animal kingdoms, cancer cells display marked similarities. The crown gall disease in plants, for example, results in a disorganized, uncontrolled tumor growth like the malignant neoplasms observable in higher forms of life. Cells from this tumor can grow in complete autonomy from the parent plant, flourishing in a minimal culture medium which proves quite insufficient to the needs of normal cells. This independence, showing a relative independence of the integrated economy of the whole organism, characterizes cancer cells in all organisms. With care and certain precautions, cancer cells can be made to propagate themselves indefinitely, even when transferred from one host to another. This host-to-host transfer usually succeeds only between individuals of the same species; but human cancers have been implanted successfully in the anterior chamber of a rabbit's eye and in the cheek pouches of hamsters. These locations are places where the foreign tissue seems to be shielded from the animal's immune reaction, the mechanism an organism uses to reject foreign bodies.

Cancer cells may be placed into two groups in the most simple form of classification: *carcinomas* and *sarcomas*. A carcinoma originates in epithelial tissue—tissue made up of contiguous cells with little intracellular material, usually constituting a lining or covering, e.g. the skin, linings of hollow organs, tubes and passages of the respiratory, gastrointestinal, and genitourinary tracts, and the lining of blood and lymph vessels. A sarcoma, on the contrary, originates in the nonephithelial tissues—structural tissues such as muscle, bone cartilage, and fat. In a larger sense, however, there are as many varieties of cancer in humans as there are kinds of tissue in the human body. Each can be identified by microscopic study because of its characteristic microscopic anatomy, or histology. A given species or even a specific breeding line sometimes seems to be peculiarly susceptible to a certain variety of cancer; for example, melanoma of the anus in gray horses, and certain skin cancers in Scottish Terriers.

Selected inbreeding of laboratory mice has produced animals in which the same type of cancer recurs, generation after generation. The phenomenon naturally raises the question of heredity in cancer. Do certain kinds of cancer "run" in certain families? Demography (the study of vital statistics) shows what seems to be racial or at least geographical patterns in cancer. Statistically, the Chinese are conspicuous for the frequency with which they are afflicted with cancers of the upper part of the pharynx. Cancer of the liver occurs more frequently among the Malaysians and West African Bantus than in Caucasians. Malignant melanoma of the skin developing from existing moles is rare in Negroes. Cancer of the cervix is infrequent in Jewish women, and cancer of the penis occurs somewhat less among peoples practicing childhood circumcision. Epidemiological research has frequently shown that extrinsic factors are probably more important than genetic susceptibility. Bantus placed on nutritionally adequate diets rather than their normal, notoriously poor diet show a sharp drop in the incidence of cancer of the liver. Icelanders, who have a high rate of cancer of the stomach owe this to carcinogenic (cancer-causing) substances in the smoked fish that constitutes a major portion of their diet.

In balance, then, current thought is reluctant to name any specific factor of inheritance except in a few rare and atypical cases, such as glioma of the eye in childhood, a tumor of special cells of the nervous system which is definitely inherited. In general, cancer itself is not inherited. Even if a degree of susceptibility could be shown to be passed along genetically, the presence of an immediate inciting cause—some trigger extrinsic to the tissue to be affected—must be weighed more heavily. A piece of steel does not cause a fire unless someone strikes it with a piece of flint.

The crown gall disease in plants, already mentioned, provides a simple example of the necessity for extrinsic irritation. The disease is caused by infection of the plant by a certain bacterium. However, the bacterium and its tumor-inducing principle alone will not transform the plant's normal cells into the uncontrolled, cancerous cells that characterize the disease. There must first be a wound—the extrinsic irritation—inflicted upon the plant's tissues. To be sure, the bacterium itself is an extrinsic cause in this case, but the wound is the necessary factor in the creation of a plant cancer. The length of time between the infliction of the wound and the transformation of a given cell into the tumorous state is also a factor in the rapidity of that cell's uncontrolled growth and division. Between 60 and 72 hours after the wound, the plant's normal cells will organize for rapid growth and division in order to repair the damage. Cells transformed by the presence of the bacterium between 60 and 72 hours after the wound has been inflicted grow most rapidly and are wholly autonomous. That is, they can be removed completely from the presence of all the bacteria, transplanted from the parent plant into a culture or a healthy plant of the same kind. They retain the power to grow and reproduce themselves, even, as noted, in a culture quite insufficient for the growth and reproduction of normal cells.*

In higher animals a single accident, a blow or abrasion, is not a likely cause of cancer. Severe burns may cause scar tissue which later becomes cancerous, but the burn is not the cause of the cancer. On the other hand, consistent, chronic irritation definitely seems to play a role. The Icelander's smoked fish might be a chronic irritation; so might a poorly-fitted dental plate or a hot pipe-stem resting by the hour day after day in the same spot of a man's lip. Since the eighteenth century cancer of the scrotum has been associated with chimneysweeps and exposure to soot. This was an occupational hazard, as was cancer of the bladder among workers in aniline dye industries. Industrial reforms and special precautions have nearly eliminated certain of these extrinsic causes, thereby stopping cancer before it starts. Cancer of the skin is often associated with constant exposure to sunlight. Such exposure cannot be eliminated for some occupational groups, as seacaptains, but an awareness of the danger encourages checkups which can catch the disease early.

In many instances of chronic irritation, the case for calling either a substance or an activity *carcinogenic* begins as a largely circumstantial one. One of the greatest public medical and legal debates in recent American history concerns the variety of cancer which the American Cancer Society calls the fastest-growing cause of cancer mortality today. This is cancer of the lung and the debated cause, for which only strong circumstantial evidence has been produced, is cigarette smoking. The mortality rate from lung cancer in men has increased ten times in thirty years; it is rising also among women. It kills nearly twice as many men each year as the next-ranking killer among cancers in men, those of the colon and rectum. Lung cancer killed 32,698 men between the ages of 35 and 74 in 1963; it has one of the lowest survival rates among major types of cancer. And in 1966 an estimated 5,000 new cases will be reported in California alone, another 5,900 in New York.

Lung cancer rates soar in smokers as compared to non-smokers. Laboratory rats and mice, treated with substances derived from cigarette smoke, develop cancers. But scientists, like lawyers,

* See "The Reversal of Tumor Growth" by Armin C. Braun, in SCIENTIFIC AMERICAN (November 1965), Vol. 213, No. 5, pp. 75–83.

demand more than circumstantial evidence. Rats and mice will not smoke cigarettes, despite ingenious devices to force them to inhale the smoke. Some researchers at Harvard have recently theorized that particles in the smoke are made radioactive in the process of burning, and that these particles are the culprits. Others have said it is arsenic in the cigarette papers. So far nothing has been proved beyond doubt. Circumstantial evidence, however, has induced physicians in this country and in England to cut their smoking considerably: in both countries an estimated 30 percent smoke compared to some 52 percent of the total adult population. There are many specific compounds that are known to be carcinogenic compounds. Among these are hydrocarbon compounds found in soot, coal tar, mineral oil, and pitch. Some amines used in dyestuffs, and alkylating compounds, including a nitrogen mustard used as a therapeutic drug against cancer, are capable of triggering the change of a cell from normal to malignant.

Cancer and Viruses

Viruses must also be considered among the possible causative agents in cancer. Numerous oncogenic or tumor-causing viruses have been discovered, and malignant tumors have been induced in laboratory animals, apparently through viral activity.

Viruses have been described as tiny balls filled with DNA or RNA, depending on the species (*see* the chapter on "Control of the Cell's Architects . . ."). DNA, or deoxyribonucleic acid, is the so-called "key to life." A biological Rosetta Stone, the strands of DNA are found in every living cell. These strands carry the genetic directions that determine the life and development of the cell. A protein molecule "reads" this chemical hieroglyph and sets it down in a new language. This translation is a strand of substance called RNA, or ribonucleic acid. Each strand of RNA copies the strand of DNA, using a complementary "alphabet." The RNA proceeds to factories of protein synthesis found in every cell. These factories are called ribosomes.

When a virus invades the body, it carries its characteristic DNA or RNA. The virus attaches itself to the victim cell and injects its DNA or RNA into the cell, like a hypodermic syringe. The protein-producing machinery of the cell unknowingly accepts the viral DNA or RNA and uses it to produce the faulty design and structure. Viral DNA or RNA fouls the cell's original genetic code, scrambles the components and effects the malfunction of the entire cellular process. A virus seizes control at the most fundamental level of life processes.

Since the controls that regulate cell growth, function, and reproduction are poorly understood, it is impossible to speak with certitude, or to describe a model instance. But if the cellular controls are wholly or partially connected with the DNA code, or if they require specific functions of the proteins and enzymes produced by RNA, it is apparent that an exchange of DNA between a normal cell and an invading virus could possibly result in changes within the cell, which could be described as "cancerous."

If viruses *can* cause cancers in humans, however, why doesn't everyone have cancer? All manner of viruses surround us; they are unavoidable. The virus that causes viral pneumonia is always with us. Yet people contract pneumonia only when their body's resistance to infection is lowered by exposure or by a long lasting or debilitating disease. The factor of susceptibility, then, remains a paramount consideration. However, as we noted in the case of the crown gall tumor in plants, presence of the bacterium associated with the tumor-inducing principle is not enough to cause a tumor; a wound, the extrinsic irritation, is an indispensable prerequisite.

Basic research into the cause or causes of cancer continues today in laboratories across the country. All possible leads are being studied exhaustively—genetics and heredity, extrinsic irritants and carcinogenic substances, and oncogenic (tumor-producing) viruses in men and beasts. In the process scientists have gained insights penetrating to the basis of life itself. Many aspects of the complex chemistry of the cell and even of subcellular particles have yielded to man's continuous probing; but the central practical problem—the cause and the cure for cancer—remains elusive, hidden.

Clinical Treatment and Techniques

In elementary terms, three modes of attack upon cancer are available today. One can cut it off, another burn it out, yet another poison it. Cancer presents a critical threat to life, but all three counter measures are not without hazard in themselves.

With our present knowledge, surgical removal of the affected area is the most generally applicable means of attack on cancer. Technical advances in recent years have altered the surgeon's capabilities no less than the development of new weaponry has revolutionized modern warfare. Patients can survive with only 20 to 25 percent of the liver intact after surgery; the bladder can be removed and an artificial replacement constructed. The major portion of the stomach and intestines can be removed. Deprived of their normal outlets by the surgical knife, body wastes can be rerouted to artificial outlets with minimal disruption of the patient's normal life. People whose larynx and vocal cords have been surgically removed can be taught to talk again; portions of damaged arteries and veins can be replaced by plastic pipes. It is possible to remove an entire lung. Only within the past year a right-handed patient has survived the removal of the entire left hemisphere of his brain. The left hemisphere controls the right-hand side of the body, and, in right-handed people, plays the dominant role in those processes of reasoning, memory, and communication—capabilities which we think of as most typically human. Yet the patient, far from becoming a vegetable, has begun a long process of rehabilitation, with the right-hand side of the brain learning to take over functions formerly dominated by the removed left hemisphere.

Nevertheless, surgical excision of the offending member has certain obvious limitations. Certain organs are simply not expendable. Even in those organs least likely to be impaired by some surgical pruning, a very large cancerous tumor may be inoperable. Because of the malignant character of many forms of the disease, excision is an all or nothing proposition. One cancer cell left behind may be sufficient to start a new growth and a new threat to life. Likewise, surgery is helpless against cancers of the blood, most cancers of the bone marrow and widely metastasized cancers of the lymphoid tissues. One cannot remove all the lymph nodes, as might be considered necessary in Hodgkin's disease. Advances in radical surgery have made it possible to remove regional lymph nodes which may provide avenues for the metastasis of primary cancers in contiguous tissues, as, for example, the lymph nodes in the shoulder and armpit region in cancer of the breast. Advanced cancer, in which the cancer cells have spread and established themselves throughout the patient's body, is almost inevitably fatal, far beyond the surgeon's skill. A cancer which has begun to metastasize but in which the metastases are still trapped in regional lymph nodes may yield to dramatic surgical expedients, although radiation is the more likely treatment in most cases. Localized invasive cancer or carcinoma *in situ* is the best candidate for surgical cures.

Since the cancers that are treatable by surgery are, generally speaking, the least serious and least advanced, surgery appears to have a better record of success against cancer than do other expedients. Tables released by the American Cancer Society showing five-year survival rates for patients with cancer of the thyroid, which has a high survival rate even with regional involvement, indicates survival rates for victims with localized cancer nearly twice as high as those for victims of similar cancers with minimal spread into the immediately adjacent areas. Sometimes the ratio is even higher. Once a cancer has progressed beyond the comparatively limited state treatable by surgery, the prognosis becomes rapidly poorer.

Radiation treatments with either X-rays or radium, or with a combination of both, are the most familiar alternatives to surgery in most cases of cancer which are, for one reason or another, inoperable. Sometimes irradiation is used in conjunction with surgery. As a properly set camera lens focuses an image precisely and sharply on the light-sensitive emulsion of a photographic film, so an X-ray machine can be used to focus or concentrate its rays upon a specific organ or tissue. Thus a miniscule area affected by cancer but otherwise unreachable may be accurately treated with minimal damage to surrounding tissues. Human tissue must absorb radiant energy to suffer damage or destruction. Cells that are transversed by energy "focused" elsewhere remain relatively unaffected. Consequently X-rays can be made effective at various depths within the human body, as well as on its surface. The generating voltage on the X-ray machine can be stepped up or turned down; the higher the voltage, the deeper the X-rays. Timing allows normal cells in the affected area as much time as possible for recuperation, while providing maximum destruction of cancer cells. Dramatic treatments have been tried on patients with widely metastasized cancers or with generalized cancers like leukemia and Hodgkin's disease. The patient is virtually "bathed" in low intensity X-rays emanating from the ceiling of a special room. Deep-seated cancers may be treated by placing the patient on a kind of rotisserie on which he is turned. In this way normal tissues are only briefly and intermittently exposed to radiation, while the seat of the malignancy, remaining always at the turning center of the revolving body, is constantly and intensely irradiated. More extensive therapy of solid tumors can be achieved by placing capsules of radium salts, radon gas, or radioactive cobalt in the patient, either imbedded in tissues or located in a body cavity, such as the uterus. A radioactive material is often encased in a heavy metal such as lead, mercury, gold, or platinum to filter out some of the *beta* rays that could cause excessive destruction of immediately adjacent tissue, and permit only the *gamma* rays to reach the target organs or tissues. One of the most common applications of the combination of X-ray and radium treatments is cancer of the cervix in women; other forms of cancer also respond well to this technique.

Leucocytes or white cells produced in bone marrow and lymphoid tissues are highly sensitive to radiation. Various forms of leukemia, characterized by a high leucocyte count in the blood, are being treated experimentally by extracorporeal irradiation. The patient's blood is channelled from his body through a machine which irradiates it. The blood is then directed back into its normal course in the patient's veins. The temporary artificial extension of the circulatory system exposes the leucocytes to the lethal rays, while other tissues remain unaffected.

Radiation therapy is potent. Exposure to the effects of X-rays, radium, and other radioactive isotopes may initiate the development of cancer. Doctors, dentists, and technicians who do not take adequate precautions in the use of X-ray machines, radium, or the fluoroscope over long periods of time may develop radiation dermatitis that may progress to an invasive cancer. A group of American women employed by a watch manufacturer in the 1920's painted radium dials on wrist watches. On their tongues they moistened and pointed the brushes used for the handwork. Since that time, all have died, the last victim some thirty years after her fatal employment, from cancer of the jaw or of the bone marrow and blood. The minute amounts of radium ingested from these tiny brush-tips concentrated in the bones of the young women.

Citizens of Nagasaki and Hiroshima who survived the immediate anguish and disfigurement from exposure to high levels of instantaneous radiation from the atomic bombs dropped twenty years ago still suffer from the consequences of this holocaust. Doctors studying the survivors have discovered a grim, if postponed, casualty list that accompanies nuclear war. The incidence of leukemia and other cancers is very much higher among these people than among the general population.

Radiation treatment of cancer is fighting fire with fire; however, the considerable data that have already accumulated show that within the great variation in response, cancers originating in lymphoid tissues, such as Hodgkin's disease, are quite responsive to radiation. Because these are precisely those cancers against which surgery is impractical, radiation treatments are a valuable weapon in man's battery of anticancer weapons and provide hope for cures in certain cases.

Chemotherapy is the third major weapon in that arsenal. It is also the least developed and probably the least familiar to the public. There are three basic ways of adding to the number of available, effective anticancer agents in the chemotherapy stockpile. The oldest, the most widely used, the best supported program is random screening. This kind of research requires more money and involves more researchers than any other program. The program costs because it is big; it has to be big because it is essentially a blind, random groping. A tumor of a given type is induced in a laboratory mouse or rat. Portions of this malignancy are then distributed and introduced into many other mice or rats, providing a large number of test subjects. Naturally occurring and synthetic chemical compounds as well as extracts from all forms of plants, animals and microorganisms are then tested against the transplanted animal tumors to see which, if any, inhibit the growth or destroy the cancer. Hundreds of thousands of compounds have been screened in the United States.

In using this method, investigators are always troubled by the question of "false negatives". A false *positive* is a compound that inhibits cancer in test animals, but later proves ineffective in humans. This is unfortunate, but the false positive does not represent an irretrievable loss. A record of its effectiveness in laboratory animals remains as a possible lead to later researchers. On the other hand, compounds which have been found to be ineffective against cancers in laboratory animals, might be effective against human cancers. But since a compound that fails to prove useful in the laboratory is never tried on humans, such potentially useful drugs are lost to oblivion. This is the "false negative" that troubles the scientists.

The random-screening program is obviously rather primitive and crude. As one researcher puts it, "What we're doing is taking any old compound off the shelf and putting it into ten rats and seeing if their tumors grow more slowly than those of the control group . . . It just doesn't arouse much enthusiasm in me." Intellectual stimulation is minimal or nonexistent in the program, and one problem is getting people to do it.

Yet several anticancer compounds have come from this random screening program, and a glance at the history of medical advances attributable to antibiotics reveals that all of our antibiotics are the result of this kind of research. The stroke of genius in this medical revolution was the initial observation that a certain compound, penicillin, inhibited the growth of certain organisms in a petri dish. After that discovery, subsequent advances were the result merely of replication with modifications of the same technique. One pharmacologist has contended that anyone instructed in the applied method of random screening, regardless of any real scientific training, could find four new antibiotics tomorrow. The work is unexciting, mechanical; but so far, it has proved a valuable resource in research.

Two other methods of conducting research are classified as "rational" research. In this approach the investigator attempts to prove in the laboratory a carefully-reasoned theory which he has developed on the basis of known facts and previous observations. One of these methods begins in the laboratory, with test tubes and diagrams of molecular structures; it follows biochemical leads into new areas. The other starts with the observation and study of actual patients, whose plights may often seem totally unrelated to the end product of research. This is research based upon physiological and clinical experience. In the next chapter we shall survey briefly the major subdivisions of cancer chemotherapy and review some of the most important drugs currently in use.

There is another kind of chemotherapy, effective against some cancers. It is based upon the tendency of certain organs and tissues of the human body to absorb and concentrate certain chemicals. The actual effective agent in the treatment is, however, radiation. This method is treatment with radioactive isotopes. After treatment in a nuclear accelerator or an atomic reactor, certain chemical elements are transformed into unstable isotopes or forms of the same or another element that decay with the accompanying generation of radioactive rays. An example of the application of this principle is the use of radioactive phosphorus to palliate malignancies of the lymphoid system. The ingested phosphorus concentrates in lymph and bone tissues. Cancerous lymphoid tissue absorbs it two and one-half times as fast as do normal lymphoid tissues. The unstable atoms of radioactive phosphorus decay with the release of highly energetic β-particles.

Similarly, it is well known that the thyroid gland preferentially takes up iodine. Radioactive iodine, then, will be concentrated by the thyroid, and will have minimal effect on other body tissues. Furthermore, the radioactive iodine is selectively absorbed and concentrated in the rapidly growing and dividing neoplastic thyroid cells; fortunately in some cases, it destroys not only the primary lesion in the thyroid, but also destroys metastases in bone and lung tissue, that retain the ability to concentrate iodine. Radioactive gold, chromium orthophosphate, and yttrium (a rare-earth metal) can be used to dry up accumulations of fluids in the chest and abdominal cavities caused by certain forms of cancer in these regions. In recent experimental studies an attempt is being made to palliate metastases in the lungs by the intravenous injection of radioactive yttrium-90 ceramic microspheres 60 microns in diameter.* These tiny spheres are carried to the lungs, where they become trapped in the capillary bed and afford long-term radiation treatment.

Hormone treatments of cancer may also be classed as chemotherapy. Hormones are useful only in an extremely limited number of cancers, mainly those derived from tissues associated with the

* One micron = the millionth part of a meter, which is a little more than a yard.

primary or secondary sex characteristics. Moreover, their effect is usually only palliative. Cancer of the prostate, however may be controlled either by surgical castration or by "chemical castration"—dosage with female sex hormones or their synthetic analogues. Some cancers of the breast in women are palliated, and in some cases death postponed, through removal of the ovaries, removal of both adrenal glands or the pituitary, or by administration of the male sex hormone, testosterone, or the female sex hormones, estrogens. The treatment can be effective even when the breast cancer has metastasized from its primary site to neighboring bone tissue. Of course, if the pituitary or adrenal glands are removed, synthetic substitutes for certain of the hormones produced by these glands must be provided to maintain life.

The final and perhaps most important branch of cancer chemotherapy concerns treatment with chemical compounds designed to starve the malignant cell, poison it, or prevent its division (in which case it will die). This field lays claim to the subcellular world; it lives daily with DNA, attempting to learn all it can about the most basic and least understood processes of life. The objects of its study are subcellular particles, enzymes, proteins, complex hydrocarbon groups; its idiom is the language of the most advanced and complex biochemistry being researched today. This line of chemotherapy is working at the foundations of all biological knowledge; it may prove the key to the elusive cure for cancer or it may accidentally open locks of totally unrelated disease states. Great promise lies within this approach but the course to the ultimate goals is not one that can be directly charted at this time.

SUPPLEMENTAL READING

Braun, Armin C., The Reversal of Tumor Growth, Scientific American, November, 1965.

Karnofsky, O., Cellular Effects of Anticancer Drugs, Annual Review of Pharmacology, *3*, 357, 1963.

Krementz, E. T., Kokarne, G. M., and Iglesias, F., Current Status of Chemotherapy of Cancer, Postgraduate Medicine, *35*, 384, 1964.

Chapter 17

Chemical Warfare Against Cancer

Part II

Every year a newspaper will report that *the* answer to cancer has been found in some basic research laboratory, and each time it turns out to be a false hope. Because most of the important anticancer drugs have a high toxicity to normal cells, quantitative differences really present an inadequate basis for chemical attack. For a long time scientists have sought the qualitative difference between the neoplastic cancer cell and the normal cell. For example, bacteria have a cell wall that is not possessed by mammalian cells; antibiotics can attack this bacterial wall without harming the mammalian host organism. The ideal chemotherapeutic agent is directed at some *qualitative* difference between normal cells and the cancer cells that it is designed to attack. We want to be able to tell the "bad guys" from the "good guys" by their hats. All we now know are such things as the bad guys have somewhat larger appetites. Poisoning the waterholes may get some of the bad guys first, but it will make the good guys pretty sick too.

Chemotherapy aims to find and learn the use of agents which operate in cells in any one of three ways: 1) inhibition of enzyme systems, the catalytic machinery essential to growth and reproduction; 2) alteration of the template molecules essential to the transfer of genetic information; or 3) alteration of the permeability of biological membranes.

The human body presents a seemingly endless array of hurdles and stumbling blocks to successful chemotherapy. To become an effective inhibitor of the neoplastic cells, some drugs must undergo a chemical change within the patient's body, perhaps within the target cell itself. Other organs, like the liver, may convert the drug into inactive compounds before the desired reaction can take place. Similarly, the active excretion of compounds by the kidney into the urine may vitiate the potential of a drug by preventing the achievement of adequate levels in the blood and target cells. Several chemotherapeutic agents potent enough to be useful against cancer, and

275

of great promise in experimental systems, are so highly toxic to other normal body tissues as to be clinically useless. Nevertheless, certain of these toxic agents can be used to considerable advantage by the careful physician, with supporting strength of extensive clinical laboratory facilities.

Finally, there is the problem of drug resistance. Sometimes the body itself manufactures agents antagonistic to the action of a drug. But, after long exposure, the cancer cell may develop new metabolic pathways or shift from a usual system of chemical reactions to a little-used but always available substitute in order to circumvent the drug's specific action. It is difficult to knock out all cancer cells at one blow. For example, some drugs affecting nucleic acid synthesis are ineffective against cells not *at that moment* making nucleic acid. Since DNA synthesis occurs only during a relatively small portion of the total life of the cells between cell division, it is virtually impossible to wipe out an entire cancer population at one time with these drugs. Long periods of treatment with the drugs might do the job, but the increasingly serious effects of toxicity to normal cells limit such an approach.

One of the most common causes of failure in the use of the currently-effective drugs lies in the existence of maybe one cancer cell in a million that is constitutionally different in such a way as to render it insensitive to the action of the particular drug. This is a circumstance similar to that being observed with alarm in bacterial types heretofore completely controlled by antibiotics. Some bacteria are resistant to the drug that kills their fellows; they survive and reproduce. Eventually the whole strain consists of the resistant descendants of the original immune individuals. For this reason, chemotherapy can often produce a temporary remission of cancer, but within a finite period the resistant cells multiply to produce an entirely new population. Subsequent treatments with the initially-successful drug are less and less effective. One possible solution that holds promise is the chemical cocktail, a package deal in which several drugs are combined. In one dose the cocktails may include both of the necessary components in that perilous balance mentioned above. They provide the toxic anticancer compound, and also the palliative or antagonist drugs designed to minimize the harmful effect on normal body tissues. It is possible also, however, to combine various anticancer compounds in a cocktail; this could eliminate more cancer cells, since many cells that are immune to the one drug will be affected by another (see Table 1).

Methotrexate, a folic acid antagonist, is one of the best understood and most successful chemotherapeutic agents known today in the fight against cancer. Folic acid, a vitamin derived from leaves of plants from the Latin (*folia*, leaves), was discovered almost twenty years ago. That story will be found in the chapter, "Testing the Drug."

All vitamins are necessary for life, and many are required for specialized functions. Vitamin A, for example, is necessary for

TABLE 1

The most important clinically useful anticancer agents.
(Grouped according to category of origin or action)

CATEGORY	AGENT	CLASS	DISEASES TREATED
Antimetabolites	Methotrexate	Folic Acid Antagonist	Acute Leukemia Choriocarcinoma Mycosis Fungoides
	6-Mercaptopurine	Purine Analogue	Acute Leukemia
	5-Fluorouracil	Pyrimidine Analogue	Carcinomas of breast, colon, other carcinomas
Alkylating Agents	Mechlorethamine Cyclophosphamide	Nitrogen mustards	Hodgkin's Disease Lymphosarcomas Other sarcomas and carcinomas
	Chlorambucil	Nitrogen mustard	Chronic Lymphocytic Leukemia
	Triethylene Melamine (TEM)	Ethylenimine derivatives	Chronic Lymphocytic Leukemia
	Triethylene Thiophosphor-amide (Thio-TEPA)	Ethylenimine derivatives	Ovarian Carcinoma Breast Carcinoma
	Busulfan	Alkyl Sulfonate	Chronic Granulocytic Leukemia
Natural Products	Actinomycin D	Antibiotic	Wilms' Tumor Rhabdomyosarcoma Ewing's Sarcoma
	Vinblastine	Plant Alkaloid	Hodgkin's Disease Choriocarcinoma
	Deacetylmethyl-colchicine	Plant Alkaloid	Chronic Granulocytic Leukemia

(Adapted from "Chemotherapy of Neoplastic Diseases," by P. Calabresi and A. D. Welch, in ANNUAL REVIEW OF MEDICINE, Vol. 13, 1962)

278 TAKE AS DIRECTED—OUR MODERN MEDICINES

vision and Vitamin D for bone development. Folic acid and Vitamin
B-12 seem to be important in the growth and replication of cells.
Most vitamins are transformed into chemically active coenzymes in
the body. The coenzyme is the metabolically active form of the
vitamin that does the work. The active form of folic acid is tetra-
hydrofolic acid—created by enzymatic reduction via addition of four
atoms of hydrogen. Folic acid cannot be synthesized by man from
its three component parts. Like some of the other vitamins, it must
be obtained from food: in the case of folic acid, this means primarily
through leafy vegetables, fruit, and liver. It is a potent substance;
only 50 millionths of a gram per day is required by the normal
human being to assure normal functioning of his body.

Since folic acid could give temporary relief of certain symptoms of pernicious anemia including malnutrition of the "blastic"
precursors of red blood cells, it was reasoned that similar effects
might be obtained on the "blastic" white blood cells of leukemia.
It was learned, however, that treatment with folic acid aggravated
leukemia; much higher counts of the blastic, undeveloped white blood
cells typical of the disease were found after treatment with folic
acid. Undaunted by this failure, chemists and clinicians reasoned
that if folic acid stepped up the progress of the disease, an antagonist
of folic acid might block progress of the disease. In 1948 and 1949,
scientists working on folic acid antagonists developed methotrexate.
Methotrexate has a great affinity for a particular enzyme, folate (or
dihydrofolate) reductase, which is the catalyst necessary for the formation of the coenzyme, essential in the formation of DNA and
RNA (see chapter on "Control of the Cell's Architects . . .").
Therefore, a reduction of the available tetrahydrofolate in a cell
interferes markedly with cell reproduction. The inhibition either prevents or slows cell division drastically by curtailing the causation
at its source. In cases of human choriocarcinoma, methotrexate has
proved highly successful. It is very selective, and has secured cures
in almost 7 percent of cases treated. However, choriocarcinoma
is not a "typical" cancer. The disease is a hormone-producing neoplasm arising from a membrane surrounding the fetus in a pregnant
woman. Hence choriocarcinoma may in some sense be considered
a tumor of foreign origin. Nevertheless, it is encouraging to see this
form of cancer, with a high mortality rate, being brought under control.

In acute leukemia in children, methotrexate has initially dramatic effects, but proves, in most cases, ultimately disappointing. The leukemia cells seem to take up the drug much more rapidly than normal cells—thus it is selective, one of the first requirements for successful chemotherapy. However, after the initial remission the disease usually returns to its earlier virulence, and is progressively less responsive to the drug. Some researchers have theorized that the drug does not affect cells having an abnormally high level of folate reductase. These cells are genetically stable, and by reproducing themselves become the basis for a resistant population.

Recent research on tumors in mice also has indicated another possibility, namely that the problem of resistance may be one of transport. Once methotrexate crosses the cell membrane, it becomes tightly bound to the intracellular enzyme and is extremely difficult to displace, insuring long-lasting effects. However, in aberrant cells from the mouse tumors the mechanism for active transport of the drug across cell membranes is quite inefficient. These aberrant cells are also genetically stable; they can pass this unfortunate (for the host) capability to their progeny as they divide, so that they become the basis of a resistant-tumor population. Finally, methotrexate cannot cross the blood-brain barrier. It does not go from the blood into the cerebrospinal fluid or the central nervous system, so that any leukemia cells that have gained access to the central nervous system escape the effects of the drug and survive to provide a source of subsequent "reinfection" of the body. Physicians have learned a very effective counterattack, however, by directly infusing the drug into the fluid that bathes the brain.

Methotrexate also has been moderately successful on another cancer front, one with international implications. A tumor found in Africa, called Burkitt's lymphoma, affects the jaws of children, causing gigantic jaw growth and malformation of the bone structures of the lower face. Similar cases have been found in the United States. The geographical pattern of its incidence corresponds to the environment and range of certain insects in Africa, and thus many researchers feel this may be the first human cancer demonstrated to be caused *by a virus*. About 20 to 30 percent of the cases have been cured by chemotherapy, notably with methotrexate.

Methotrexate, however, like all the important tools of chemotherapy, has the problem of toxicity. Large enough doses will produce bone-marrow toxicity, which decreases the production of both the white and red blood cells. Also, side effects on the gastrointestinal mucosa (lining membrane) will cause diarrhea, ulceration, bleeding, nausea, and vomiting. Although the mucosa normally is replaced by cells every few days, it cannot reproduce and replace itself because of the drug's interference. In some patients, loss of hair and skin rashes have been noted, although usual dosage ordinarily will not have these effects.

Owing to the seriousness of these toxic effects, sufficient amounts of a drug such as methotrexate can rarely be used to cure a cancer. Much research today is being devoted to the hunt for newer, more effective folic acid antagonists that may possess greater selectivity for the cancer cell. In these studies the target enzyme, folic reductase, is being purified and its interaction with the new inhibitors tested.

The action of 6-mercaptopurine, an analogue of a naturally-occurring component of DNA, cannot as yet be entirely explained. It appears to be converted to a ribonucleotide by cellular enzymes. In this form, it interferes with the utilization by the cells of pathways essential to the formation of nucleotides, the building blocks of nucleic acids. Some cells are resistant to 6-mercaptopurine because of an apparent defect in their capacity to form the fraudulent ribonucleotide. These eventually may become the source of a resistant population. Other mechanisms, however, appear to be responsible for much of the clinical resistance observed with mercaptopurine.

5–Fluorouracil and 5–Fluoro–2′–Deoxyuridine

Fluorouracil is one of the antimetabolites used most widely in the treatment of solid tumors. As an antimetabolite or analogue of a natural metabolite it tricks the cell: fluorouracil, rather than the natural and essential substance which it resembles, is introduced into the metabolic machinery.

There are two pathways by which cells get the nutriments they need to function and grow. One is the so-called *de novo* pathway, in which the cell makes everything it needs, in effect from scratch, from basic molecules. The other is called the preformed or salvage pathway. Here the cells simply rely on material in the diet or material released in the normal turnover of other cells. This duality of routes exists for most key intermediate steps in biosynthetic processes. Some researchers several years ago believed that their observations had shown that cancer cells were inherently lazy and preferred to utilize the preformed pathways rather than build compounds themselves. If an agent could be designed that would seem to a hungry cell to be one of its essential nutrients, and if this agent could be placed on the preformed pathway, it would presumably have greater specificity for cancer cells than for normal cells. The toadstools, so to speak, would find their way into the cancer cells' stew, while the normal cells would grow their own mushrooms rather than be poisoned by toadstools from outside. Dr. C. Heidelberger at the University of Wisconsin decided to replace a hydrogen atom on the uracil molecule, a pyrimidine base with a fluorine atom, thus producing a kind of chemical guerrilla. This is an example of the rational approach in research at work. If you visualize an atom as a sphere, the radius of a hydrogen atom is nearly the same as that of a fluorine atom. If you wished to build a child's model of the compound with tinker toys, you could not tell the difference unless you colored one red and the other yellow. This was not an easy synthesis to achieve, but after some years of work Dr. Heidelberger succeeded in preparing 5-fluorouracil and found that it was extremely active against a variety of experimental tumors.

As administered, the compound was inactive; but in the human body it undergoes a series of anabolic alterations, being converted to the ribonucleotide, 5-fluorouridylic acid, and then to 5-fluoro-2′-deoxyuridylic acid. In this form it blocks a critical step in the formation of DNA. This series of intermediate forms of the original compound presented a confusing number of opportunities for the drug to affect normal metabolic reactions, rather than the desirable specific one-site, one-time, one-manner of attack by the ideal chemotherapeutic agent. Thus, attempts were made to synthesize a more specifically effective and more active derivative. Also, 5-fluorouracil had no apparent significance in the treatment of leukemia and was so highly toxic that concern about the effect of the drug on normal reproducing cells restricted its use in man. Nevertheless, a hopeful indication was the effectiveness of the drug against selected forms of solid tumor—about 25 percent effectiveness. Most other chemotherapeutic agents were relatively useless against solid neoplasms.

Since fluorouracil was inactive until metabolically converted into certain derivatives, the logical approach for the chemists was to perform that conversion in the laboratory and administer the ultimate inhibitor directly from the test tube. This effort resulted in the synthesis of 5-fluoro-2'-deoxyuridine. The new compound was expensive to make, but looked promising in experimental systems. However, once again the human system proved more complicated than the laboratory testing apparatus. In men, and for that matter in most experimental animals, the precise portions of the complex molecule, put on with such great care and expense in the laboratory, are knocked off just about as fast as the substance can be introduced into the body. The only way to fool the body's mechanism is sneaking the 5-fluoro-2'-deoxyuridine (FUDR for short) into the system through a very slow intravenous infusion; FUDR seems much more stable this way than when given as a single injection. Both fluorouracil and FUDR are highly toxic; in fact some deaths among very ill, poor-risk patients have been attributed to therapy with both drugs. Considerable care with strict supervision are required for their use clinically. Their great importance is their apparent success against solid tumors, the type of cancer least affected by most other chemical agents.

Alkylating Agents

> Gas! Gas! Quick, boys!—An ecstasy of fumbling,
> Fitting the clumsy helmets just in time;
> But someone still was yelling out and stumbling
> And flound'ring like a man in fire or lime . . .
> Dim, through the misty panes and thick green light,
> As under a green sea, I saw him drowning.

At the second battle of Ypres in 1915, the German army for the first time in the history of warfare used poison gas (sulfur mustard) in combat. Public opinion throughout the world registered shock; poison gas was subsequently banned in international agreements. Wilfred Owen's poem is ironically entitled "Dulce et Decorum Est." It captures with extraordinary vividness the horror felt by those troops who were exposed to the monstrous new weapon, as Owen wrote, "obscene as cancer."

Today, fifty years after that battlefield experiment, and over one hundred years after its initial synthesis, the descendants of "sulphur mustard" are aiding man in his fight against cancer. All these compounds, known collectively as "alkylating agents," are highly reactive chemicals. This is because their end groups are alkyl derivatives, such as bis-β-chlorethylamines which are strongly attracted to electrically charged sites. They react with amino, phosphate, sulfhydryl, hydroxyl, imidazole, and carboxyl groups found in human cells.

Despite considerable investigation, the mechanism of alkylating agents' action against cancers remains unclear. Little need be said concerning specific drugs within the group. Nitrogen mustards were the first synthetic agents found to inhibit tumors in human tissue not under the control of the endocrine system. The earliest report on these studies came in 1946. A later chapter, dealing with drug testing, tells how it was discovered that nitrogen mustards suppressed the production of white blood cells. Mechlorethamine retains much of the character of the original poison gases, unlike chlorambucil, which is built from mechlorethamine by a series of chemical substitutions and derivations. It causes nausea and vomiting, and has a vesicant (blistering) effect upon exposed and subcutaneous tissues. It palliates malignant effusions in body cavities, particularly when they are of pleural origin, so well that direct intracavitary administration of mechlorethamine has largely supplanted the use of radioactive gold, mentioned previously in the discussion of radiation therapy in the treatment of cancer.

Cyclophosphamide is the result of continuing efforts to achieve a zeroing-in on neoplastic tissues through modification of the chemical structure of the alkylating agents. Its effectiveness is similar to that of mechlorethamine. Frequent alopecia (loss of hair) is an unfortunate side effect, coming from differences in tissue specificity achieved with cyclophosphamide. It also commonly causes nausea and vomiting, whether administered orally or intravenously. TEM (triethylenemelamine) does not at present seem to offer any important reasons for choosing it over mechlorethamine. TEM has an inconsistent and unpredictable rate of absorption when introduced into the human body. The most important drawback encountered in the ethylenimine derivatives is the depression of bone marrow. Nausea and vomiting also occur. Busulfan, the most useful sulfonic acid ester for clinical purposes, was developed at the Chester Beatty Research Institute in London. Its selective action against granulocytes (a type of white blood cell) led to its use against chronic granulocytic leukemia, producing remissions in some 85 to 90 percent of patients after the start of therapy. Its initial effect is often an improved appetite and sense of well-being. Primarily valuable for reduction of the morbidity of the disease, it also appears to prolong life significantly.

The alkylating agents have been prominent in experiments that combine drugs and radiation. The aim of these efforts is to find a drug that would reduce the threshold of susceptibility to radiation in neoplastic cells. Alkylating agents have also been particularly successful in regional chemotherapy (which will be dealt with shortly) because their rapid inactivation reduces the duration of toxic effects.

Recent Experiments

Actinomycin A, the parent of a whole genus of antibiotics extracted in the laboratory, was the first crystalline antibiotic derived from a streptomyces (a soil organism). It was isolated in 1940. The mechanism of action of actinomycin D (dactinomycin) against biological systems is not known. It is usually given intravenously, since oral doses equivalent to those possible through the circulatory system are precluded by the resulting severe damage to the digestive tract. Subcutaneous or intramuscular injections are impossible because of the drug's local vesicant action. Actinomycin D appears to be very toxic.

The story of the vinca alkaloids, vincristine and vinblastine, will be considered in another chapter. Particularly in the case of vinblastine, it is too early to predict its possible ultimate usefulness in the clinic.

The agent o,p' -DDD (its full designation is 2,2' -bis (2-chlorophenyl, 4-chlorophenyl) -1, 1-dichloroethane) is of general interest mainly because it is closely related in structure to the common insecticide DDT. The drug selectively cells of the adrenal cortex, destroys both normal and neoplastic; it has been used with some success against adrenocortical carcinoma.

6-Azauridine, developed by a group at Yale University, deserves mention here primarily because it is the first agent that does not cause serious toxic effects upon any normal human cells, but has selective destructive effects on certain types of leukemia cells. However, the drug's antineoplastic effects are very transient. Perhaps the drug's greatest importance to cancer research will be as a biochemical lead in the continued search for an anticancer drug with selectiveness for cancer cells, and low or nonexistent toxicity for normal cells and tissues.

Regional chemotherapy presents an interesting means of lessening or eliminating the toxic effect of most chemotherapeutic agents. A malignancy too widespread in an extremity to be operable may be treated by isolating the entire arm or leg by tourniquets and controlling the whole circulation of that limb with external equipment, i.e., an oxygenating pump. The chemical agent chosen for the course of treatment is continuously introduced into the affected area through the feeder artery, which is connected to both the supply of the drug and the oxygenating pump. The used blood returns through the vein draining the limb, to be refreshed and re-circulated by the pump. By this means, a high concentration of the antineoplastic drug can be achieved and maintained for a considerable period of time without the usual drawback of toxic effects on normal body tissues elsewhere.

Palliative chemotherapy is also given to certain internal organs by infusion into an artery supplying such an organ over prolonged periods of time—so-called infusion therapy. Perfusin therapy, in contrast, fills a body cavity with a drug and drains it out at another site; or the term may be used to describe arterial introduction of a drug with isolation of the treated area. Antimetabolites such as methotrexate can be introduced by the arterial route without isolation of the regional circulation. Encouraging results have been noticed using such regional chemotherapy on melanomas and soft-tissue sarcomas (malignant tumor of connective tissue origin) of the extremities, as well as on advanced tumors of the head and neck. At the same time systemic administration of the proper metabolic antidotes cuts down the toxic effects of the drug on tissues other than those in the target area. Folic acid has been used systemically with regional intra-arterial infusion of methotrexate. Conversely, selected regions may be protected by intra-arterial introduction of the normal metabolic agent while the antimetabolite is circulating systemaically. The latter approach has been used with high local concentrations of thymidine while the corresponding antineoplastic agent, 5-iodo-2'-deoxyuridine, was circulated systemically.

Research must first demonstrate preferential metabolic pathways that can be blocked selectively to allow biochemical discrimination between normal cells and malignant tissue. Perhaps this will prove to be an empty hope in itself, but work and development in the field of regional chemotherapy appears to be most promising for delivery of effective dosages of the presently available antineoplastic drugs—with maximum protection of the patient's normal tissues from serious and even fatal toxicity.

In the Future

For the scientists working today in cancer chemotherapy, the world is, literally, "all before them, where to choose." The possibilities to be examined by random screening are infinite, and daily new insights from basic research into the structure and life of the cell open up new opportunities for a more rational approach by means of chemistry and biology. It is a difficult field, for the most exciting and important research is being carried into borderline areas between the physical and biological sciences. A combination of very special training and competence, unusual alertness, and a rare breadth of knowledge is needed by the researchers. Today, the field of cancer chemotherapy stands in a position analogous to that of the medical measures against syphilis some four hundred years ago. Long before Dr. Ehrlich's "magic bullet," our ancestors treated syphilis with quicksilver—mercury. Their insight was accurate, for sufficient amounts of mercury *would* have cured syphilis, that is, killed the spirochete responsible for the disease. The sufficient amount of the drug would also surely have killed the patient.

This problem is not unlike the dilemma of the cancer chemotherapist today. Dr. Ehrlich sought a "magic bullet"—a specific agent that would attack the organism responsible for the disease, but not affect the cells and tissues of the human host. His discovery of Salvarsan was an important milestone in a search that ultimately led to penicillin, a highly effective agent for the treatment of syphilis. No such weapon has been found thus far by cancer researchers. As the brief survey of the major drugs discussed previously will show, the compounds in the cancer-fighter's arsenal suffer in part from the same flaw as the sixteenth century apothecary's mercury. Revolutionary medical techniques and great care in their application make these compounds useful allies against cancer; but for the ideal compound—or, as most researchers today would agree, the ideal *compounds,* each one tailored to a specific variety of cancer—we look to the future.

Ideal chemotherapeutic agents could eventually come from a better grasp of how the genetic information in DNA is translated (see chapter on "Control of the Cell's Architects . . ."). Since cancer is believed to be the introduction of faulty information into the DNA code, the spurious portions are read by the cell as uncontrolled growth. Better selectivity could be achieved if preferential pathways were found. In this way the neoplastic cells could be nourished on fatal drug-poisons, while normal cells will continue to function normally. Or perhaps qualitative differences between normal and cancerous cells will be determined.

In the field of medical research, it may be a pleasant task to undertake the study of diseases that are relatively minor threats to life or for which some reasonably effective therapy already exists. Research in the field of cancer is, on the other hand, one of the assiduous tasks that one could undertake. This is particularly true in the clinical area. Future programs in this field will depend not only on the extensive development of our basic understanding of the chemistry and biology of cancer, but also on the recruitment of talented young investigators who will extend these findings to the difficult but immediate problems in the care of patients with cancer.

SUPPLEMENTAL READING

Ambrose, E. & J., and Roe, F. J. C., D. Van Nostrand Co., Ltd., London, 1966.

Chapter 18

Control of the Cells Architects:

The time has come, it may be said,
To dream of many things;
Of genes—and life—and human cells—
Of medicines—and kings . . .

E. L. Tatum
*Reflections on Research and
the Future of Medicine.*

In 1942 and 1943, U.S. military officials became increasingly concerned as "casualties" from malaria mounted among soldiers in the South Pacific. In fact the toll from malaria far exceeded the number of casualties from bullets, high explosives, and bayonets. Quinine and synthetic substitutes developed by German chemists proved to be too limited for suppressive therapy. Besides, these drugs required daily dosage—obviously unrealistic under wartime conditions. Scientists on the Board for the Co-ordination of Malaria Studies began a series of tests involving 14,000 chemical compounds and countless monkeys, chickens, ducks, canaries, and turkeys. The 7,618th drug tested, chloroquine, was found to be an effective cure and, just as important, a preventative in the case of jungle fever, the second most common form of malaria and the most lethal. This drug, known as SN7618, remains the drug of choice in treating malaria.

DNA

By the end of the war, problems created by malaria throughout the world were still great enough to merit the investment of further research, time and money. A drug for the other three forms of malaria was still needed. SN7618 had only suppressive effects against the parasites in the blood, driving them out of the bloodstream and back into the body tissues, but failing to eliminate them completely. Anti-mosquito campaigns, relatively effective in the civilized portions of the world, were futile in the jungles and in underdeveloped countries.

One approach, pioneered by Dr. George H. Hitchings of Burroughs Wellcome Laboratories, centered on the nucleic acid, DNA (deoxyribonucleic acid). Its chemical nature was then becoming more and more clear. Hitchings reasoned that if DNA is responsi-

291

ble and necessary for cell multiplication, an attack on the hardy and elusive members of the genus *Plasmodium*, the malarial parasites, might well be undertaken via the nucleic acid route.

DNA carries the genetic code, and is basically responsible for what all of us are as we exist today; RNA (ribonucleic acid) acts as the transmitting agent, DNA determines who has blue eyes or brown, whose hair is curly and whose is straight, and to some extent who is tall and thin or short and fat. Yet it has been calculated* that the amount of DNA immediately responsible for the immense diversity of the human race as it exists today—every individual now alive—all the genetic information behind this vast, varied, polymorphous and teeming world of men and women, could be contained, not in the Lincoln Center, nor beneath the dome of St. Peter's nor in a boxcar or a bank vault—but in one aspirin tablet.

Moreover, there are only four "code words," as the chemists call them, contained in the nucleic acid. They are the four chemical groups denoted by the letters A, B, C, and D, and it is only the arrangement of these four groups that determines the nature of the information transmitted by the genes. All four code groups are strung together on a sugar called ribose, which is the same in all individuals and carries no information. The phosphate molecule that travels down the string and in effect "reads" off the information is relatively uninteresting in itself. It is the groups that rest atop the sugar platform and provide chemical interchanges within the cell that provide the opportunity for molecular modification.

Hitchings went to work on that point. He sought a chemical group which would look enough like a natural compound to fool the cell's metabolism and chemistry, yet would be sufficiently different to interfere with the parasite's machinery of cell nourishment and DNA synthesis. He decided to substitute an iodine atom for a methyl group in a key molecule. The alteration was accomplished in 1945 and studied in various bacterial systems as well as in other

* By taking the amounts of DNA found in each egg cell and sperm cell that unite to make up a new individual, adding the two figures, and multiplying times the present population of the earth. For fun, carry this calculation further and multiply the sum of egg and sperm DNA times the estimated number of people who have lived and bred on the earth since man's emergence as a species. (For further discussion, see the chapter on "Heredity and Drugs.")

organisms. Interesting properties came to light, but the compound did not really go very far as it then stood.

It was quite some time before anything useful against malaria came out of Hitchings' research, but eventually the important anti-malarial drug Daraprim resulted. In any case, it was immediately apparent that if nucleic acids were important for the multiplication of the protozoan parasite and if the acids provided a convenient avenue of attack on this very difficult microscopic foe, then similar drugs designed to interfere with DNA synthesis and function might be effective against the replication of cancer cells. Subsequent carefully directed testing, using drugs as inhibitors of the growth of experimental tumors, proved the validity of the idea. The research has produced one of the most important compounds in use today against forms of childhood and adult leukemia, 6-mercaptopurine or Purinethol. Much work has since been done to modify this drug, and many derivatives now exist, but the original compound is still the most potent against selected forms of cancer.

Fooling DNA: Useful "Fallout"

The compound prepared by Dr. Hitchings that appeared to have very little future was called iodouracil. It showed no significant activity when used against any experimental animal tumors. Study of its career in the human body showed that this analog could not be converted into the potentially useful inhibitory compound. Yet it could be incorporated into bacterial cells, because these lower forms of life had special mechanisms for such a conversion. These mechanisms, however, were lacking in the mammalian cells treated for malignancy. So the idea of using iodouracil in cancer chemotherapy lay fallow for some fifteen years until 1960 when Dr. William H. Prusoff and Dr. Arnold D. Welch of Yale applied to Hitchings' compound a new method of synthesis which had been discussed in chemical literature. Dr. Prusoff produced a new compound called 5-iododeoxyuridine, or IUDR for short. Far from being inert when given to laboratory animals, IUDR proved to be extremely toxic. It also showed some distinct activity against experimental tumors. The researchers were back on the right track.

IUDR was incorporated into the DNA of a cell in the place

of one of the groups mentioned earlier as an interesting site for specific chemical substitution. This substitution gives "fraudulent" information, when incorporated into the cell's DNA code, causing cells that have incorporated much of the chemical either to die or become so debilitated that they cannot reproduce normally. Against most forms of cancer, however, it was useless because of its high toxicity. Because damage to normal tissues equaled damage to neoplastic tissues, the drug could not be administered systemically to human beings. Consequently, most scientists lost interest in it.

If IUDR were given directly into the arterial circulation supplying a tumor, scientists reasoned, the infusion of the chemical would affect the tumor much more than it would poison normal body tissues, because the highest concentration of the drug would be at the target site. Some work was done on this admittedly crude quantitative approach to selective chemotherapy with IUDR, but even here success was limited. However, Dr. Prusoff's work had made it possible to identify the specific site at which IUDR was effective. Knowing the specific target of the antimetabolite marked a notable advance in our knowledge of the mechanics of the cell's DNA synthesis, and provided a new lever for further research.

Seizing this lever, other scientists in the Midwest considered that a chemical taken into and inhibiting DNA should do the same thing to DNA viruses. Testing showed that this indeed was the case, but, to permit clinical use, the drug was still too toxic for the normal cell. One more interesting observation had been made, but it apparently led up one more blind alley. IUDR lay dormant for several more years.

Then Dr. Herbert E. Kaufman, a resident physician in opthalmology in Boston, came across the data showing the results of tests of IUDR against DNA viruses, and was struck by a possible application in his own field, the treatment of eye infections. The drug was, to be sure, far too toxic and nonselective for systemic use. It happens, however, that there is an infection of the outside of the cornea caused by a herpes virus (the virus of the common cold sore), which is often resistant to topical medicines (that is, medicines applied to a particular surface of the body). Herpes keratitis, the resulting disease of the eye, is one of the major causes of blindness in America. Since the eye is like a microcosm, all to itself in the body and relatively isolated as a whole, it offers in the cornea an enclave not reached by normal channels of the circulatory system.

Dr. Kaufman decided to try eye-drops of IUDR to treat the condition. It was known that the herpes virus was a DNA virus, and it seemed reasonable to hope that the virus, bathed in a solution of the drug, would incorporate enough of it into its own DNA to be killed. He induced the typical ulcerating condition of the cornea in the eyes of rabbits. The resulting lesions caused blindness in an untreated eye. Yet if the other infected eye in the same rabbit were treated with IUDR, the disease was cured. Experimental treatment of herpes keratitis in humans was equally successful, and today, IUDR is the standard form of therapy for this disease. Because of the cornea's practical isolation, and the small doses needed, little of the drug enters the body and the toxic effects—loss of hair, damage to bone marrow, intestinal ulcers—do not occur.

For researchers, Dr. Kaufman's work has been highly exciting, giving meaning to a long and at times discouraging program of testing and development of what appeared to be an ineffective drug. This is "fallout" from research directed originally at cancer therapy. Similar forms of treatment are now suggested for other topical viral diseases. This form of therapy has entered upon areas never before approached.

In another program, still in the pioneering stages, scientists In India contemplate treatment of smallpox with IUDR. Vaccination, as a preventive measure, is always preferable. Vaccination, however, cannot keep pace with the growth of the world's population, particularly in underdeveloped countries, and some form of treatment for the disease itself is needed. IUDR appears to have some possibilities of use as such a countermeasure, although its high toxicity remains a problem. Another drug which has recently received considerable newspaper publicity, isatin-thiosemicarbazide, is good for preventing development of smallpox in persons known to have been exposed to the disease, but in whom the symptoms have not yet been manifested. Once the disease begins to develop in the body, no drug is now effective. Further study of drugs with a target similar to that of IUDR, the DNA inhibitor, may uncover new approaches to the problem.

Purine Analogues for Gout

Recent research and experimentation have produced a whole series of purine analogues. Purine, a white crystalline compound, is regarded as the parent substance for a number of compounds including uric acid and xanthine. One of these purine analogues in which two atoms have been switched around is called allopurinol—technically hydroxypyrazalopyrimidine (HPP). When this compound was tried against a wide variety of experimental tumors, it was found to be absolutely inactive. Since HPP represented a logical derivation of basic structures and required a clever bit of chemical synthesis, the original developer of the drug, as well as other interested scientists, were reluctant to let it be written off as useless. Even though it could not inhibit tumor growth, there was indication that further study of the behavior of HPP would be worthwhile. The drug inhibited an enzyme called xanthine oxidase, the enzyme that converts the purines in the body into the urinary product of purines, uric acid.

Uric acid is one of the waste products when cells die a normal death, or are killed by chemicals or infection. Since everyone has a vast number of cells dying and being replaced each day, uric acid is continually excreted. But when people with cancer are treated with a chemical that dissolves a tumor, or when they are subjected to extensive radiation, a large mass of tissue is killed in a very short time. The same situation occurs with victims of extensive burns. Massive cell death puts an enormous strain on the kidneys, for they must remove uric acid from the blood and excrete it in the urine. Unfortunately, uric acid is highly insoluble and consequently, when too much uric acid is to be excreted at one time, crystallization in the kidney itself or in the ureters may occur—with the formation of a painful kidney stone. After radiation or certain types of chemical treatment, an actual shutdown of the overworked kidneys may take place. Because functioning kidneys are necessary to life, work stoppage here has been a serious problem accompanying certain forms of cancer therapy. Once it was determined that HPP inhibited the enzyme that converts purines in the body into uric acid, researchers decided to try the drug to see if it could cut down on the rapid formation of uric acid after massive burns, radiation, or drug therapy.

Indeed, HPP was found to work well in this role. Moreover, in an area completely unrelated to cancer research, HPP has proved useful in relieving the discomfort of gout. In this chronic disease state, characterized by high levels of uric acid in the blood, crystals of this acid are deposited in the joints where they form painful inflammations. By preventing the formation of uric acid, HPP has proved useful in treating people who tend to overproduce uric acid and are unable to eliminate sufficient quantities of the substance rapidly enough.

The story of HPP points to the necessity of alertness and imagination in research. Narrowly-confined goals in experimentation are likely to produce a greater number of washouts and "useless" substances. Unexpected possibilities for applications beyond the original design of the testing program are missed. Although the massive expenditures of effort and time put into the cancer research program have produced only a few agents effective in the control of cancer, the "fallout" from that program has been invaluable, and in addition, our basic understanding of biology and biochemistry has been vastly increased.

Pursuing research along the same lines followed in the development of 5-fluorouracil, a group of scientists at Yale under Drs. Robert E. Handschumacher and Arnold D. Welch further modified the chemical structures of uracil.* Instead of adding to the molecule, a procedure that produced 5-fluorouracil and FUDR, these researchers chose to remove a carbon atom from the basic uracil molecule and to replace it with a nitrogen atom, giving a structure known as 6-azauracil. This new compound was somewhat active as an antineoplastic substance, but not effective enough to be really exciting to the scientists. Very large doses could be given without curing an experimental tumor. Nonetheless, it was of unusual interest that very large doses *could* be given without resulting in the toxicity characteristic of all other anti-cancer drugs. Further intensive study of the biochemistry of the drug showed that it had to be converted to a ribose derivative known as 6-azauridine before it exerted its antitumor activities. Moreover, this derivative was some twenty times as potent as the original compound and had even less toxicity for normal tissues.

* *See* the two chapters on cancer, 16 & 17.

Laboratory tests of 6-azauridine looked promising enough to encourage tests in humans, and in preliminary trials on a limited number of cases of human leukemia, the drug was found to affect several forms of acute leukemia in adults. The initial enthusiasm began to fade, however, with the realization that the drug's beneficial effects lasted only for a few weeks or months. Although it is possible to define with some certainty the reasons that the compound ceases to be effective, so far no means of overcoming the problem have been devised.

A breakthrough will be necessary to translate an understanding of the biochemical reason for resistance into a mechanism for effective implementation of 6-azauridine. Until—or unless—some new information is obtained, the drug will remain practically useless in the therapy of human leukemia. Nevertheless, the drug is important; when given to humans, it shows some activity, however transitory, against cancer and yet it is not severely toxic to normal tissues. Knowing the biochemical locus of the inhibition of cellular metabolism by 6-azauridine may provide a significant lead for future development of a chemotherapeutic agent that would be nontoxic to the host but lethal to cancer cells.

During the experiments in the treatment of leukemia with 6-azauridine, it became apparent that the compound was particularly effective in treating leukemic lesions in the skin. This observation led scientists to wonder if other types of hypertrophy of the skin could be controlled by a similar kind of chemical, possessed of minimal toxicity. Researchers in Czechoslovakia who had participated in the development of 6-azauridine were the first to try the drug in another neoplastic disease, mycosis fungoides. Although this drug does not cure the disease, it does provide an effective form of management and control.

A logical extension of this work was the treatment of the nonmalignant skin disease, psoriasis, which is characterized by scaly red patches on the skin. In severe cases of this disease, use of the drug at nontoxic dose levels has effected a complete remission in a short time. Previously psoriasis had responded to treatment with other anticancer compounds, since psoriasis lesions, like neoplasms, represent a form of relatively uncontrolled cell growth. With other anticancer drugs, however, the attendant risk of toxicity makes such a course of treatment hazardous at times. It is too early in the testing program to say definitely whether 6-azauridine will be a widely-applied, effective therapy for psoriasis, but initial results are promising.

"Fallout" from basic work on 6-azauridine led toward a possible treatment of the parasitic disease typanosomiasis, characterized by fever and anemia. An accidental observation made in a medical school teaching laboratory began this line of inquiry. At one time it was decided to test all the compounds being used in cancer studies against a trypanosome infection in mice which was used as a model for the chemotherapy of parasitic disease in the medical student laboratory. To the surprise of the tester, the original compound, 6-azauracil, was found to prolong the life of the test animals.

From this observation and extensive biochemical studies, the reason for the sensitivity of the parasite to 6-azauracil and *not* to the derivative compound 6-azauridine was established to be a qualitative difference between the biochemistry of trypanosome and mammalian cells. Discovery of such a qualitative difference between a parasitic organism and its host is a long step toward the development of some effective means of chemotherapy. Although 6-azauracil itself is not the answer, some other derivative that mimics the uracil molecule could prove to be an effective means of therapy for trypanosomiasis, a major cause of economic hardship and death throughout the world.

The story of 6-azauracil and its derivatives is an interesting example of international cooperation in drug research, testing, and production. The American group discovered 6-azauridine but then synthesis involved a process which was too expensive for mass production and mass marketing. The Czech researchers who had done complementary work on the same compound, devised a fermentation method for the large scale preparation of the compound. The East European scientists also contributed in a significant way to an understanding of the mechanism of action of the drug. The American scientists found the Czech method of preparing the compound much cheaper than any means they had. In an international exchange of scientists and information the two groups of researchers found mutual benefit. Exchanges of information across national lines by members of the scientific community are only a logical extension of the cooperation and mutual assistance that have long been the rule among researchers in all countries despite sometimes sharp ideological differences in their governments.

Organ Transplants and Auto-Immune Diseases

Everyone knows that organ transplantation and replacement is made almost impossible by the body's immune reactions. The reactions cause the rejection of foreign bodies, including tissues not originally from the intended host. Much publicity has been given lately to kidney transplants, including one of a chimpanzee kidney to a human. So far, success in organ transplant attempts has been attained only when a very close genetic relationship exists between the donor and the recipient, as in the case of members of the same family, preferably identical twins. If these immune reactions could be overcome, the wornout, diseased, or damaged human organs might one day be replaced from organ banks as easily as blood transfusions are made today. The surgeons are ready to transplant; the techniques have been mastered and the instruments have been designed; but the organ will nonetheless be rejected unless the production or attack of antibodies against the foreign tissue is withstood.

The source of the antibodies is well known. The hypersensitivity of the tissue is a host idiosyncrasy; and it is difficult to estimate. For chemotherapy the obvious objective would be the suppression of the cells responsible for antibody formation and rejection or chemical interference. To date, the most effective means of inhibiting antibody synthesis and tissue rejection in human beings is the use of chemical agents developed for use in cancer chemotherapy—the nitrogen mustards and the derivative of 6-mercaptopurine, Immuran. The high toxicity of these agents is always a problem and it appears certain that the ultimate development of organ and tissue transplantation requires more effective suppressors of antibody synthesis than are now available. The door has at least been opened and the test systems have been developed for an effective selection of such compounds. Until they are found, substances like 6-mercaptopurine will be the mainstay of therapy designed to suppress the immune reaction. Even in the present primitive state of this branch of medicine, it is possible to maintain transplanted kidneys in some patients for many years. It is hoped that if such a graft or transplant can be maintained long enough, the body will become adjusted to the presence of the foreign tissue and refuse to reject it even though the anti-immune therapy is stopped.

The obvious extension of research on the immune response in organ transplantation is the study of a group of diseases in man known as auto-immune diseases. In this somewhat ill-defined and little understood category are such diseases as auto-immune thyroiditis, certain forms of encephalitis, lupus erythematosus, and possibly rheumatoid arthritis. In these states, for some reason yet unknown, the patient becomes allergic to some of his own tissue and responds by a vigorous inflammatory reaction. It can range in intensity from states of minor disability to a cause of death. Research is being done examining the possibilities of chemotherapy in these diseases. The concept is quite new, however, and the conditions themselves are little understood. In most cases real progress in the field lies in the distant future.

As for other areas to which chemotherapy may extend in the next few years, Drs. Henry G. Mautner and Robert E. Handschumacher conclude:

> The application of chemotherapy to management of hereditary defects, such as diabetes and muscular dystrophy, requires as precise as possible a characterization of the aberrant area of metabolism and the design of agents that through metabolic control can restore these (sufferers) to a more normal state. Similarly, impaired function of certain organ systems in degenerative disease, typified by arteriosclerosis, rheumatism, and multiple sclerosis, present major challenges for elucidation of their etiology (causes) and the development of suitable therapy. Such approaches must also extend to those forms of mental illness that are organic in origin. Population control is another field where chemotherapy may be expected to play an important role.*

* In "Some Current Approaches to Chemotherapy," *Yale Scientific,* February, 1966.

DNA, RNA, and Memory

Among older people, events long past may be remembered in precise detail though what happened yesterday might not be re-callable at all. Memory is highly developed in humans and our civilizations depend upon it. But strange as it seems, memory is possessed to some degree by everything that lives. Scientists are just getting around to understanding why.

Some of the implications of the growing knowledge of the nucleic acids, common to all life, are now beginning to bear fruit. The nucleic acids may be the key to memory and, with the complex feedback mechanisms of brain nerve cells, to the process of recall as well. Molecules of DNA may act like "tapes" of the sensory recordings which constitute memory; molecules of RNA, the trans-mitting agent of DNA, may furnish the playback systems of recall, triggered by the sensory input of the moment with all its associational potential. Since DNA and RNA are the essential factors in genetic phenomena, heredity and growth, it would be expected that all living things would possess these functional potentials, even including what we call memory. There actually is a considerable chain of verifiable evidence connecting RNA with memory.

In the 23 November 1962 issue of *Science,* Dr. C. E. Smith of San José State College reviewed experimental studies suggesting that the basis of a form of biological memory lies in an increase of enzyme concentrations associated with transmitter substances as "long-lasting effects of stimulation." Concerning the enzymes, Drs. E. L. Kropa and Chauncey D. Leake considered that while one part of an enzyme might be protein, another part might be a porphy-rin. As shown by Dr. H. Klüver of Chicago, there are increasing amounts of porphyrins in the central nervous system with increasing evolutionary development. Porphyrins may combine with metals and become semiconductors. On the basis of provocative analogies be-tween computers and brains, any factor involving semiconduction might be an important aspect of the phenomena of "memory." In fact, memory may reside in the arrangement, stacking, and interplay of enzymes in the brain associated with nerve cells.

Meanwhile, in 1960 and 1962, respectively, Drs. H. Hyden and Francis Schmitt indicated that learning and memory are related to the DNA and RNA content of brains. Dr. Leonard Cook and his colleagues reported in 1963 that daily injections of RNA into experimental animals would increase learning and memory. Other scientists (T. I. Chamberlin and associates) found that administration of tricyano-aminopropane increases nucleic acids in the brains of experimental animals and, at the same time, increases rates of learning. Indeed, Dr. D. E. Cameron and his associates showed in 1964 that daily RNA injections into presenile patients would enhance learning and memory. Are the statistics sound? Memory-testing does involve *subjective* phenomena. Perhaps the elderly patients remembered because someone cared about their memory for a change. Later, reports issued from Abbott Laboratories and the Illinois State Pediatric Institute at a Berkeley symposium on "Behavior, Brains, and Biochemistry" during the annual meeting of the American Association for the Advancement of Science. Two biochemists, Drs. A. J. Glasky and L. N. Simon, presented evidence that the rate of enzymatic synthesis of RNA was increased threefold by administration of the chemical compound magnesium pemoline to animals. This compound is a mild central nervous system stimulant.

Dr. Nicolaus Plotnikoff, studying conditioned avoidance responses in rats, found that giving magnesium pemoline enhances the acquisition and retention of such responses. Both groups of scientists are properly cautious in noting that their results do not establish a causal relation either between learning and RNA synthesis, or between "magnesium pemoline" enhancement of learning and memory and its biochemical effects. Yet at face value the data suggest that magnesium pemoline may have clinical usefulness in the improvement of learning and memory.

Actually, Dr. D. Ewen Cameron, of the Veterans Administration Hospital in Albany, New York, has found on double-blind clinical trials in old patients that magnesium pemoline measurably improves memory, as tested by the standard Wechsler memory scale. Those patients whose age was around 60 showed better gain than those over 75. Dr. Cameron, who followed the RNA work of Dr. Paul Weiss, has found memory improvement after RNA injection. Whether or not magnesium pemoline may be helpful in treating older people in order to prevent loss of memory or ability to learn remains a long-term clinical problem. Since magnesium pemoline is relatively non-toxic, cautious clinical trials are in progress. Improvement in memory would certainly seem to be a blessing to many older persons frustrated by a failure to recall recent happenings.

Drug Combinations

One area of research today does not try to develop new drugs, but investigates a more intelligent use of existing drugs. Work in cell kinetics is an example. Scientists in this field examine the rate at which cells reproduce and study the development of resistant populations. Many investigators feel that a lack of understanding of cellular reproduction rates is the major obstacle to the development of effective cancer chemotherapeutic agents. The parallel problem—the appearance of strains of bacteria resistant to all commonly used antibiotics—has been noted by some scientists as a development that could push medicine back a hundred years.

Cell kinetics can be illustrated by the work done on leukemia therapy. When treatment of a person with leukemia is begun with a drug like methotrexate or 6-mercaptopurine, a seemingly thorough destruction of cancer cells appears to result. The remission may last for considerable periods of time—many months and even, in some cases, years. Eventually the disease rallies, however, and in turn the same drug in the same dosage becomes ineffective. This may be due to two different things. First, the cells which compose the resistant leukemic population may be circumventing the inhibition of the particular metabolic pathway blocked by the antimetabolite or drug, destroying the drug by reacting with it chemically, or converting the drug into inert derivatives. Alternatively, the drug may have selected a population of cells which are growing at the same rate and in the same generation as certain crucial normal cells in the body—cells such as the bone marrow, or the intestinal mucosa. Consequently, the chemotherapist cannot move in with his drugs to hit the malignant cells without doing lethal damage to normal cells essential for the maintenance of life.

Some researchers today are studying the rate of replication of cancer cells. The aim is to devise a dosage schedule that would more effectively encompass the whole or the greater part of the replication cycle of the malignant cells without increased damage to normal cells with similar time-growth cycles. A compound that affects DNA synthesis will not do anything to a cell not synthesizing DNA at the time of administration; furthermore, synthesis of DNA occurs only during a comparatively short time span in the life of a cell. The researchers want to devise some way of getting all the cancer cells into the stage of making nucleic acid at once, and then administer the proper inhibitory drug.

Another possibility in cancer therapy is the "drug cocktail," a combination of chemotherapeutic drugs. Each drug attacks the same cancer cells, though, perhaps, in slightly different ways. But each drug in the cocktail also differs from the others in its effect on normal tissues. Thus three or four shots at the same cancer are afforded by a relatively small dosage of each drug, with toxic effects to normal cells distributed widely enough to make them negligible. Programs working on this approach are being pressed by the National Cancer Institute. Names of the programs are based on the initials of the chemicals used in the cocktail. For instance, the VAMP program uses vinblastin, which exerts undesirable side effects on the brain and nervous tissue; amethopertin (methotrexate), which affects the lining of the intestine and the bone marrow; mercaptopurine, which is toxic to the bone marrow as well; and prednisone, which interferes with adrenal function. Thus the toxic side effects of the drug are scattered, while a concentration of the effects of the four drugs on one cancer can be attained by proper administration of the cocktail.

Whereas remissions in acute leukemia in children used to be achieved in only 30 to 50 percent of cases treated, use of VAMP or other combinations, either in a one-course heavy dosage or in quick successive doses, has raised the complete remission figure in children to some 80 to 90 percent, and longer remissions are achieved. Although it is too early to tell whether these children are actually cured (and it is very likely that they are not), a jump in the remission rate is still a significant step in control of the disease. The more we know how the human body works, and the more we know how a specific drug works, the greater the possibility of using known remedies to best advantage and finding new and better ones.

Most of the projects and experiments just discussed are based upon finding a chemical that attacks a biochemical process or pathway peculiar to cancer cells without damaging normal cells at the same time. Another area of attack, distinct from the biochemical approach, is the study of physiological differences that may exist between certain types of cancer cells and normal cells. It is known that a number of tissues in the body have transport systems that concentrate certain chemicals within those tissues. Knowing this, researchers try to design a compound based on, or attached to, those readily transported and concentrated chemicals. Thus, an extra dose of an antineoplastic agent can be tracked directly to the target organ with its cancer cells—just as switches in a railroad yard arrange the distribution of freight to the proper sites. Although effective therapy has not resulted from this approach as yet, the concept may prove much more important in the future.

SUPPLEMENTAL READING

Carlton, Peter L., ed., Memory Transfer and RNA, summation of experiments quoted in general summation, Science, *153*, No. 3736.

Gaito, John, ed., Macromolecules and Behavior, Appleton-Century-Crofts, Div. Meredith Publishing Co., New York, 1966.

Chapter 19

Hormones as Drugs

For when the Prince hath now his mandate sent,
The nimble posts quick down the river run,
And end their journey, though but now begun;
But now the mandate came, and now the
mandate's done.

Phineas Fletcher *The Purple Island* II

T he endocrine system consists of glands that spill their products, the hormones, directly into the bloodstream. These glands have no channels, entrances or exits except those provided by their blood supply. For this reason they are called the "ductless glands"; they are to be distinguished from such glands as the salivary and the tear glands, which do possess "ducts."

In the past two or three decades the field of endocrinology has been raked again and again. Endocrinology, as it stands today, bears little resemblance to the same field forty years ago. Actual knowledge about sexual processes and pregnancy, of course, dates from the earliest civilizations. Only since the late nineteenth century, however, has much solid scientific work been done with the endocrine glands. The advances in biochemistry are largely responsible for this progress. We have come a long way from Théophile Bordeu who in 1775 suggested that these glands produced a secretion, and from Arnold-Adolph Berthold who in 1849, by implanting testicular tissue in fowl, reversed the effects of castration. Even further behind us is the man who has been called the first endocrinologist, Ruggero di Salerno; in the 12th century he burned seaweed and used the ashes (high in iodine) to treat goiter.

As many as eleven glands have been proposed for the endocrine system. But the usually accepted number is eight: the pituitary or hypophysis, often called "the master gland," the hypothalamus, a recent addition to the roll, the thyroid, the parathyroids, the adrenals, the islets of Langerhans in the pancreas, and the gonads—testes in the male, ovaries in the female. (The location and a brief indication of the hormonal production of each is given in Figure 1.) Differences in function and effective activity suggest the division of the pituitary into three areas: the anterior pituitary, the posterior pituitary, and the intermediate lobe. Likewise, the adrenals have two parts, which are apparently unrelated and function separately. These

309

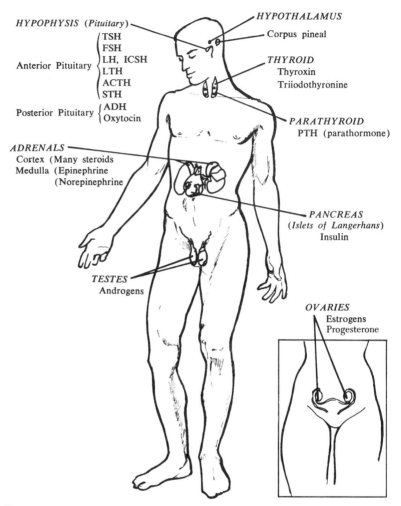

FIGURE 1. *Location of major endocrine organs in the human male and female, together with the chief hormones produced by each. The pineal body has been suspected of endocrine function relating to light-controlled reactions, pigmentation, and aldosterone secretion, but complete evidence is lacking*

are the adrenal medulla and the adrenal cortex. The placenta, a vascular organ within the uterus, is ordinarily considered an intermediary between the fetus and the mother; it is, so to speak, an environment for the fetus. But the placenta also possesses many endocrine functions that sustain pregnancy.

Definitions make any discussion of the endocrine system difficult at the outset. Perhaps even the word "system" seems odd. The endocrine glands interrelate in various ways, but they are not clearly linked and bound together like the nervous system, the circulatory system, or even the lymphatic system. The endocrines are an aggregation of diverse tissues, scattered throughout the body, secreting various substances that serve diverse purposes in the organism as a whole. As their name indicates, the endocrine glands are all similar in that their hormonal secretions are internal and yet disassociated: endocrine is derived from the Greek *endon,* within, and *krinein,* to separate. Their secretions, called hormones (from the Greek *hormạo,* "to excite"), are released directly into the bloodstream. In Bayliss's classic definition a hormone is simply a "substance normally produced by specialized cells in some part of the body and carried to other parts by the bloodstream where it affects the body as a whole."

In certain cases hormones are initiators; in others, regulators. Some of the processes they control would go on without them, but at a level of efficiency too low for the normal life of the organism. The hormones are, in essence, modifiers: they contribute nothing to a process but a control, speeding up, slowing down, sometimes raising, sometimes suppressing each other's production. The two major types of hormones are classified by their activity. *Trophic* (sometimes called *tropic*) hormones are chiefly secreted by the pituitary. These hormones regulate certain other endocrine glands. The second group is composed of hormones produced by other glands to control body development, mineral balances, metabolic rate, and other such organic processes directly. In addition to regulating the body's internal environment (e.g. metabolism, salt and water balance, etc.), hormones function in two other ways in the body. First, they control the individual's rate and type of growth, contributing notably to the development of secondary sex characteristics at puberty. Secondly, they integrate the body's functions and responses, reaching every cell in the body affected by the bloodstream. Insulin and many slower-working steroid hormones also appear to reach all or most cells and affect them.

The quantity of activity generated by a hormone stimulus depends on the amount of hormone present (and utilized) at the site. This is called a dose-response relationship. The concentrations of a given hormone may also affect the relations between endocrine organs, particularly between the pituitary and other endocrines. The amount of one hormone in the bloodstream influences the activity of one or more endocrine glands, and so on. The pituitary, for instance, normally secretes a small amount of a given hormone, say ACTH (adrenocorticotrophic hormone), which stimulates secretion of a small amount of a hormone from the target organ—in this case hydrocortisone, among others, from the adrenal cortex. Circulating in the blood, the hydrocortisone in turn "holds down" the activity of the pituitary. This is a feedback or servomechanism. Disruption of normal function or introduction of outside interference upsets the delicate balance. A pituitary tumor, for example, may produce ACTH in excessive amounts, undeterred by the hydrocortisone "brake"; this will result in an increase both in the size of the adrenal cortex and of its hormone production, including production of hydrocortisone. The latter hormone, however, cannot suppress the unnatural activity of the tumor in the pituitary. If the pituitary atrophies or is removed (hypophysectomy), the adrenal cortex will in turn atrophy in the absence of its stimulant, ACTH, and the steroid hormone production of the cortex will cease.

Administration of ACTH (exogenous ACTH) to an animal or human will stimulate the cortex and its steroid production. But the excess of hydrocortisone will suppress the pituitary so that sufficient dosage with exogenous ACTH over a period of time could make the organism dependent upon the external administration of the hormone for normal activity. The body's pituitary ceases to be active under the pressure of the massive secretions of hydrocortisone. Administration of the steroid drug hydrocortisone suppresses the pituitary directly; now deprived of its triggering mechanism, ACTH, the adrenal cortex begins to function improperly and eventually atrophies.

Finding and Evaluating Hormones

Like the shape-shifter of medieval folklore, the hormones are masters of mutability. A hormone may be manufactured by the producing gland in one form, stored or released into the bloodstream in another form, and finally altered in use and excreted in yet another form. Thyroid hormone, for example, forms in the thyroid follicles where it is part of a complex storage protein, the thyroglobulin complex. But it must be split off to be transported into the bloodstream across the thyroid walls and is then loosely bound with another protein for transport in the blood. Consequently, a researcher cannot assume that a hormone as he finds it excreted in the urine or bile is still in its original or its active form. More likely it is not; it has undergone combination with other substances, chemical breakdown, or other alteration since it began its journey. Most hormones, furthermore, have a very short life measured in minutes to hours. There are enzymes in the body that attack and completely destroy proteins in short order; steroids combine readily with other substances for greater ease of excretion.

In the case of the more complex proteins, understanding of structures is immensely difficult to achieve. The researcher must first determine the active form of the hormone, then attempt the analysis of its exceedingly complex structure, all the while working with a very "perishable" chemical subject. Active extracts of the pancreas were, for example, isolated in 1922 by Banting, Best, and Macleod, but the structure of insulin was not determined until the 1950's by Frederick Sanger of Cambridge University, who received the Nobel Prize in chemistry in 1958.

The insulin molecule, which is not the most complicated, consists of fifty-one amino acids in two chains, insulin A with twenty-one amino acids and insulin B with thirty, bound together by two disulfide bridges, with the sulfur atom links at specific places within the chains. Insulin, with unimpaired biological activity, has at last been synthesized in China, Germany and the United States—the first complex protein to be synthesized by man with success in terms of activity.

Radioisotope labeling has somewhat brightened the outlook in tracing the routes of hormones and determining their specific sites of activity. Now it has become possible to "tag" a given atom in a protein molecule with radioactive iodine and follow its progress through the chemical changes that the hormone undergoes, just as one would band one bird in a flock, or "bug" one animal in a herd with a radio transmitter. Unfortunately it is sometimes difficult to establish whether the label stays in place throughout the hormone's travels.

Establishing the existence and activity of hormones precedes the intricate matters of chemical description and analysis. In view of a hormone's elusiveness, the easiest and most common approach is a kind of functional definition: we know gland X produces a hormone that does such-and-such, because if we remove the gland, such-and-such does not occur. If in turn we supply extracts of gland X or ground portions of the gland to an animal deprived of it, such-and-such happens again, or the rate of such-and-such is stepped up. There is a classic five-step proof for the existence of any hormone:

1) The suspected secreting organ is *removed* and the effects observed.

2) The suspected organ or its supposed product is *reintroduced* (that is, the corresponding organ from another animal is transplanted, or its extract administered), and the effects noted. If researchers are on the right track, reintroduction of the organ or extract in an animal that has been deprived of the organ in question should prevent the developments observed in step 1.

3) The suspected effective extract is prepared in quantity; massive doses are used on both test groups of normal animals and animals with the suspected organs removed. The effects of this *overdosage* should be predictable from steps 1 and 2.

4) Technicians assay the extract in the laboratory to *isolate* the basic material or ingredient that has the same effect as grosser extracts or ground preparations of the whole gland. If no simple substance works, a search for more than one cause implicated in a single process is the logical step.

5) Clinical cases meanwhile are canvassed to try to locate naturally occurring, *spontaneous deficiencies* resulting from hyperfunction (overactivity) or hypofunction (underactivity) of the suspect organ in cases where some disease or trauma of the suspect organ is already known to exist.

With most drugs and chemical substances the activity in lower animals, even through the primates, cannot be assumed as proof of similar activity in man. Detection and study of spontaneous deficiencies in a given species provides the only final proof of the existence and activity of any particular hormone in that species.

The "How" of Hormones

One aspect of hormonal action that has been fairly well documented is modification of cell membranes. Certain hormones act as doormen and determine what gets inside a cell. For example, one would think that glucose or blood sugar, a major metabolic fuel, could readily enter any cell. It should certainly be welcome anywhere, but it does not find entry at all easy. Muscle and fat cells actively exclude sugar, and the hormone insulin, produced by the islets of Langerhans in the pancreas, must be present to get the sugar into the cells where it can be utilized. A transport mechanism of some sort is involved, but insulin is not the actual carrier; it merely activates the transport system. If the cell is a furnace, and the glucose is coal, insulin is not the shovel that pitches the coal into the furnace, but the fireman who "activates" the shovel. We cannot write equations or draw diagrams showing exactly how this happens; we can only describe the rate at which the hormone will facilitate the entry of the blood sugar into the cells. But Dr. Randall, chairman of the department of biochemistry at the University of Bristol, England, has proposed an attractive theory concerning this operation. Randall and his associates demonstrated a number of years ago that the cell expends energy to keep sugar out, and that if anything disrupts energy metabolism, the disruption tends to permit glucose to enter the cell. According to this theory, insulin diverts the energy output of the cell into synthetic work (e.g. building protein) so that insulin might be called an anabolic (constructive) hormone, promoting the synthesis of protein and the deposition of glycogen, the storage form of glucose.

Other hormones affect enzymatic reactions. Enzymes are proteins that act as catalysts within the cell, making possible a numberless variety of chemical reactions, so that cellular metabolism can go on at body temperature (37 to 38 degrees centigrade). The enzymes within a cell may be in either an active or an inactive form, and hormones may promote the activation of inactive enzyme forms. The hormone glucagon, a protein produced by the *alpha* cells of the pancreas, causes the breakdown of glycogen, a complex carbohydrate stored in the liver, into glucose. This breakdown, which is by hydrolysis (taking on elements of water), is easy enough to achieve, but glucagon does it in a rather indirect manner. Glucagon presumably interacts at the cell membrane with an enzyme that activates another enzyme; this enzyme in turn initiates the breakdown of glycogen, releasing glucose into the blood.

The complex mechanism suggests the analogy of a vacuum tube in a radio: a weak signal (the glucagon) is taken in by the antenna (the first enzyme). The antenna puts the electromagnetic signal on the grid of the vacuum tube (stimulation of the second enzyme by the first). Thus the weak signal can influence the rate of flow of electrons through this vacuum tube, amplifying the signal to operate the speaker (initiate the breakdown of glycogen), to produce the sounds of music or the human voice (the release of blood sugar into the circulatory system).

Another popular theory holds that hormones act directly upon the DNA or RNA in the cell, modifying the genetic information contained inside. In essence, the hormone would then control and regulate the snythesis of more enzyme by altering the reading of the cell's genetic code. The information for their production is locked in the DNA of the cell nucleus. This message, which is like a military command, is relayed by the DNA to the RNA, a kind of line officer that comes out into the cell protoplasm where the action is and synthesizes protein. There is evidence that hormones do in fact interact with this process. It has been shown that a puffing of the chromosomes occurs under certain hormonal influences. This observation suggests that the hormone is causing genetic information to express itself. One can readily demonstrate that the enzymatic activity of certain specific cells may be increased after hormonal treatment, as though the hormone had initiated the synthesis of more intracellular catalyst that would increase rates of reaction.

The third major type of hormonal function is activity as a coenzyme, a nonprotein substance that works with an enzyme. Dr. Tallalay of Johns Hopkins University has shown that estrogenic hormones may be alternately oxidized and reduced to serve as coenzymes for a transhydrogenase (enzyme) system. In this form, they act as directors of the flow of energy in the organism. Hydrogen in the body represents a source of energy no less than it does in its liquid form as rocket fuel, or employed in a thermonuclear bomb. The hormone can participate in the direction or allotment of hydrogen in the cell, either to synthetic work within the cell, or toward oxidation to produce energy.

Nerve-Hormone Relationships

Endocrine glands react to external stimuli transmitted by the nervous system, but they also appear to share certain areas of overlap in activities. The mobilization of fat from adipose tissue (stored fatty tissues in the animal body) can be influenced by both the endocrine glands and the autonomic nervous system (see Chapter 7). Nervous stimulation will cause fat mobilization, influencing fat removal and fat deposition; so will endocrine hormones such as the growth hormone, and yet no clear picture of the interrelationships between the two systems can yet be given.

Insulin release from the pancreas provides another notable example of nervous system influence on the endocrines. The autonomic nervous system will modify the release of insulin markedly. Catecholamines, e.g. Adrenalin, or increased activity of the sympathetic nervous system tends to inhibit insulin release, while acetylcholine or increased activity of the parasympathetic nervous system stimulates release of the hormone. Insulin levels may thus be influenced either by other endocrine organs or by the nervous system. Moreover, the adrenal gland is made up of two tissues of differing origin and structure, with the cortex clearly endocrine. The medulla of the adrenal gland, however, is bivalent; it has both endocrine and nervous functions. There is no more structural relationship between the two tissues than would ordinarily be expected between contiguous structures. Epinephrine is called an endocrine hormone when released by the adrenal medulla directly into the blood stream; on the other hand, nerve endings appear to emit epinephrine independently (as well as norepinephrine, the other primary adrenal medullary hormone). Here it acts directly on the cell or cells adjacent to the nerve endings, so that the "hormone" would be a mediator of the nerve impulse or "message" across a tiny junction between a nerve cell and the cell it innervates. This area of relationship is one of particularly fuzzy understanding at present.

Epinephrine (Adrenalin) is probably one of the best known hormones. When the organism is subjected to external stress—causing fright, intense anger, or injury—the adrenal medulla quickly gets the message and secretes epinephrine into the blood stream. This hormone, one may recall, immediately mobilizes the body's forces for self-defense and for survival. Some effects happen immediately: rapid heartbeat, constriction of the blood vessels of the skin and viscera, stimulation of sweat and salivary glands, rapid breathing with increased oxygen consumption, stepped-up production of lactic acid by the muscles. Many of these effects, it will be noted, are similar to or identical with effects caused by nervous stimulation. The classic reactions are reproduced: cold chill, muscular tenseness and readiness, rapid breathing, pounding heart, knot in the pit of the stomach. Stimulated by Adrenalin, men seem able to run faster, move more weight, overcome pain and injury, and conquer obstacles that normally would have seemed insurmountable. All these immediate responses are mobilized within perhaps ten seconds, enabling the animal who takes fright to flee or to stand and fight. Hence, it is called the "fight or flight" syndrome. After three or four hours, however, longer-term effects of epinephrine appear, together with the results of adrenocortical steroids released in the stress reaction but slower to act than epinephrine. These delayed effects of epinephrine are much more like normal effects.

Liver and muscle glycogen were depleted by the first action of epinephrine. The glucose formed is rapidly metabolized to lactic acid.

During the recovery phase the level of lactic acid drops and liver glycogen rises rapidly as the process of muscle glycogen→lactic acid→liver glycogen takes place, restoring the balance in the liver disturbed by the first epinephrine stress reaction. Epinephrine speeds up the rate of one step in this reaction—the conversion of glycogen to glucose-1-phosphate. Muscles treated with epinephrine show a rise in the level of hexosephosphates. One of the reasons for muscle fatigue is thought to be a decrease in the rate of conversion of glycogen to hexosephosphate, so that epinephrine, stimulating the phosphorylase enzyme that is the catalyst in this reaction, may help prevent the onset of fatigue. The longer-lasting effects of the "fight-or-flight" syndrome in terms of sustaining and supportive activity can be seen in Figure 2, a graph of relative changes in levels of important blood and muscle constituents following the injection of epinephrine (at 0):

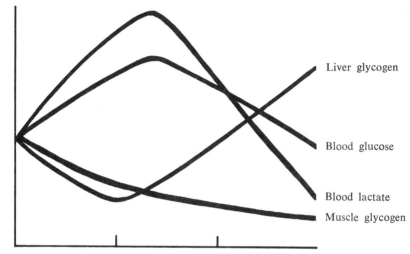

Liver glycogen

Blood glucose

Blood lactate
Muscle glycogen

FIGURE 2. *Time in hours (3-hour duration). From Brown and Barker, F. A. Davis Co., Philadelphia, 1962*

Relations between hormones can be illustrated quite neatly with epinephrine through its role in blood sugar control. Blood sugar (glucose) is decreased in the presence of insulin. Decreased blood sugar in turn causes the adrenal medulla to release epinephrine, which then effects the breakdown of glycogen, notably in the liver, into glucose, raising the level of blood sugar to normal again.

Epinephrine is an unusually rapid-acting hormone. Insulin also acts immediately upon cell membranes, allowing glucose to enter the cell. But most hormones are more like the tortoise than the hare. Effects of the gluco-corticoids (hormones from the adrenal cortex, causing an increase of glucose production) cannot be seen for about three hours after their administration. Thyroid hormone is notorious for delayed onset of action. Although the newer derivatives like triiodothyroidine act more swiftly, thyroxin in the original experiments done in the 1930's required eighteen to twenty-four hours to produce observable effects.

The Pituitary

The deeper one probes, the more complex an organ is found to be. The pituitary is a case in point. The anterior lobe, the posterior lobe, and the intermediate lobe of the pituitary may now be considered almost as *separate* glands. Each appears to have characteristic secretions that are not dependent upon either of the other lobes. The order of importance of the three lobes of this endocrine gland is as they are listed above. The anterior lobe is so important that it has been called the "master gland". This is a somewhat misleading epithet, since not all endocrine glands are responsive to the pituitary; some are affected only in the rate at which they function, and can continue to function even when the anterior pituitary has been removed. In all animals the classic results of hypophysectomy (removal of the pituitary) are:

1) Atrophy of the gonads, shrinkage of accessory sex organs and an end of their function. If the pituitary is removed after fertilization of the female animal but before parturition, lactation (milk production of the mammary glands) will not occur.

2) Shrinkage of the thyroid coupled with lowered metabolic rate.

3) Decrease in the size of the adrenal glands (only the cortex actually atrophies, however) and a resultant dramatic drop in the level of adrenal steroid production.

4) Stunted growth in immature animals, and in adults alteration of body size and hair structure.

5) Upset of protein, fat, and carbohydrate metabolism.

Surprisingly, however, hypophysectomy is not generally fatal, despite its apparent effects on so many important body functions. Balances are upset; thyroid function slowly falls, that of the adrenal cortex fades as does function of the gonads. But output of mineralocorticoids from the adrenal cortex continues. The imbalance does mean, however, that the animal may not survive stress or starvation.

All anterior pituitary hormones are related to proteins, but vary widely in actual composition. Sites of secretion for the various hormones are a matter of much dispute and intensive research today, but need not concern us here.

STH has been called the growth hormone as well as the metabolic hormone. Its main functions are to promote the elongation of the bones in the extremities. It also influences the synthesis of protein, affects carbohydrate and fat metabolism, and apparently inhibits glucose absorption by all the cells of the body. Because of this last activity, hypophysectomy has been used to ameliorate diabetes mellitus; adrenalectomy is also more or less successful in the same situation. As a growth hormone, STH is more effective in combination with other hormones, e.g. thyroxin.

Giants twice the size of normals have been produced by growth-hormone treatment of laboratory animals; yet these "monsters" retain perfect shape and physical symmetry. Hypophysectomy, on the other hand, results in dwarfism. Hyperfunction of the STH-producing cells in childhood lies behind pituitary giantism, in which the height of the individual may range from $6\frac{1}{2}$ feet to over 8 feet; accompanying disturbances of metabolism and sexual function may result, and libido (instinctual urges or desires) may be abnormally increased or prematurely lost. If the hyperfunction occurs after major bodily growth has ceased, acromegaly results. The symptoms of acromegaly are the gradual overdevelopment of terminal bones of the hands, feet, and face—the ridges and bones of the face elongate into a distorted mask—the frontal sinuses and orbital ridges are enlarged, the jaw protrudes, and the nose and lips become oversized and prominent. This is in contrast to giantism, which results in proportioned, undistorted growth. In the child or adolescent the epiphyseal junctions (cartilage bridges between bone structures that grow until finally ossified and permanently fixed to the adjoining bones at maturity) are not yet closed, and growth is merely exaggerated. But in the acromegalic, since these junctures are closed, the only available sites for growth are the terminal bones and structures. As would be expected, hypofunction (deficiency of hormone production) of STH-producing cells results in pituitary dwarfism, characterized by well-proportioned, but child-like body and normal intelligence (as opposed to cretinism due to thyroid deficiency.

The effects of TSH, thyroid-stimulating hormone, are mediated through the thyroid gland. In a normal organism, TSH regulates cellular activity and basal metabolic rate via the thyroid gland. The thyroid gland inactivates TSH after the signals have been transmitted, and consequently very little TSH is found in the blood plasma. In some species, combination with secretions of the adrenal cortex is necessary for efficient TSH action.

ACTH is by definition the pituitary hormone that stimulates the adrenal cortex. Its relationship to adrenal function and the servo-mechanism of which it is a part have been discussed previously. In addition, pituitary-adrenal relationships are portrayed schematically in Figure 3. ACTH is inactivated by many tissues besides the adrenal cortex. Recent research has also indicated that it plays a role in the rate of mobilization or release of fatty acids (fat) from adipose tissue. Pituitary basophilism, known as Cushing's syndrome, is often due to anterior pituitary hyperfunction, although the condition can result without direct implication of ACTH from such adrenal problems as adenoma (benign tumor) or carcinoma (cancer) of the adrenal gland. Pattern obesity, confined to the face and trunk, with a fat pad at the base of the neck, protruding abdomen, and skinny arms and legs, along with muscular wasting and weakness, hypertension, salt and water retention, and, frequently, diabetes mellitus which is resistant to insulin, are the common manifestations of the disease. Masculinization may occur in an affected female.

There has been some debate concerning the probability that the posterior pituitary is the actual site of synthesis of all the hormones stored there. Now evidence indicates that some hormones, including oxytocin, are the products, not of the posterior pituitary itself, but of the nerve cells of the hypothalamus, a structure located just above the pituitary in the brain, with nerve connections to the posterior lobe of the pituitary. How these hormones are released into the bloodstream is not yet fully understood. Oxytocin has as its target organ the uterus. It is apparently active both in speeding the sperm on their way within the uterus, and in expelling the fetus from the uterus. Some observers have alleged that the sex act or merely sperm in the vagina initiates a release of oxytocin in the cow, causing a uterine contraction and increased motility of the uterus.* Even more interesting in connection with the mystery sur-

* See especially the discussion of rabbit ovulation under The Hypo-thalamus below.

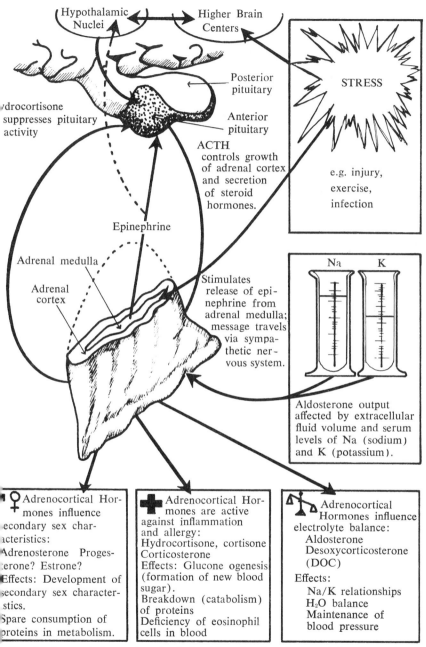

Fig. 3 Some pituitary-adrenal relationships, showing, hormonal functions of the adrenal, feedback and mutual balance systems, and effects of stress. All relationships shown are highly schematic and tentative. (The relationships shown, though not the diagram itself, owe much to *The Merck Manual*, Tenth Edition, (1961), pp. 1650–1651.)

rounding the mechanism that induces labor is the report that an enzyme in the blood of the normal female destroys oxytocin. This enzyme decreases in amount and concentration toward the end of pregnancy, perhaps even starting labor. It is known that the uterus, although ordinarily sensitive to oxytocin to an extreme degree, becomes gradually more sensitive during pregnancy, reaching the extreme of responsiveness just before delivery. The cervix (the lower portion of the uterus), on the other hand, appears to have an oxytocin sensitivity curve that inverts this, being least sensitive just before delivery.

Vasopressin, also connected with the posterior pituitary, seems to be misnamed; so far, no practical importance of the substance as an agent to increase blood pressure has been established. However, this polypeptide does play an important role in reducing urine formation. Its designation in this capacity is ADH (antidiuretic hormone). In some animals, because of a dry, hostile environment, water retention is essential to life. In the kangaroo rat, urine is highly concentrated in order to cut down on water loss through excretion; the desert rodent's urine is five times as concentrated as that excreted under normal conditions by the common dog. Likewise, the kangaroo rat's ADH excretion in the urine is measured at something over eight times that of the common dog. In comparison with the white laboratory rat, the desert rodent's posterior pituitary contains about ten times the ADH found in the former's gland. Like epinephrine and insulin, ADH is a very fast-acting hormone. The high point of the inhibition of urine flow in man may occur one-half hour after drinking a concentrated salt solution. Conversely, an infinitesimal decrease in concentration of ADH in blood plasma (ADH in solution in the liquid part of the blood) will produce diuresis through an effect on structures in the kidney that are responsible for formation of urine.

The ADH stimulator is not so easily pinned down. The primary stimulus has been shown to be the osmotic pressure of fluid within the cells of normal animals, but some researchers have also put forward a theory that volume may be the actual controlling factor. Functional failure of the posterior pituitary to produce ADH results in a condition known as diabetes insipidus, in which huge quantities of very dilute urine are excreted every day. Patients suffering from this disorder may not uncommonly excrete more than 40 liters of urine every day—a little better than 10 gallons. As long as unlimited intake of water is possible, this condition may continue indefinitely with no damage to the patient. Another hormone intimately involved in water metabolism, primarily through its control of salt balance in the body, is the adrenal cortical steroid, aldosterone. This mineralocorticoid by indirect action has the opposite effect from that of ADH: absence of aldosterone results in water retention (see below, "The Adrenals").

In some animals, the intermediate lobe of the pituitary produces a hormone that darkens the skin by dispersion of the dark-pigmented cells of the skin. The effect gives the hormone its designation, MSH (melanocyte-stimulating hormone). This role of the hormone is largely confined to lower forms of life, especially amphibians. In humans and most higher animals, the intermediate lobe is so intimately connected to the anterior lobe as to be inseparable from it, so that in these species it becomes impossible to test and define its role by standard procedures. The most accurate and dependable methods of assay available today do, however, indicate that pregnant women and victims of Addison's disease excrete about ten times the normal amount of MSH per day.

The Hypothalamus

The most recent studies in endocrinology, some of which have not yet been written into the textbooks, make it appear highly probable that the so-called master gland, the pituitary, itself is subject to a master. Various phenomena observed in the animal world suggested that a hunt for a responsible cause might produce such a master. In any case, what caused the pituitary to secrete its hormones at the proper time and in the proper levels? Since the *milieu intérieur* is by no means absolutely stable and unchanging, and since the organism is constantly exposed to stresses and changing conditions outside itself, requiring varied and efficient response, a theory of nervous control or connection seemed promising.

Two observations concerning animal behavior related to the endocrine system are revealing in this matter. In birds, the whole endocrine system has been shown to be geared to a stimulus-response relationship with the length of the day. Sexual behavior in mating season is like a built-in time clock, related to the angle of the sun and the duration of daylight. The "sundial" which reacts initially to this light stimulus must be part of the nervous system. The result, however, is stimulation of the pituitary, causing the release of the gonadotropin which makes the creatures sexually active. Thus the mating season occurs at a "right" time of the year when the light angle and duration trigger the pituitary. The sexual behavior of rabbits provides another striking illustration of nervous-endocrine relationship. The female rabbit usually ovulates only after coitus. Indeed, a virgin female will occasionally do so upon merely seeing a male rabbit, or even another female, in the same room: just seeing another rabbit may be sufficient stimulation.

The nervous stimulation, whether by sign or by the physical act of coitus, is apparently transmitted to the pituitary. Then this gland releases the appropriate hormones into the blood to set the sexual glands into activity. A site and an origin for nervous stimulation of the endocrine system were suggested in experiments by Dr. B. Vaughn Critchlow. This scientist made rats ovulate by stimulating the hypothalamus for periods of half an hour. Later it was found that pituitaries transplanted to the median eminence of the brain continued to secrete gonadotropin and maintain normal sexual activity, while transplants to the temporal lobes failed to produce hormones. It appears that pituitary release of gonadotropin was effected by the brain, that the region of the brain involved was clearly demarcated and localized, and that direct nervous pathways between the stimulating region and the pituitary were not necessary for stimulation to take place. The likely gland seemed to be the hypothalamus.

Independent research has shown hypothalamic control over other hormones. Injuries or damage inflicted on the hypothalamus cut off adrenal cortical steroid secretion in conditions of stress. Thus, the hypothalamus appears to control pituitary ACTH production, and yet, dogs with hypothalamic lesions do not develop adrenal atrophy which would be expected in the absence of all ACTH. Furthermore, adrenal atrophy *does* follow severance of hypothalamic-pituitary connections, while the stress response remains unaffected. More specific understanding of mechanisms involved has progressed only as far as the isolation of an extract of the hypothalamus, poly-peptide in nature, which is able to stimulate adrenal cortical secretion so long as the pituitary is present. This material is called CRF (corti-cotropin-releasing factor). The hypothalamus also appears to be im-plicated, along with thyroxin, in TSH and STH stimulation and release.

Finally, the hypothalamus may actually produce vasopressin and oxytocin, which are only stored in the posterior pituitary prelimi-nary to secretion. Specific regions in the hypothalamus are thought to release specific neurohumors. Hypothalamic stimulation causes the release of these neurohumors, each of which is believed to cause release of a specific hormone from the pituitary. The hypo-thalamus has many related non-endocrine functions, ranging from cardiovascular control to control of hunger, thirst and sleep, so that any lesion in this region will probably produce a massive effect. This fact greatly complicates the problem of delicate, specific ex-ploration of hypothalamic endocrine-related activities. Once again, the specific mechanisms involved in any given secretory response have eluded definition.

The Adrenals

One atop each kidney, the adrenal glands are, after the pitu-itary, the most versatile and varied of the endocrines, both in hor-mones produced and in processes controlled. Although each gland seldom weighs more than ten grams in the male and only slightly more in the female, it controls protein, fat, and carbohydrate metab-olism, and salt and water balance. It is also a member of the sym-pathetic nervous system. Each adrenal gland consists of two separate, apparently unrelated, parts: the *cortex* and the *medulla*. The medulla may actually function as a part of the sympathetic nervous system. Accessory glands—colonies or satellites—can be formed by both the cortex and the medulla in any location from the pelvis to the neck. Consequently, they can present major difficulties when exces-sive activity makes removal necessary, since the hyperplastic tissue may prove to be extremely hard to find. Likewise, in experimental adrenalectomies, the satellites that were not removed with the parent tissue may take over its function completely, confusing all experimental data. The cortex is the portion of the adrenal essential to life, but it is also a tissue that regenerates itself easily. But medullary tissue, once destroyed, is gone for good. Since it is nervous tissue, it does not regenerate.

The functions of the cortex have already been touched upon several times, notably in connection with the ACTH-hydrocortisone servomechanism (see, especially, Figure 3.). The cortex, it will be remembered, secretes steroids. Seven major ones have been distinguished in man and animals. All are built upon the cholesterol molecule, as are the steroids produced by the sex glands, such as progesterone and testosterone. The close relationship to the cholesterol structure molecule is shown in Figure 4.

The ways and relationships of the whole kith and kin are easy to trace. The blood always carries steroids to their sites of action. Degraded inactive forms are also found in the blood travelling to the kidney for excretion; pre-steroid molecules travelling to the adrenal for conversion into active forms are in the blood at the same time. The blood is the highway for all forms of the molecules, those of potential use, the exhausted, and those about to be.

A condition called "steroid diabetes" can be induced by overdosage of adrenal hormones. Gluconeogenesis (manufacture of sugar from scratch) is accelerated by the hormones, and carbohydrate oxidation is suppressed; proteins are devoured as the principal source of blood sugar. The condition is not notably improved by insulin, since the diabetes is not primarily the result of difficulties encountered by glucose in entering the body cells and being utilized, as in the usual form of diabetes, diabetes mellitus. The rise in blood sugar is so pronounced, however, that it appears that the adrenal hormones may also inhibit glucose utilization in addition to stimulating its production.

As discussed earlier the cortical steroids also control salt and water metabolism. In an animal whose adrenal cortex has been removed, the excretion of sodium (salt) increases and the sodium level in the blood plasma plunges, though plasma potassium levels rise. With salt goes water, and dehydration results. On the other hand, a lack of the adrenal cortical steroids will cause water retention—literal "tanking up"—when the organism is deliberately plied with water, since low plasma sodium levels cause overproduction of ADH, leading to water retention. The relatively recent discovery, aldosterone, seems to be the most active steroid in the correction of salt metabolism defects. But aldosterone cannot correct water retention problems, and it does not result in diabetes insipidus which is a side effect of long-term treatment with deoxycorticosterone.

The wide-ranging province of adrenal hormones—the difficulty in finding a pattern in processes they control—is suggested by a survey of the effects of adrenalectomy. The capillaries seem to become more permeable, lacking in tone, and unresponsive to sympathetic stimulation. As a result, the blood in not so readily routed to areas in stress. Muscle fatigue is common. Pronounced anemia usually sets in from depression of the bone marrow and failure of red blood cell production. The lymphatic system grows and expands. Collagen and connective tissue production essential to the healing of wounds is inhibited. Since arthritis is a collagen disease, this reaction suggests a reason for the success of cortisone in treating rheumatoid arthritis. Bone growth is slowed, and even decalcification of the bones may occur. Hair and skin growth are obstructed. The adrenalectomized animal shows much greater sensitivity to stress; thus shock, cold, and toxic substances, which a normal animal could withstand, may kill the adrenalectomized creature. Just how important the adrenal alone may be in this last matter is not yet clear; but as the adrenal is part of a highly integrated and delicately balanced system, it seems dangerous to underestimate the importance of other factors in what has been called the "general adaptation syndrome." The adrenals interact not only with the pituitary and numerous non-endocrine tissues, but also with the gonads, the pancreas, and the thyroid.

The adrenals are subject to both hypo- and hyperfunction; the former commonly produces the condition known as Addison's disease, while the latter results in Cushing's syndrome or adrenogenital syndrome. Addison's disease is usually progressive, and is characterized by increasing weakness, abnormal pigmentation of skin and mucous membranes, weight loss, dehydration, hypotension, gastrointestinal upsets, and occasional hypoglycemia or low blood sugar. Supplying the missing hormone is simply administering a drug. Here the drug is no foreign element in an ongoing chemical system (as

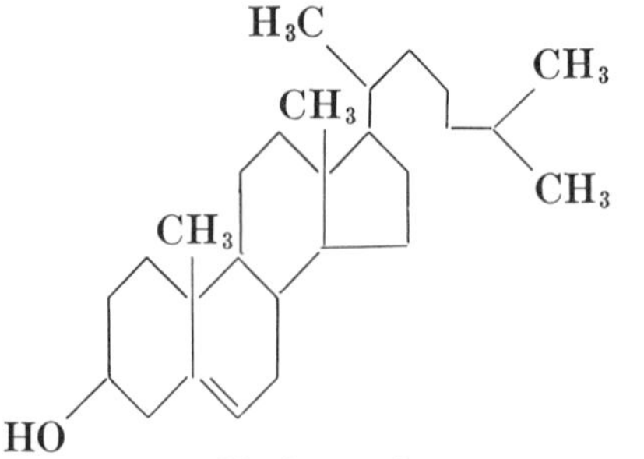

Cholesterol

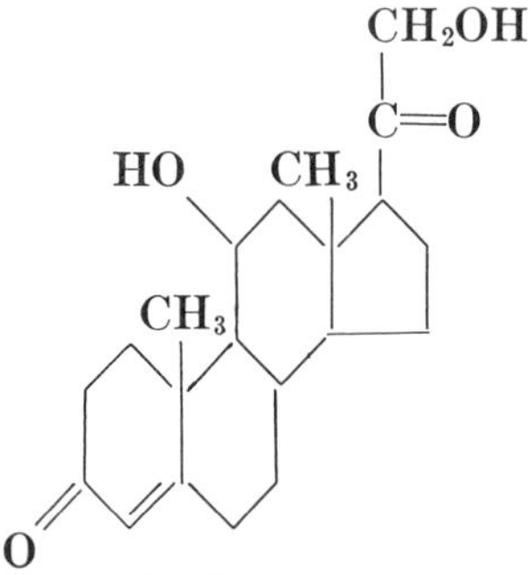

Corticosterone

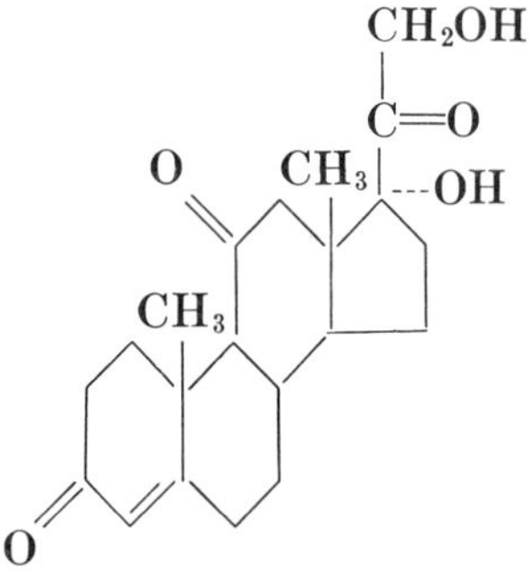

Cortisone

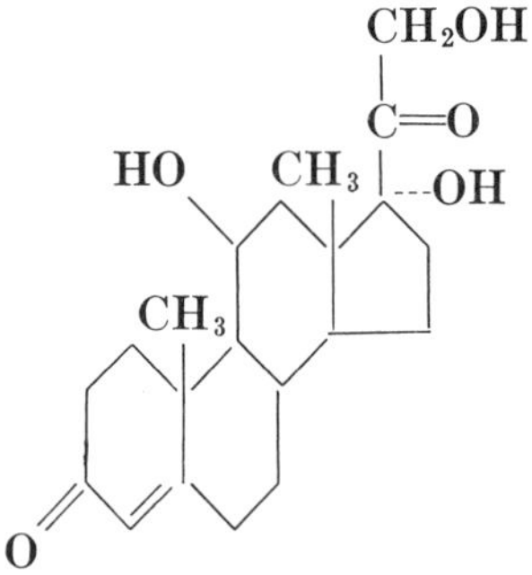

Cortisol

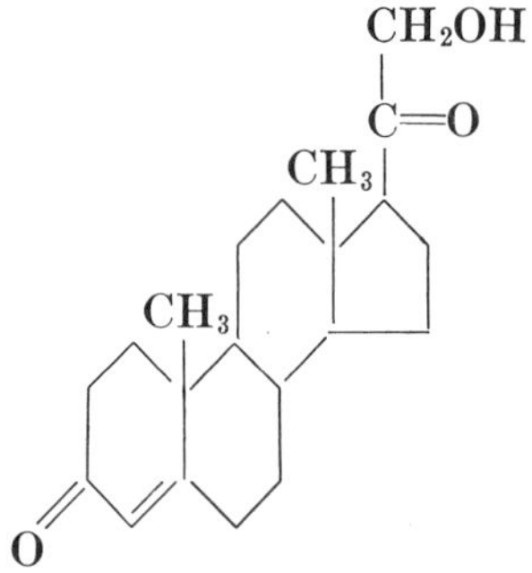

Desoxycorticosterone

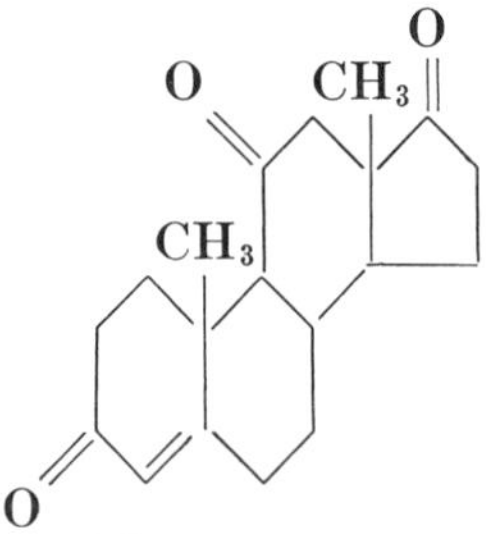

Adrenosterone

FIG. 4

Diagram of the cholesterol molecule showing close family resemblance of steroid derivatives.

FIG. 4 (*continued*)

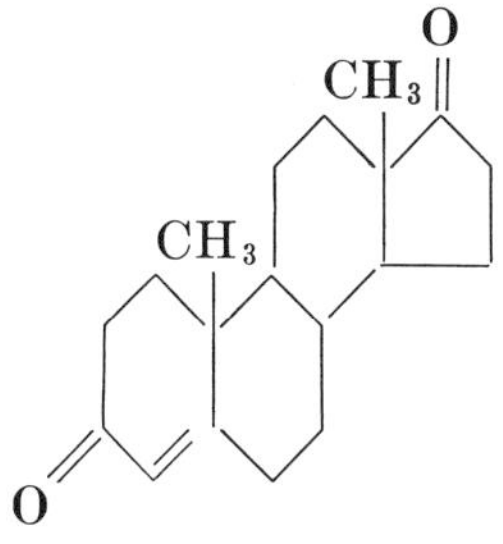

Δ⁴-Androstenedione

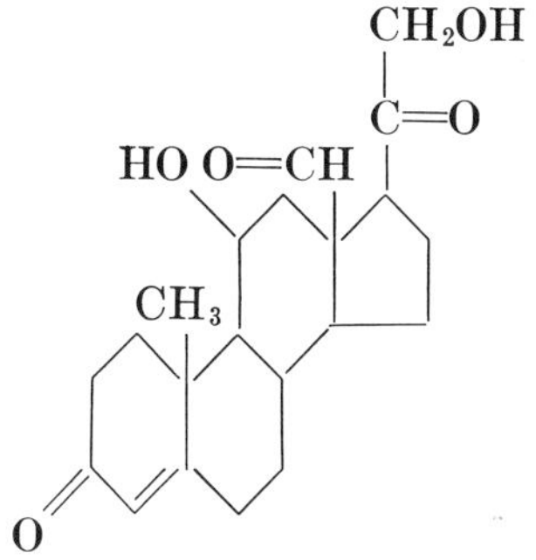

Aldosterone

some scientists consider drugs). It is a regular hormone, added to an insufficient supply in the body.

Adrenogenital syndrome occurs most frequently in children, sometimes in adults; the disorder is characterized by high production of the androgens, male sex hormones. These cause an early onset of puberty in males and virilism in females. The skeleton grows rapidly and matures early. Androgens are not part of the adrenal-pituitary servomechanism, so no feed-back to the "master gland" occurs to regulate ACTH production. Treatment with a steroid such as cortisone or one of the new steroid analogs will check the disease by suppressing the pituitary stimulation of adrenal androgen production. The level of 17-ketosteroids—products of the adrenal cortex—being excreted in the urine is watched in order to gauge dosage; if excretion of large quantities of 17-ketosteroids is not suppressed by ample amounts of cortisone or steroid analog, a tumor rather than pituitary hyperactivity is indicated.

Cushing's syndrome occurs in adults, more commonly in women. Both adrenals increase in size and number of component cells, overproducing steroids. The result is accumulation of excess fat, chiefly in the face and back, protein loss sometimes resulting in bone damage, weakness, hypertension, salt retention, and diabetes mellitus. Virilism may also occur, together with disruption of the menstrual cycle. If administration of exogenous steroids is ineffective, the disease may be classified as of adrenal origin. If patients are helped by steroid treatment, origin of the disease in the pituitary is indicated.

The adrenal medulla produces epinephrine and norepinephrine. Epinephrine has been treated at some length previously under "Nerve-Hormone Relationships." Its activity is generally greater than that of norepinephrine, except on the cardiovascular system. The influence of epinephrine upon metabolism is far greater, although some of this influence may be indirect. Hyperglycemic (high blood sugar) activity, for example, may stem from adrenal steroid activity set off by the anterior pituitary when it is stimulated by epinephrine, rather than result from epinephrine alone, working directly on elaboration of blood sugar. As already noted, the medulla of the adrenal gland is bivalent in its function. Nevertheless, some of the activities of epinephrine and norepinephrine are clearly endocrine; these substances have metabolic effects that cannot be attributed to nervous-system stimulation. Thus the two main medullary hormones are both endocrines and mediators in the autonomic nervous system.

The Thyroid

To most people, the thyroid means goiter and metabolic derangement; and that is, in fact, just about what it *does* mean, in clinical terms. This gland incorporates iodine into the thyroid hormones, thyroxin and triiodothyronine. The thyroid's activity in taking up iodine is regulated by pituitary TSH and a low concentration of iodine in the thyroid which accelerates uptake. Some researchers have suggested that a very active thyroid may in some cases inactivate and destroy TSH as quickly as it can be produced. TSH would then be given no chance to cause the production of hormones in the thyroid, which would in turn suppress pituitary TSH production. Without this feedback mechanism, continuous stimulation of the thyroid would result. It is apparent that the thyroid is involved in a feedback cycle with the pituitary. For example, abnormal "thyroidectomy" cells are produced in the pituitary after removal of the thyroid. Similar effects are typical when the pituitary or the adrenal gland is denied a customary stimulus or control by an endocrine organ that has been removed. "Castration cells" appear, for instance, in the pituitary after removal of the testes. In this case, as in the case of thyroidectomy cells, the abnormal histological phenomenon seems to arise from the basophil cells of the pituitary.

The thyroid is a great overseer for metabolism. It secretes a general metabolic hormone, so that its effects are widespread and diverse. The external characteristics of the victims of thyroid hyperfunction and hypofunction are fixed in the popular imagination. Obesity, sluggishness, physical weakness, and mental dullness result from under-production (hypothyroidism). Extreme skinniness, constant nervous activity, bulging eyes, and quickness of manner result from over-production (hyperthyroidism). The reason for some of these characteristics concerns specific metabolic activity of the thyroid hormone. Thyroxin increases metabolism in the majority of the body's tissues. This requires more oxygen and, hence, a greater oxygen consumption by the body. Knowledge of this led to the oldest test of thyroid function, the BMR (basal metabolic rate), which is based upon measurement of oxygen consumption during the stabilized metabolic period that occurs sometime after feeding. Young organisms have a higher metabolic rate (calorigenic activity) than older ones and the hypothyroid animal is highly sensitive to the thyroid hormone. This adds yet one more example to a pattern often observed in endocrinology: target tissues appear to become extremely sensitive to a given hormone in its absence.

Also possible, the normal hypothalamus-pituitary-thyroid system or feedback may inactivate thyroxin, decreasing the effect of a given dose in normal animals, while animals lacking or low in the endogenous production of the hormone would have no such feedback control to cushion the effect of administered hormone. Thyroid failure in a young animal causes cessation of growth, apparently by interfering somehow with STH's effect on anabolic activity. The antithetical malfunction, overproduction of thyroxin, increases the body's demand for fuel to burn for energy, causing increased gluconeogenesis which depends on cannibalism of body proteins. This self-consuming production of energy may be so intense that loss of weight occurs. Liver glycogen is also raided for the extra glucose needed in the increased metabolism. Water and electrolyte balance is affected by thyroxin as well. The excess of the hormone may cause minerals in the bone to be leached out, with increased calcium excretion, while deficiency of the hormone prevents synthesis of the organic foundation and building blocks for normal bone production. Thyroid malfunction also affects other endocrines extensively. The greatly increased metabolism due to thyroid overproduction or administration of exogenous hormone leads to increased stress on the organism; one result is stepped-up adrenal cortical steroid release and increased size and activity of the adrenal cortex itself. Decreased thyroid activity has quite noticeable effects on the sex glands and their operations, depressing sperm production in the male, disrupting the normal menstrual cycle in the female, and generally impairing the sex drive, perhaps as much through non-specific metabolic slowdown as through direct and specific interference with the gonads. The combination of easy oral medication and its effects on the gonads has made thyroid therapy a frequent resort in medical treatment of complaints relating to the reproductive system, especially in the female.

Goiter is—or was—among the commonest malfunctions of the thyroid. This disease is a symmetrical enlargement of the gland owing to dietary deficiency in iodine or to enzymatic failure. The great inland areas of the U.S.A., including the Mid-west and Great Plains, were once known as the Goiter Belt, so common was the unsightly distention of the neck resulting from the lack of iodine that the thyroid uses as raw material for its secretions. With insufficient raw materials present, the overworked cells enlarged themselves and expanded in an effort to keep up with organic demands. The patient was treated with iodine, but that mineral is most useful as a prophylactic or preventative measure. Scientists noted that people living near the sea coast and eating fresh seafood regularly do not suffer from the problem. The general use of iodized salt has now made it possible for inland dwellers to enjoy this health advantage formerly confined to those on the coasts. Still, some regions seem to be plagued by specific "goitrogens" in certain vegetables growing there; thus iodized salt is no all-purpose preventative. Long exposure to stress, including adolescence and pregnancy may induce thyroid enlargement even with adequate dietary iodine by causing the body's need for thyroid hormone to mushroom far beyond the normally-sufficient, available supply of hormone and hence iodine.

Hyperthyroidism in contrast to goiter (endemic goiter), may produce some enlargement of the gland, but the more characteristic symptom is exophthalmos, protrusion of the eyes caused by accumulation of fatty substances behind the eyeball. When treatment of the gland is indicated, it may be by anti-thyroid agents, surgery, or radiation, the latter two especially if malignancy is present or likely to develop. The exophthalmos is extremely difficult to treat, however, and often persists after the apparent cause, thyroid derangement, has been corrected.

Underproduction of hormone by the thyroid can result in cretinism or myxedema. Deficiency of thyroid hormone during fetal or early infant life will result in cretinism, a condition of physical and mental underdevelopment with characteristic physical conformation in the victim. Developmental failure without thyroid stimulation can be illustrated by the thyroidectomized tadpole, which fails to metamorphose into a frog). The thyroid may be congenitally absent in cretins, or greatly reduced in size. The mental state varies "from helpless imbecility to that of a dull but happy moron," according to the *Merck Manual* (Tenth Edition, p. 421). Treatment with desiccated thyroid or sodium levothyroxine and maintenance of adequate dietary intake of iodine can bring about normal growth and greatly improved mentality, although normal intelligence and complete mental development are probably out of the question for the congenital cretin. Juvenile myxedema is the name given to essentially the same symptoms encountered in cretinism, but occurring later in life. The cause may be failure of enzymes essential to iodine metabolism. The prognosis for the victim of juvenile myxedema is generally better than that for the congenital cretin.

In adults, myxedema is found primarily in women, usually about the menopause. Stress appears to contribute to its appearance.

Toxic goiter or an exhausting illness may eventuate in myxedema. Other causes include prolonged treatment with anti-thyroid drugs, overdosage of radioactive iodine in clinical procedures, excision or atrophy of the thyroid itself, or hypofunction of the anterior lobe of the pituitary, which of course secretes TSH, the thyroid-stimulating hormone. Puffy facial configurations, mental apathy, thickened skin, sensitivity to cold, and sometimes cardiac problems are commonly seen. The hyperthyroid person tends to be warm and to sweat easily, while the hypothyroid person is cold and dry. Administration of desiccated thyroid or thyroid hormones or hormone-analogs is the standard treatment, and such maintenance therapy must be continued for the duration of life.

The Parathyroids

The secretion of the parathyroid glands, PTH, is necessary for life. The glands, small and easily overlooked, commonly lie close to the thyroid. In fact, careless removal of the thyroid without steps to save the parathyroids led to the belief, which persisted for years, that thyroidectomy was fatal. Although the parathyroids usually lie in the dorsal portion of the thyroid, they may be distributed anywhere from the bottom of the skull to the chest region. There are always two or more. Little is known about the mechanism and control of parathyroid secretion, and much speculation exists concerning the action of PTH. The hormone was not obtained in workably pure form until recently.

Currently, the dominant theory holds that a decrease in the level of calcium in the blood plasma arouses parathyroid activity. Some studies also point to a possible phosphate-ion-level relationship. Calcium intake in the diet and size of the parathyroid glands show an inverse relationship; it will be remembered that some endocrines, like the thyroid, increase in size as availability of their raw materials or stimulants decreases. Calcium and magnesium ions decrease tissue excitability, while potassium ions support and sustain it. Lowered calcium concentrations in the blood plasma produce neuromuscular hyperreactivity resulting in tremor and even tetany (severe intermittent muscular contractions and pain). Shifts in the pH (the acidity) of the blood can produce rapid changes in plasma calcium. Hyperventilation is a good example: a baby crying violently discharges carbon dioxide from the blood through the lungs, causing the blood pH to rise to an important degree, diminishing calcium concentration in the blood even to the point that muscle tremor may set in. The condition has its own control of sorts, for a sufficient increase in uncontrollable muscle activity interferes with pulmonary activity as well as bringing about increased accumulation of lactic acid in the blood and thus lowering blood pH (the lower the pH, the greater the acidity). In this way the ionization of calcium may be stepped up enough to relieve muscular hyperirritability and spasms.

It is not clear exactly how PTH accomplishes its regulatory function, but removal of the parathyroids in an animal results in a decrease in serum calcium and an increase in serum phosphorus. Normally, about 80 percent of the body's phosphorus is situated in bone tissue. The animal loses alertness and tautness, loses appetite, then develops the uncontrollable twitching of the muscles which grows into convulsions of apparently nervous origin. Death comes with tetany of muscles controlling respiration. PTH's site of action is still vigorously debated, one theory favoring a major effect on the reabsorptive processes of the kidney, the other arguing that the major effect is on dynamic relationships relating to bone resorption and deposition. Recent evidence may cause a search for clear proof of tissue effects more general in nature than those accounted for by either competing theory.

Calcium-phosphorus metabolism has close relationships with other portions of the endocrine system. The gonads, particularly, affect bone deposition, with testosterone increasing bone size and calcium and phosphorus retention. Estrogens stimulate bone-forming cells and accelerate bone formation and maturation. Parathyroid-gonadal relationships should be a particularly fruitful area of exploration in the chicken, which can draw off 25 percent of total bone weight for the production of eggs when on a low-calcium diet. Calcium goes both into the shell and into the egg itself. It has also been remarked that the calcium needs of the human fetus will be met in one way or another, and that insufficient dietary calcium results in the fetus absorbing calcium directly from its mother's bones and teeth.

The Gonads: Testes

Compared to the varied activity of the ovaries and the female hormones through the menstrual cycle and during and after pregnancy, the testes seem quite steady, workaday, and unspectacular in the performance of their endocrine functions. The organ consists of two major types of specialized tissue: the tubules which produce the sperm cells essential in reproduction, and the interstitial cells of Leydig. The tubules, in turn, contain two types of cells: spermatogenic cells ranging in development from immature spermatogonia to mature spermatozoa ready to play their role in reproduction, and the so-called Sertoli cells which are thought to be nutrient cells servicing the actual sperm-producers. Mature sperm cells are developed by a process that begins with a simple cell division of a spermatogonium, the primary cell. The new cells formed from that division are called spermatocytes and already have the genetic material arranged as it must be to determine the sex of the offspring produced by union with an egg cell in the body of the female (see Chapter 2).

The spermatocytes are still only a short way on the course of their destiny. They must divide again to form spermatids, which mature through a step-by-step process, finally becoming the mature sperm cell. The spermatids appear to spend part of their time inside the very cytoplasm of the Sertoli cells; as they mature, they are forced out and a new generation of immature spermatids enter the cell. Thus the Sertoli cells seem to serve as some sort of *alma mater*.

Besides producing sperm, the testes trigger the development of male secondary sex characteristics through their hormones. In this process, they are responsible for a characteristic male psychological pattern. The male sex hormones are collectively called "androgens." While the tubules, as noted, produce the sperm, androgen is produced by the interstitial cells. Normal androgen production may continue without sperm production, but a modicum of androgen is necessary to mature sperm cells, so that in the absence of the former, the latter do not develop. The androgens are steroids; the two most important ones produced by the testes are testosterone and androsterone. They resemble some andrenocortical steroids, and most of the 17-ketosteroids.

Androgen production begins at puberty, stimulating growth of the male reproductive organs and development of the adult male hair pattern on the head and body. The beard develops, the boy soprano loses his place in the choir, the sweat glands develop, and deposition of muscle protein increases, resulting in the tall, gangling teen-ager. Control of the new mass of muscle is usually slow. A male castrated before puberty does not undergo these changes, and the post-pubertal castrate may show regression of some of the secondary sex characteristics. On the other hand, a female with an adrenal tumor or one dosed with androgens will usually develop typically-male secondary sex characteristics. In the male, androgen production appears to relate to the development of an adult male psychic outlook, the sex drive, and ability to perform the sex act (although, contrary to popular opinion, the castrate can both erect the penis and perform the sex act, probably because of conditioning). Ejaculation is closely tied to the presence of androgens; the seminal vesicles and prostate, where much of the emission fluid is formed, are maintained by androgen.

Lack of proper levels of androgen secretion and failure to produce sperm may result in male infertility, which is not always the same thing as sterility. Recently, an approach similar to that employing oral contraceptives as "conception pills" in relatively infertile women has been used with some success. This approach relies upon the "rebound" phenomenon: treatment of the male patient with large doses of androgen inhibits sperm production and release, but when the treatment is withdrawn, the "rested" glands bounce back with higher-than-normal sperm output.

It is not clear just why puberty begins at the "proper" time, between 12 and 15 years of age. Furthermore, substantial amounts of gonadotropin, the gonad-stimulating hormone, exist in the pituitaries of young people and animals, and children are capable of reacting to injections of gonadotropin long before puberty ordinarily sets in. Nevertheless, when the time is ripe, the seminal vesicles, prostate, etc. become highly sensitive to gonadotropin, androgens are produced, and sexual maturity gradually develops. Quite recently, the hypothalamus has been given the ultimate responsibility as the trigger that sets off pituitary activity; it had been observed earlier that certain lesions and injuries to the brain could cause precocious puberty, and this was seen as contributory evidence for the theory. This observation and theory merely pushes the search back through one more secondary cause; the prime mover remains shrouded from our understanding.

Feedback systems between the gonads and the pituitary clearly exist. For example, in tubule deficiencies where little or no sperm are produced, pituitary output of FSH is high in spite of androgen output, while the normal individual with normal sperm production has a characteristically low FSH output. So FSH controls and regulates sperm production but the exact nature of the feedback that keeps FSH production at a level neither too high nor too low for normal sperm production is only guessed at today. The testes affect other endocrine organs: atrophy of the thyroid and adrenals usually accompanies castration.

The androgens also affect general metabolism—notably nitrogen, salt, protein and water retention. As we shall see shortly when we glance at what can be done to hormones in the laboratory, the androgens have been very interesting in altered forms, so that, for example, their effects on secondary sex characteristics are eliminated and only their effect on nitrogen retention and metabolism remains. They are used both for fertility control in the female by virtue of their capacity to suppress ovulation, and for boosting deficient fertility in both men and women through the "rebound" effect mentioned above. Almost anything you do to the structure of testosterone, as Dr. James Ashmore of the Indiana University School of Medicine comments, will decrease its biological activity as a male hormone. Hence, it was very easy to make a number of different derivatives, all having much less androgenic activity than the original hormone, and to test these in various disease states and abnormal conditions. These devirilized male hormones were found, in some cases, to retain an ability to suppress pituitary gonadotropins and thus to shut off estrogens supplying a mammary carcinoma (cancer of the breast) in women, while not inducing undesirable masculine characteristics as a side effect. Conversely, estrogens apparently act through the pituitary to shut off the supply of gonadotropins in men, so that decreases in the growth rate of prostatic cancer can be obtained in males through estrogen treatment, which cuts off at their source the hormones that stimulate prostatic tissue.

Female hormones are discussed in the chapters "Contraception and The Pill" and "Drugs and the Unborn Child."

The Role of Hormones

The endocrine system seems to be shorter-lived or to have less staying power than many other systems and tissues in the body. Perhaps this is to be expected. The endocrines are responsible day by day for the balances in the delicate chemistry of the body. With age the various endocrine functions begin to break down. If one lives to be 75 or 80, there is a very high probability of mild diabetes coming from decreased pancreatic activity. The same is true for prostatic carcinoma, a cancer related to endocrine malfunction. The probability of developing prostatic cancer increases markedly above the age of 65, and if one lives to be 90, it is almost certain that the prostate will suffer some hypertrophy. Many famous men in public life—MacArthur, Churchill—suffered late in life from this condition.

Through specialization during the course of our evolution, man has lost the ability to synthesize vitamins within himself. Consequently, we take vitamins in our diets, often supplemented by vitamin pills from the drugstore. We consider them essential for our survival. One scientist noted that a projection 30 or 40 thousand years into the future may find man in the same situation with hormones in which he now finds himself with vitamins. Diabetes, for example, is known to be, to some extent at least, a hereditary disease. Since we now can keep diabetics alive through the reproductive period, it is likely that they will pass the trait along to their offspring. If estimations prove correct, over 30 percent of the people alive today carry the diabetic trait. So one might gloomily project a time in the future when nearly everyone would require some insulin to stay alive. If the source remains beef and pork pancreatic tissues, it is not difficult to see that with an exploding world population the supply of the drug will become strictly limited. We would have to find other means to make the molecules synthetically, from scratch and in quantity. The problem lies with synthesis of insulin today. It cannot compare very favorably with the fermentation of other hormones in huge 50,000 gallon vats seeded with microorganisms.

Perhaps research will come up with a smaller, easily manufactured molecule that will perform the same function. Such progress has occurred with the steroids. Twenty years ago, all the steroids were laboriously extracted from beef adrenals, and to treat an arthritic patient with cortisone to lessen pain and inflammation would have cost $50 to $75 per day. Today, the same hormones are made from the Mexican sweet potato by a fermentation process; and the cost is only $5 to $7 a day.

Finally, hormones may play a role in the auto-immune diseases, discussed in the chapters of this book dealing with cancer. The glucocorticoids, cortisone in particular, are very effective in treating all these diseases, including arthritis, for they knock out the body's ability to make antibodies. The conditions result from the body's becoming allergic to its own tissue and manufacturing antibodies against it. Cortisone is a protein catabolic agent—it increases the break down of proteins—proteins which are the body's immunizing agents.

Treatment with massive doses of adrenal steroid will reduce the ability of the body to make antibodies against organs transplanted from donors and prevent the death of the patient or the rejection of the transplanted organ for a time. Some cases have been treated with the steroids for years. Theoretically, treatment could go on until the patient's natural death, although some scientists hope that after prolonged steroid treatment the body may relax its hostility and accept the originally rejected organ without struggle. The undesirable side effect of this line of treatment, at this time unavoidable, is the body's lowered resistance to infection. In most cases of organ transplants that have been initially successful with hormone maintenance treatment, death has ultimately come from pneumonia or some such infection which the body, with its resistance lowered, cannot combat.

The hormones have been used in many ways; athletes with painful injuries, like football quarterback Joe Namath of the New York Jets and Mickey Mantle of the New York Yankees, or Sandy Koufax of the Los Angeles Dodgers, may have cortisone injections directly into a muscle, ligament or joint that gives chronic trouble.

The effect may be partially psychological. Yet these hormones are very potent, even when not used systematically, breaking down proteins, fighting inflammation and decreasing pain.

But relatively little is known today about many hormones and the details of how they work. Advances like the synthesis of biologically-active insulin, studies of hypothalamic relations and controls, hormone-enzyme relationships and similar areas of dark understanding, can open up new clearings in this dense difficult wood.

SUPPLEMENTAL READING

Karlson, P., editor, Mechanisms of Hormone Action, A Nato Advanced Study Institute, Academic Press.

Von Euler, U. S., & Heller, H., editors, Comparative Endocrinology, 2, Academic Press.

Williams, R. H., editor, Textbook of Endocrinology, 3rd edition, W. B. Saunders Company.

Chapter 20

Insulin and the Diabetic

Violent lightning storms raging over the primordial seas probably sparked the creation of early complex molecules, the precursors of life. Recent experiments starting with electricity, air, and cold salt water have simulated the earth's ocean and atmosphere a few billion years ago. These experimental conditions have led to the formation of amino acids, the building blocks of protein. Of course, making amino acids from a few loose atoms and molecules requires large amounts of energy—intermittent energy from the sky happily sufficed long ago. But now biochemists under highly-controlled conditions can modify the natural hormones with much less difficulty. Alteration of steroid hormones, for example, can be readily achieved by a few deft chemical maneuvers, especially since the basic steroid structure is wide-spread in nature. In fact, the structure of most body steroids—adrenal, androgenic, and estrogenic—are found in the Mexican sweet potato.

The process of synthesis begins with a molecule already formed in its basic structure, and the biochemist modifies it as the body itself would in developing the various derivatives in a hormone family. A group of atoms is added here, another removed there, this or that existing group is altered. Instead of having a thirty-eight step synthesis, it may be possible to achieve the end product in no more than four or five steps. Unfortunately, steroids are the exception rather than the rule in setting standards for ease in the chemical modification of hormones. The steroids are relatively simple, compact structures, and their major activities are not much changed, in many cases, by tinkering with peripheral groups.

The classic example of steroid alteration concerns the activity of a male sex hormone, androgen. This steroid shuts off production of gonadotropin by the pituitary; and this reduces the levels of estrogen feeding a carcinoma in the female breast. An androgen does this job well, but its other effects are highly undesirable cosmetically:

347

its virilizing property may cause growth of beard, baldness, lowering of the voice, and cessation or interruption of the menstrual cycle. It has now become possible to alter androgens chemically so that they retain their ability to suppress the pituitary, but lose all virilizing tendencies. Desirable side effects including decrease of pain associated with a breast tumor and its metastases, and improvement of appetite and a general sense of well-being, can sometimes be accentuated by chemically modified androgens. Such modification is not done at someone's desk, by abstractly considering, "Well, if we knock off this hydrogen group and alter that carbon group, we'll get more improvement of appetite and less stimulation of male secondary sex characteristics." It is done largely by trial and error.

The only way the scientist can be sure any idea on paper will work *in vivo* is by trying it, first on laboratory animals such as rats, rabbits or dogs, to see if it does anything effectively or adversely at all; then on human patients to see how far it works across species lines. A hormone made or modified is always tested first on animals, but success there is only a clue, a hint, as to whether it will be effective in humans. The differences in the cellular chemistry from species to species may make one hormone work perfectly in the rabbit's system, yet have no more effect than sugar water when placed in the system of a human being. Once again, the steroids provide safer ground. Simple in structure, quite similar from species to species, they are often almost universal in their effectiveness. An example is the industrial usefulness of the Mexican sweet potato's steroids in the production of synthetic steroids for humans.

While steroids are easy to synthesize and generally uniform in their effects throughout the great chain of being, the more complex the molecule the more diminished the occurrence of these estimable traits. When amino acids join together in large numbers, they form proteins. Thyroxin, an amino acid containing iodine, is in effect on about the same level of difficulty as one of the letters that go to make the word "antidisestablishmentarianism," with the word standing for a not-too-complex protein molecule. Thyroxin itself was synthesized in 1926; the first adrenal cortical steroid was synthesized in 1943. But it was not until the summer of 1963 that researchers achieved the synthesis of ACTH, the pituitary polypeptide—a kind of subprotein—consisting of 39 amino acid units in a single chain.

Insulin is yet another step in complexity, for this pancreatic hormone is a small true protein.

What Diabetes Is

All the body's life and activity depends upon the burning of carbohydrates by the individual cells to produce energy. Energy is used for metabolic processes of building and tearing down chemical entities. The carbohydrate fuel is supplied to the cells by the blood stream in the form of glucose (blood sugar), which is maintained in the blood at a relatively constant level by the liver. The liver responds to various hormones from several endocrine glands in playing its role in this process. Quite simply, the liver converts the glycogen stored within it to blood sugar when the blood sugar level drops, and synthesizes glycogen from blood sugar and lactic acid when the levels of these substances rise in the blood. Thyroid hormone steps up sugar absorption from the intestine; epinephrine increases the breakdown of glycogen to glucose in the liver. Increased blood sugar is produced by an adrenal cortical steroid which promotes the formation of sugar from amino acids or fats, a process called gluconeogenesis; and utilization of glucose appears to be suppressed by pituitary STH (somatotropic hormone—somatotropin). The hormone most immediately involved in the control of blood sugar is a product of the pancreas, insulin.

In 1899 Joseph von Mering and Oskar Minkowski took out the pancreas of a dog and showed that its removal led to diabetes mellitus. Active extracts from the pancreas were first obtained in 1922. They were used in treating diabetes, which at that time was still classifiable as fatal. By 1925, the pancreatic tissues involved were localized still more; it was found that the drug alloxan destroyed the beta cells of tissues in the so-called *islets of Langerhans* in the pancreas, thereby inducing diabetes. Finally, the responsible pancreatic secretion was identified as insulin.

Removal of the pancreas or deficiency of insulin causes the rapid development of hyperglycemia, an excess of blood sugar. When the blood sugar level becomes so high that the tubules of the kidney cannot completely reabsorb it, glycosuria occurs. In this condition sugar appears in the urine—glycosuria was once another name for diabetes mellitus. Glycosuria in severe diabetes may reach the point at which the entire daily sugar intake may be passed from the body with the urine, augmented by sugar produced by gluconeogenesis. This sugar accumulates in the blood and finally is excreted in the urine because the diabetic's body cells are unable to utilize it. Since glucose in the blood is thus useless for the body's normal metabolic needs, fat must be burned as a source of energy instead. The diabetic maintains life by "cannibalizing" fat and protein from his own body. This results in weight loss, increased appetite, polyphagia (over-eating), high urine volume (polyuria) to rid the blood of the high levels of sugar, and thus great thirst (polydipsia) resulting from rapid and continuous loss of fluid.

Insulin's primary role seems to be that of enabling cells to use glucose at lower concentrations in the blood than would be the case in the absence of insulin. The central nervous system is an exception to the whole process, needing no insulin at any time for the metabolism of glucose. Insulin's main site of action, the cell membrane, and the manner of action, either on a transport mechanism or to increase permeability, need not be discussed in any detail here. Insulin secretion is seemingly controlled, not by the pituitary or hypothalamus, or any other endocrine gland, but simply by the level of blood sugar itself. When the blood sugar level rises, the beta cells of the pancreas simply release insulin, thus lowering the blood-sugar level through cell use of the glucose.

Differences Among Diabetics and Methods of Treatment

Back in 1935, H. P. Hinsworth of London classified diabetics as either sensitive (i.e., responsive) to insulin or not sensitive. The distinction would have been important in determining proper clinical treatment of given patients, but Canadian and U.S. researchers were unable to confirm his findings. It was not until 1954 that Dr. George Anderson of the State University of New York College of Medicine announced such confirmation. He attributed earlier failures of scientists in this country and Canada to duplicate Hinsworth's results to the fact that insulin available in the Western Hemisphere contained the hyperglycemic (blood-sugar elevating) factor glucagon, not present in European commercial insulin.

Anderson's work produced a "6-minute" clinical test that gauges a patient's efficiency in utilizing available insulin. A patient who does not efficiently utilize insulin may have plenty of the hormone available in his system naturally; what he needs is not more insulin, but something to help him use it. Conversely, much more careful control of sugar intake allows the fuel to be burned in time for the body to accommodate it. The examination of obese non-diabetics from diabetic families revealed a resistance to insulin that, Anderson reasoned, would result in an increased demand in the body for greater production of the inefficiently utilized hormone. These demands ultimately "bankrupt" the intrinsic insulin producer, creating another diabetic.

The islets of Langerhans are particularly sensitive to over-work. When adrenal cortical steroids are over-administered, increased gluconeogenesis may cause "steroid diabetes", a condition of hyperglycemia originally unrelated to the pancreatic problem. Long continuation of such hyperglycemia stimulates insulin production. This might exhaust the islets of Langerhans, resulting in permanent diabetes. Consequently, insulin-resistant fat people from diabetic families constitute probable "high risk" cases for the development of diabetes. Their early recognition could be greatly helpful to physicians. The "6-minute" test showed this tendency of resistance clearly in persons whose glucose-tolerance test was normal, and who had normal blood-sugar levels.

In 1958, Dr. Henry Dolger, Chief of the Diabetes Clinic at Mt. Sinai Hospital, New York, declared that diabetes mellitus could no longer be considered a single disease, to be treated with insulin. Research with the new drug Orinase, taken orally rather than by injection, showed that the drug was effective in more than 50 percent of cases of adult diabetes. Dr. Dolger was led by his observations to divide diabetics into two groups: 1) those with no insulin available at all, and 2) those who have some insulin available, but suffer from some interference with its proper liberation and use. The second appeared more often responsive to Orinase.

About a year ago, Dr. Jerome W. Conn of the University of Michigan suggested to the New England Diabetes Association that more than one million Americans who have been diagnosed as diabetics may actually be victims of an adrenal disorder requiring, not insulin, but surgery. Dr. Conn was working with a form of high blood pressure caused, it was discovered in the early 1960's, by an excess of adrenal aldosterone resulting from adrenal tumors. The disorder brings with it imbalances in the body's delicate chemistry— lack of proper potassium levels in the system and usually an excess of sodium—which may result in intermittent paralysis, uremia, and high blood pressure.

Dr. Conn noticed that 40 percent of those suffering from this disorder, studied in the University of Michigan Hospital at Ann Arbor, showed the classic sugar metabolism problems that characterize adult diabetics. Fourteen of twenty-seven victims of aldosteronism tested closely had a reduced ability to metabolize sugars. What proportion of adult diabetics actually suffers from aldosteronism? Unmistakable onset of diabetes in childhood or adolescence is not noted in many who develop diabetes later in life. In fact, Dr. Conn considered whether there were such a thing as mature-onset diabetes at all.

Such a sweeping question seems to be going a bit far on the relatively little data and study so far done on the matter. Nonetheless, Dr. Conn's theory does relate interestingly to the two groups of diabetics discovered and described through the use of the drug Orinase in the late '50's by Dr. Dolger. Dr. Conn would be inclined to consider the adrenal cortex, rather than the pancreas, as the source of the difficulty.

Orally-Effective Hormones

Protein molecules, including insulin, are large molecules made up of what chemists call polypeptide chains; one amino acid is hooked to another in a "peptide bond." A "polypeptide," like ACTH, consists of a long chain of these amino acids, but a protein may contain two or more chains bound together in various geometric arrangements. Some chains have spiral structures called *alpha* helics. This complex spiralling structure of amino acids then folds back upon itself in various ways to form the protein molecule. The biological activity of most proteins depends upon the integrity of the whole spatial configuration of this huge molecule. In addition, each protein molecule has somewhere a *sine qua non,* its active center. The biological activity of a protein may be changed without alteration of its chemical composition, that is, without taking away or adding or substituting for any of the component amino acids, simply by altering the way the molecule typically folds.

Some hormones can be administered orally; the glucocorticoids are among them. Naturally-occurring estrogens (female sex hormones) are not, for they are absorbed from the gastrointestinal tract directly into the portal circulation, which carries them straight to the liver, breaking down the hormone. A hormone cannot be camouflaged to fool the liver, but it can, in effect, be armored to protect it from the liver's destructive action. The "armor" is some protective group that can be placed on the molecule to cover the sites that the liver attacks in breaking it down. Of course the protective group must be carefully chosen, or it may alter all the chemical relationships within the intact molecule to which it is attached. The choice of a protective group to be added to any given molecule is like the selection of an electrical component to be inserted into an already carefully balanced and tuned circuit. The male sex hormone testosterone was one of the first natural hormones to be successfully altered; methyl testosterone, for example, is active orally.

Other possibilities for hormone treatment are varied. The androgens (male sex hormones) can be absorbed directly into the lymphatic system by holding the hormone pill under the tongue without swallowing. If, however, a hormone is destroyed by the digestive enzymes or broken down by the liver, it cannot be expected to be effective when ingested orally. All proteins are thus automatically excluded from oral administration, because the normal digestive enzymes dismantle the complex structures and chains immediately, breaking them down into their component (and inactive) amino acids.

All proteins and some other hormones must consequently be given by injection. Except in the most unusual circumstances, however, they would not be injected intravenously, for drastically acute effects are not generally desired. Most hormone treatments are termed "replacement therapy," substituting for the products of a gland that has been removed or lost through accident, or supplementing inadequate natural secretions, or suppressing another endocrine function that is overactive in a particular individual. Long-term effects are usually sought; hence the hormones are injected intramuscularly or subcutaneously, often in an oil solution to insure slow absorption. When insulin is given intramuscularly, it is usually in combination with another protein, protamine, and sometimes bound in a preparation with zinc. Both of these methods insure longer activity per injection than shots of undiluted, pure insulin. The latter is extremely short-lived in the blood. Pure injected insulin can expect a "half-life" of only an hour, at least partly because of the destructive action of the enzyme insulinase in the blood and other body tissues. The exact nature of this supposed enzymatic destruction is unknown, and the problem now stirs much controversy in scientific circles. Insulin with protamine may be effective up to twenty-four hours, compared to a fifth or to a third that time for regular insulin. The effects of protamine insulin with zinc may extend beyond thirty-six hours.

Insulin presented a major problem for many years in its role as controller of diabetes. Of course it was far better than nothing. Exemplary figures such as Bill Talbert, the tennis star, afflicted with diabetes, gave new hope and inspiration to millions of diabetics who before would have been condemned to a slow course toward virtually certain death, and a weakened physical condition and inactive life along the way. Talbert was a success in a most vigorous and competitive sport, and he did much to spread understanding on the use of insulin. But the amount of insulin in any dose had to be very carefully controlled. It is the nature of insulin to be dangerous in excess as well as in deficiency. Excess insulin, from careless injection as well as from natural hyperfunction, causes the blood sugar to drop to hazardously low levels, depriving the cells of the nervous system of energy needed for ordinary function. This may result in hypoglycemic shock, accompanied by convulsions and coma. The countermeasure is quick introduction of glucose into the system—the reason for the diabetic's rule: always carry a candybar.

The effects of undersupply of insulin have already been noted, in part, as the symptoms of diabetes. However, the extreme result is diabetic coma, requiring instant treatment with insulin, and other measures as well, to return the metabolism to normal. Diabetic coma was the cause of death in over 50 percent of cases before insulin was developed and put into general use. Furthermore, the very process of injection was uncomfortable, inconvenient even to the point of being a social stigma, causing diabetics to become confused with drug addicts. At times injection was harmful as a possible cause of infection, localized degeneration of tissue, and other complications.

Experiments showed that small amounts of insulin could be absorbed from the intestine when massive doses of the hormone were given orally, but the procedure was too haphazard and costly for general use. In addition, a fear for a time, although it is generally discounted now, was the possibility that the number of diabetics might exhaust the store of insulin. The disease is still one of the major medical problems. The disease rate is increasing twice as fast at the population rate. More widespread overeating and higher percentages of carbohydrate in the diet may be factors. And there is the simple statistical fact that more people are living into and beyond the fourth and fifth decades of life—the time of life showing the maximum incidence of diabetes.

Sources of Insulin

Fortunately, entirely adequate supplies of insulin for the five to six million diabetics in this country are apparently available through the use of a mixture of beef and pork insulin. Also, fortunately, there are very few allergic or immune reactions when beef or pork insulin is used in human beings. All variations in the hormone between species are confined to amino acids in the middle of the molecule. These variations are so insignificant that all purified insulins are equally active in all animals. Pigs and steers taken to the slaughterhouse thus perform a service to man beyond putting meat on his table. Their pancreases are collected and shipped to chemical and drug firms to be processed for insulin to be used by human diabetics. Much of the insulin made in the United States is manufactured in Indianapolis, Indiana, where Eli Lilly & Co. receives frozen pancreases shipped from the great stockyards and slaughterhouses of Chicago, as well as the same by-products from the meat-packing firms in its own backyard, so to speak, in Indianapolis. In countries where the meat-packing industry would not provide a sufficient source of supply, other shifts are employed. Most of the insulin used in Japan, for instance, is made from fish.

Despite the apparent abundance of the supply of animal insulin and the operation of other factors, such as the improvement of diabetes control in some obese persons by purely dietary regulations, scientists pressed the search for some effective insulin substitute. The discomfort, hazard, and inconvenience of insulin injection was sufficient spur. Furthermore, the operation of all the factors outlined above was not fully appreciated at the time much of the work was done. Some success has been achieved with oral hypoglycemic agents.

Sulfanilimide and its derivatives had been developed in the forties and used to control bacterial infection. These drugs provided a starting point. A French physician treating patients with these particular agents found that they became hypoglycemic, that is, their blood sugar levels were lowered. The idea was not much developed during the war, but by about 1950 research was well underway. One particularly successful group of drugs, the sulfonylureas, has descendants and modified versions on the market today. These substances presumably act by causing insulin's release from the pancreas. So they are effective only in those diabetics who do have some insulin but are either not producing enough or are not liberating it freely from the pancreas . . . about 30 percent of the cases, perhaps. These persons are most frequently found in Dr. Dolger's second group: usually they are the overweight, often middle-aged persons who develop diabetes late. These sulfonamide-like compounds, the sulfonylureas, can be taken effectively by mouth, making them far preferable to insulin injections once or twice a day. Some concern arose, however, over the problem of *beta* cell exhaustion from overwork, a problem already noted in long-continued maintenance of cases of steroid diabetes. The overstimulation of already patently inadequate insulin-secreting machinery must be considered a possible danger, although no general tendency in that direction resulting from sulfonylurea treatment has yet been noted.

Phenformin, another widely-used compound, has a mechanism of action that is not at all understood. This drug induces hypoglycemia in animals and humans with neither exogenous nor endogenous insulin, indicating that its effect is not upon insulin release and utilization at all. In fact, phenformin and other diguanides may not correct any defect fundamentally and specifically *diabetic* at all. They are most useful in cases of mild diabetes to prepare the organism to be more receptive to exogenous insulin, an area where the sulfonylureas also are most successful. The principal disadvantage of phenformin is its high toxicity. None of the oral hypoglycemic agents are really substitutes for insulin. Their primary role is to improve utilization of existing endogenous insulin, or to prepare the body for the most efficient use of exogenous insulin used in conjunction with them, in quantities much lower than would otherwise be possible.

The Structure and Synthesis of Insulin

Although many of the factors mentioned above have combined to relieve the practical pressure to develop a synthetic insulin or insulin substitute, the search has gone on. Today, synthetic insulin is important primarily for advancing the understanding of diabetes and hormone actions.

The basis for synthetic insulin was laid down by Frederick Sanger of Cambridge University, who received the Nobel Prize in chemistry in 1958 for first elucidating the structure of the insulin molecule. The basic principles of protein chemistry had been firmly established in 1943: all proteins are built from amino acid residues bound by peptide bonds to form long chains. It was known that twenty different amino acids were present in most mammalian proteins, and chemical analysis could generally determine how many residues of each were present in a given protein. And yet, scientists remained in the dark about the order of these "beads" on their "chain", and it appeared that most of the biological and chemical properties of the proteins were dependent more upon the *order* of amino acids than upon the mere quantity of various amino acids in the chains. Sanger's work clarified the existence of two chains of polypeptides that together compose the insulin molecule, and the existence and location of the sulfur bridges that hold the two chains together.

This definition of structure paved the way for efforts by P. G. Katsoyannis in this country, H. Zahn in West Germany, and a group of Chinese scientists in Peking and Shanghai, all of whom began a lengthy series of experiments in an attempt to give a final proof to Sanger's definition by taking an insulin molecule apart in the laboratory and then putting it back together again, piece by piece, according to Sanger's plan.

This is no easy task. Consider dropping two strands of a necklace on the floor of a darkened theater. All the pearls slide off the strings and scatter. In addition, the few links that held the two strands together in the first place have also been broken and you have a hard time remembering the order in which the pearls came. Now make the pearls on the floor gummy or sticky—these amino acids can and readily do recombine in all manner of possible combinations besides the desired, essential, and only biologically active one. The pearls keep sticking together in random clumps. It is absolutely necessary that the pearls go back on their strands, each one to its proper place on the proper strand, but the sticky things resist being separated, and the house lights cannot be turned on to make the process any easier. Size is not much help in arranging the little things either since they are all about the same size.

If your strands of pearls really were the two chains of insulin there would be twenty-one amino acid "pearls" in the A-chain, which is acidic in composition, and thirty in the B-chain, which is basic in composition. The two links holding the two chains together would be composed of sulfur atoms, and another sulfur atom linkage would compose a "superstructure" or "bridge" in chain A. Highly sophisticated chemical procedures and processes are required first to align the fifty-one amino acids properly in their two chains, then to link the two and create the disulfide superstructure in the A-chain.

Dr. Panayotis G. Katsoyannis was the first to announce a limited success, crowning five years of hard labor by his research team at the University of Pittsburgh. The new product developed by Dr. Katsoyannis and his associates closely resembled the natural animal product, and it had some—although, as it later turned out, disappointingly small—biological activity. It was the first synthesized chemical to produce *in vitro* biological activities connected with naturally-occurring proteins. At the time of his initial announcement,

however, Dr. Katsoyannis and his co-workers had synthetically constructed but only partially purified the insulin B-chain, although total
success had been achieved in assembling the A-chain from component parts and purifying it. Before the work could be acclaimed
a total success, the purification of the B-chain and recombination
with the A-chain were required.

The synthetic A-chain from Dr. Katsoyannis' laboratories
was sent to G. H. Dixon at the University of Toronto, another pio-
neer in the field. Dixon combined this synthetic A-chain with a natural insulin B-chain to obtain an insulin with full biological activity.
At the stages of purification then possible, the synthetic B-chain
derived by Dr. Katsoyannis showed only slight hormonal activity
in combination with either natural or synthetic A-chains. Nor could
Dr. Katsoyannis himself report more than slight chemical activity
when, using Dixon's method, he joined his two synthetic chains.
Anyone who has labored hours, days, or months over anything mechanical or functional, a hot-rod, a hi-fi component system, model
trains, cabinetry where doors and drawers must fit and work, can
share to some degree the disappointment that must have swept over
these researchers who, after years of thought and effort, trial and
error, partial failure and partial success, had their apparently per-
fectly-formed synthetic molecule before them, only to find that it
would not work.

That was 1963. In 1965, Chinese scientists from Peking and
Shanghai reported their findings in the low-circulation English language journal *Scientia Sinica*. The November issue of this journal
first reported the total synthesis of bovine insulin possessing the
full biological activity of natural insulin.

The scientific community in the world at large, however, was
forced to wait for the April, 1966 issue of *Scientia Sinica* for detailed
descriptions of the methods used by the groups from the Academica
Sinica, Shanghai, and Peking University. In this article there was
more than the desired scientific account of methods used and results
obtained, which would enable Western scientists to duplicate procedures and check the validity of results. The communist regime in
Peking, apparently fully satisfied that the Peking-Shanghai group's
methods can be reproduced successfully and that their conclusions
are correct, has seemingly decided to stake its prestige on the scien-

tists' discovery. The April article teems with political slogans: "Holding aloft the great red banner of Chairman Mao Tse-Tung's thinking and manifesting the superiority of the socialist system, we have achieved, under the correct leadership of our party, the total synthesis of bovine insulin." The achievement is cited as fulfilling the prediction of Engels ninety years before to the effect that, once man knew what the protein molecules of life were, he would make them himself; and the pathway to the synthesis of life itself from organic compounds is regarded as opened by this discovery. What will surely cause considerable controversy in the scientific community is that Dr. Katsoyannis of the U.S.A. is attacked directly and rather unnecessarily.

In any case, the tone of the April *Scientia Sinica* article soon becomes considerably cooler, less jargon-ridden and one more worthy of competent scientists who are fully aware of the significance of their work. Kung Yueh-ting and his associates, many of whom were trained in the West and hold Ph.D's from universities in the free world, claim ten-to-fifty-fold increases in specific activity of the synthetic insulin they have produced. The synthetic protein in crystalline form possessed insulin activity greater then 20 insulin units per milligram, by the mouse-convulsion method of assay, according to Kung and his co-workers.

The Chinese work is the result of seven years of concentrated effort. The publications of these scientists reveal their complete awareness of Western work and thinking on protein structure and function. A paragraph in their account even echoes the comments made by the English student of the structure of whale myoglobin, John Kendrews, when he received the Nobel Prize in Stockholm in 1962:

> The success achieved in the synthesis of crystalline insulin, first from its natural chains and subsequently from its synthetic chains, proves that once the amino acids are in correct sequence, the formation of the *alpha* helix and its coiling or folding into the proper conformation will follow if suitable conditions are provided. In other words, the primary structure of the protein is able to determine, to a large extent, its higher-ordered structure.

The successful synthesis of insulin has paved the way for the synthesis of larger proteins and of proteins with multiple polypeptide chains linked through disulfide bonds.*

Whether these reports from China will indeed be proven valid remains to be seen. It is apparent that the scientists and their political masters are quite sure of themselves. If the results claimed are indeed valid, the synthesis of insulin with biological activity is a landmark in the history of endocrinology.

SUPPLEMENTAL READING

Weber, G., Editor, Advances in Enzyme Regulation, *1, 2, 3,* and *4,* Pergamon Press, New York.

Gorman, A., Editor, Comparative Endocrinology, John Wiley & Sons, New York.

Gardiner-Hill, H., Editor, Modern Trends in Endocrinology, 2nd series, Paul B. Hoeber, Inc., Medical Book Department of Harper & Brothers, New York.

* For this and other quotations directly from the hard-to-acquire *Scientia Sinica* April article, a great debt is owed to the magazine *Science,* a journal of the American Association for the Advancement of Science, Vol. 153, 281–83, 15 July 1966, which reprints large portions of the scarce original.

Chapter 21

Allergies and Sensitivities

Making a drug means taking a chance, but the odds are by far in your favor. Sometimes, however, adverse and anomalous reactions will occur. These are the price of effective drugs. Unless a chemical is pharamcologically inert (and thus useless), some unwanted effects in some patients are inevitable, assuming the drug is taken by enough people. Even a therapeutically-inert chemical—foreign to the body—may be "sensitizing" to some people, acting to elicit an allergic reaction. The unparalleled number of drugs introduced and distributed in the past ten years has only confirmed scientists' fears, fears of adverse reactions coming from the simple matter of statistical probability.

A sampling of the literature on adverse drug reactions involves a risk of error. But an idea of the frequency can still be obtained by reviewing the kinds of reactions that physicians feel constrained to report. Curiously, reactions of unknown cause head the list. They account for about 35 to 40 percent of severe reactions. Allergic reactions account for 20 to 30 percent, and direct toxic reactions resulting from undesired pharmacological effect, 15 to 20 percent.

A trend toward a phenomenon known as polypharmacy—the simultaneous use of a number of drugs—increases the likelihood of adverse interactions between and among drugs. Polypharmacy, of course, obscures the relationship of any one drug and a sensitivity. A recent survey in the Johns Hopkins Hospital showed that among patients treated with a particular antibiotic a minimum of six and maximum of thirty-five other drugs were being administered simultaneously. When a patient is desperately ill, many drugs may be needed. Using the minimal number at any one time is the best way to avoid unexpected complications due to interactions between drugs.

Adverse Reactions: Types and Causes

An adverse reaction is quite simply one that is both unexpected and undesired. Although dealing with uncertain numerators

365

and unknown denominators, one can make several generalizations about the types of these reactions. Drugs that are used primarily because they are known to be toxic in the first place—such as drugs used for treating cancers—will almost always produce toxic side effects. Drugs that have a wide range of effects other than the desired therapeutic effect will also produce undesired, though usually minor, reactions in most patients. The phenothiazines, for example, may not only induce a state of tranquilization, but lower the blood pressure as well. This becomes serious in some patients for whom lowering of blood pressure brings on fainting spells.

There are several factors which contribute to reactions of the person taking the drug:

1. Generally, the older the patient, the more susceptible he is to unexpected or exaggerated drug effects. Infants and very young children present special problems because they may not be able to metabolize drugs as well as adults do. Some infants have died from doses of the antibiotic chloramphenicol; in proportionate amounts this drug would have been innocuous to adults. Young adults, who are least likely to need drugs, are most resistant to adverse reactions.

2. Although the science of pharmacogenetics—genetic differences between people in the way they respond to drugs—is still relatively new, heredity is known to play an important role. A personal history of allergies such as hay fever, asthma or eczema, does not mean allergic reactions to drugs are inevitable, but it increases the probability. A usual dose of isoniazid, a drug used for treating tuberculosis, may produce a toxic reaction, neuritis, in a patient who is genetically unable to metabolize the drug at the normal rate.

3. The part played by racial variables is undetermined; few reports specify the race of the patients studied. One racial hereditary trait, prominent in many people of Negro, Mediterranean, or Japanese ancestry, is manifested by a deficiency of a certain enzyme in the red blood cells, a deficiency that under ordinary circumstances is harmless. When such patients get certain drugs, chiefly those used for treating malaria, or certain sulfa drugs, the precarious balance is tipped and a rapid destruction of red blood cells may lead to severe anemia (see the chapter on "Heredity and Drugs").

4. Distribution of adverse reactions according to sex is

equally uncertain. Some types of reactions do tend to occur predominantly in males, while others are seen more commonly in females.

5. Reactivity may also be influenced by nutritional state, concurrent illness other than the one for which a drug is given, or other therapy.

6. The pathway of administration also influences the type of untoward effect.

Anaphylaxis is a severe allergic reaction which may occur within minutes after the injection of a drug like penicillin. The skin is reddened, breathing becomes difficult as in asthma, and shock ensues. Unless promptly treated with an injection of epinephrine (Adrenalin), these reactions may be fatal. Many people sensitive to penicillin, however, develop such reactions only when given a later injection.

If a drug is applied to the skin repetitively, a local allergic reaction may occur in the skin, manifested by peeling and weeping lesions (eczema).

The longer the treatment and the larger the dose, the greater is the likelihood of adverse reactions. Some reactions are the result of a build-up of toxic levels of the drug over a period of time. This This is due to accumulation of the drug in the body when it is given more rapidly than it can be inactivated or excreted. Even allergic reactions are dependent to some degree on the dose of antigenic material. Some preparations of drugs, especially those designed for slow absorption following an injection into tissues, contain substances such as oils and waxes which either increase the possibility of allergic reactions or may be directly damaging to tissues. Also, administration of one drug along with others, as well as contamination of drugs or deterioration into different compounds, may produce adverse reactions which may be erroneously attributed to the initial drug. Some orally-taken drugs cause less severe reactions, perhaps because they are absorbed slowly from the gastrointestinal tract.

Allergies to Drugs

An antigen is a large protein foreign to the body; upon entering the body, the antigen stimulates formation of a defensive "antibody." If the antigenic material is a disease-producing bacterium, such as the one which causes typhoid fever, previous immunization by typhoid vaccine will have elicited antibodies that protect against the disease. However, the body's recognition system is too good—all foreign antigens are perceived as potentially harmful. When a drug becomes an antigen by combining with a body protein, it produces allergic reactions. These reactions to drugs resemble allergic reactions to the naturally-occurring protein antigens in a number of ways:

1. A brief induction period is needed for the formation of the antibody.
2. Reexposure to the antigen (specifically readministration of the drug) usually evokes an acute, immediate response from the body.
3. Clinical reactions are basically similar.
4. Antiallergic agents may influence the immediate response.
5. Tolerance or desensitization may develop.

The differences, however, are as striking:

1. The incidence of allergies to drugs is relatively low considering the vast number of drugs presently being administered.
2. Antibodies are difficult to demonstrate.
3. Readministration of the simple chemical often fails to reproduce the same response.
4. Anaphylaxis is comparatively rare.
5. Allergic reactions may be localized in a single organ, like the liver, or a single cell type, such as the thrombocyte (blood platelet).

To become antigenic, a drug must be reactive enough to form a strong bond with a protein. A sufficient amount of a suitable protein "carrier" must be available to the drug to form the antigen. Then, the resultant complex must be recognized as "foreign" and elicit an antibody response. In this way, the body can protect itself with an army of antibodies against the invading army of the drug-protein antigens.

There are clinically two kinds of allergic responses—the immediate and the delayed. An immediate reaction arises when the exposure has occurred primarily by injection, ingestion, or inhalation, and when the antigenic complex is both soluble and rapidly absorbed. Topical contact or injection directly into the skin is more likely to lead to a delayed reaction, because it takes longer for the drug to be absorbed. Immediate reactions may be manifested by signs and symptoms characteristic of anaphylaxis, as for example: serum sickness (fever, lymph node swelling, pains in the joints, rash, a decrease in the number of white blood cells, or neuritis); or atopy (asthma, running nose, hives, or other rashes). Delayed reactions are usually manifested as a contact dermatitis or a persistent patch of skin eruption which is always associated with taking a certain type of drug.

Sensitivity to light represents a different kind of allergic mechanism, one evoked by an external stimulus. A true photoallergic reaction involves a chemical change of the drug or metabolite produced by exposure to ultraviolet light. The altered product forms a complex that may be locally or systemically antigenic. On the other hand, a phototoxic reaction is an exaggeration of usual effects of light due to the presence of the drug. An example is severe sunburn in patients taking certain phenothiazine tranquilizers; other drugs that may provoke such phototoxic reactions are sulfa drugs, oral antidiabetic drugs and some of the newer diuretics—all somewhat related chemically.

Therapeutic Effects and Adverse Reactions

The therapeutic range of a drug is broadly the range of dosage within which the drug exerts its optimal effect. Sometimes the therapeutic range is very close to the toxic range. Digitalis is an example of a drug which, in order to be used properly, *must* be given virtually to the point of producing minor toxic reactions. Toxic effects most commonly represent extensions of useful therapeutic actions. The customary dosage of a drug is at best a *compromise,* representing the center of a considerably wide range of normal variation. Exaggerated responses may reflect the extremes of individual variations in absorption, metabolism, excretion, or susceptibility to the action of a drug; for example, an unexpected excessive sedation can be produced by a customary dose of barbiturate; and excessive hypoglycemia may follow the use of tolbutamide. The rate of absorption of hexamethonium, a drug lowering blood pressure, varies widely, and different patients may display an eightfold variation in the rate of metabolism of coumarin anticoagulants.

A therapeutically-useful drug may be harmful when it affects an organ other than the target organ. Most drugs that affect the autonomic nervous system are used for an effect on a selected part of this system, but all these agents act on the entire system to a greater or lesser extent, such as the salivary glands and bowels, producing side effects of dry mouth and constipation. All but the desired action may be considered undesired actions. Anticancer drugs may impair the growth of normal cells—the bone marrow and mucous membrane—as well as the growth of malignant cells. Vasoconstriction of cranial arteries effected by ergotamine is useful when treating patients with migraine attacks, but if the constriction occurs in a narrowed coronary artery, one may have a heart attack as a complication.

Concurrent disease other than the one for which a drug is administered may influence the metabolism or excretion of the drug or a person's susceptibility to its action. Genetic predisposition may cause similar effects. Swelling of the liver with accumulated blood, associated with congestive heart failure, may completely change the requirements of anticoagulants administered for coronary arteriosclerosis by altering the liver's metabolism of the drug. Impaired function of the kidneys may lead to a greatly increased blood concentration of antibiotics and to direct toxic effects.

Combinations of drugs, or combination with another form of therapy, may alter the toxic potential. Some antidepressants are called monoamine oxidase inhibitors because they impair the action of this enzyme in the body. This enzymatic impairment may be essential to their therapeutic value for treating mental depression, yet it will severely alter the action of certain other drugs, such as barbiturates, the analgesic meperidine, and various drugs which increase blood pressure, such as epinephrine. Even some items of the diet, ordinarily quite harmless, such as cheddar cheese, pickled herring or wine may become toxic in the presence of this enzymatic inhibition, resulting in acute attacks of high blood pressure, sometimes associated with brain hemorrhage. Simultaneous administration of monoamine oxidase inhibitors with other types of antidepressants, such as imipramine and amitriptyline, may produce a combined effect *greater than the sum of both drugs taken separately;* patients may become overexcited, suffer convulsions, develop high fevers, lapse into coma or die from such combinations.

Nondrug therapy may also influence a drug's toxic potential. X-ray treatment is often used along with certain drugs for treating cancers. As both types of treatment depress the blood-forming functions of the bone marrow, their concurrent use makes this depression all the more severe.

The Nontherapeutic Effects of Drugs

Drugs rarely act in just one way, or have just one pharmacodynamic effect. Sometimes a separate action that constitutes a side effect in one situation, as drowsiness from the antihistamines, may be turned to advantage: antihistamines as sedatives. Pharmacological doses of adrenal steroids used for treating inflammatory or allergic disorders are much larger than the usual amounts of such steroids physiologically secreted by the glands. Such pharmacological doses may produce a clinical pattern (Cushing's syndrome) closely resembling that seen in tumors of the adrenal gland, or a simple exaggeration of the physiological functions of the steroids. Diphenylhydantoin, one of the most effective drugs for treating epilepsy, is also—unavoidably—an antagonist of folic acid, a vitamin necessary for the proper development of red blood cells. Some epileptics being treated with this drug may develop an anemia very much like that of pernicious anemia.

Diuretics eliminate excess sodium from the body, and thus are useful in treating heart failure and high blood pressure. Unfortunately, some diuretics, e.g. thiazides, cause increased potassium excretion and may produce muscle weakness or increase the possibility of digitalis toxicity. Morphine kills pain, but may adversely affect the intestinal tract.

This list of unusual adverse reactions could go on for pages; only a few more will be presented. Coma associated with liver failure, as in advanced cirrhosis of the liver, may be aggravated by the use of nitrogen-containing drugs such as thiazide diuretics. Atropine or epinephrine may precipitate an attack of narrow-angle glaucoma in a patient who is genetically predisposed to this disease. Acute porphyria is a genetic disease in which there is a tendency for the body to overproduce the red blood pigment. A single dose of a barbiturate to such a susceptible individual may further aggravate this tendency, causing an acute, and possibly fatal, attack of the illness.

Other Types of Adverse Reactions

The largest group of toxic reactions to drugs are from an "uncertain cause"—drug reactions without any explanation. Sometimes these reactions seem to be allergic, while some appear to be more directly attributable to drug toxicity. They may or may not be associated with the size of the dose or the duration of treatment. An anaphylaxis-like reaction following administration of the first dose of meprobamate suggests an allergic reaction. But it may reflect only the usual capacity of this drug to release histamine in some persons. Many features of jaundice (from impaired outflow of bile) following the use of phenothiazines suggest an allergic reaction: fever, narrow time range of onset, frequent appearance on rechallenge. But the case is far from proved.

On the other hand, a syndrome somewhat like rheumatoid arthritis, or systemic lupus erythematosus, may occur during long-term treatment with the antihypertensive drug, hydralazine. Quite possibly, this reaction represents a latent genetic predisposition to the disease which, in some manner, is aggravated by the drug.

Massive death of liver cells, associated with the use of iproniazid (an antidepressant drug no longer available for use), pyrazinamide (a drug employed rarely in the treatment of tuberculosis), or the sulfa drug sulfamethoxypyridazine, is probably due to toxic metabolites of these drugs.

Older doctors and their patients well remember the small kidney stones associated with the use of the sulfonamides; these are still observed occasionally. Chloroquine, used for treating rheumatoid arthritis, and some phenothiazine derivatives, which have a strong affinity for melanin-containing structures, may be deposited in some parts of the eye, damaging sight. Gold salts and silver proteinate also may be deposited in the cornea.

Recording Drug Reactions

Unless a patient dies or the disease from which he suffers becomes quite seriously complicated, an adverse reaction—one that is both unexpected and undesired—is likely to be forgotten. Consequently, published reports of adverse reactions to drugs represent only a small fraction of the total that occur. Moreover, such data in outpatients are even less complete than reports of unusual reactions in hospitalized patients. Minor reactions, such as the nausea or bloating that some women experience from oral contraceptives, are often tolerated. The physician seldom reports such reactions, although the medication may be stopped.

The Food and Drug Administration (FDA) and the American Medical Association (AMA) are currently sponsoring programs to obtain more adequate data. These programs show considerable promise. Through its Division of Research and Reference, the FDA solicits reports of adverse reactions and publishes a weekly compilation of abstracts from the literature. The Council on Drugs of the AMA now includes a section on Adverse Drug Reactions. This is an extension of a section formerly concerned only with abnormal blood reactions resulting from drugs. Periodically, brief review articles concerning special problems of drug reactions appear in the Journal of the AMA. Doctors are asked to report any suspected adverse reaction to either of these agencies—a liason now exists between them—and to use their resources to learn of current developments. Reporting mechanisms like these should serve as an "early warning radar." If any new drug had a totally unexpected complication, such as the deformities in unborn children produced by thalidomide, the relationship would be quickly detected and only a few, rather than many, individuals would be affected.

All physicians would like to have effective drugs without serious side effects. Pharmaceutical chemists and pharmacologists are constantly striving to produce drugs which are effective but carry less risk of toxic reactions. We can only hope those continuing efforts will result in safer agents for the treatment of disease.

Chapter 22

Our Response to Drugs

No rule is so general, which
admits not some exception.

Robert Burton
Anatomy of Melancholy, Part I,
Sect. 2, Memb. 2, Subsect. 3.

T he more scientists learn about the biological processes of life, the more they may appreciate the truth of Burton's classic rule of thumb. In nature, paradoxically, the rule is often variability rather than sameness; to find a better example of this than the response of an organism to a foreign chemical would be difficult. The pharmacologist and the physician seek for or base their treatment of disease on similarities of human reaction to drugs, yet they continue to be plagued by the differences.

Some factors that account for variability in responses of individuals to drugs have been defined, but many more remain to be identified. Some of those which have been already recognized and investigated rather thoroughly include: (1) the relationship between the dosage of a particular chemical and the biological effect produced, (2) the effect of the route of administration, (3) the form in which the drug is administered, (4) the influence of other environmental factors (such as other drugs, foods, physical conditions, socio-economic influences), and (5) variables within the organism which are either difficult or impossible to alter or to control.

Dose—Response Relationships

Even in antiquity it was realized that there is a relationship between the amount of a drug that is given a person and the intensity of its effect. This dose-effect relationship was implicitly sensed for several millennia before any attempt was made to quantify it. Indeed, the solid establishment of pharmacology as a quantitative science did not come until 1927. At that time the English mathematician J. W. Trevan (1887–1955) published his classic report on "Statistical methods for estimation of biological variations in toxicity determinations." A consultant for a well-known drug company in London, he had much to do with the development of methods for biological assay and standardization.

Trevan showed that there is a Gaussian (normal) distribution of variations in the intensity of response by biological material to a given dosage of a drug, and that if these intensities are summated for increasing dosage in accordance with the percentage of the total number of living specimens responding, the resulting relation is expressed graphically as a sigmoid (S-shaped) curve. Many refinements are possible with this sort of graphic representation, but the essential features were established by Trevan and extended by A. J. Clark (1885–1941). Clark not only analyzed various aspects of the dose-effect relationship but also established quantification in time-concentration relationships. Time is often a crucial biological factor.

It is rather remarkable that it took so long for a firm scientific basis to be provided for such an ancient idea as the relationship between a dose of a drug and the effect it might produce. There still, in fact, remain many aspects of dose-effect and time-concentration relationships that are not ordinarily understood by those who employ chemicals for their biological effects—physicians, dentists, or members of other health professions, or by agriculturists, or indeed by scientists in general. The matter is of practical importance when a physician tries to evaluate the relative merits of similar chemical agents which may be recommended for the same purpose. The "safety factor" is involved. The idea is to develop a drug with as wide a spread as possible between the dosage which will produce the effect desired and the dosage which may produce some unwanted, even lethal, effect.

Even for scientific purposes, drugs are often compared on the basis of the ratio between the dosage that will produce 50 percent of the effect desired and the dosage that may kill 50 percent of the samples of living material. This is the familiar ratio of ED_{50} (effective dose 50) to LD_{50} (lethal dose 50). In a practical way, however, no physician is interested in the dosage that will give the effect he desires in only half of his patients, and certainly no physician in his right mind gives a rap about dosage that will kill half of his patients. Much more significant, in practice, is the relationship between ED_{99} and LD_1. However, since this is not as readily obtained by experimental methods, new drugs are often introduced clinically on the basis of a "safety factor" represented by the ratio of ED_{50} to LD_{50}. This is dangerous.

Those who use chemicals to produce an effect on living material are concerned with the factors which determine the intensity of activity. These factors can be expressed in a shorthand manner:

$$i = (f) \, D \, \frac{rA}{rE} \, PS$$

This statement indicates that the intensity of action of a chemical on biological material is determined by dosage (D) in terms of mass of chemical per mass of living material; the ratio of the rate of absorption and distribution of the chemical through the living material (rA) to the rate of detoxification or excretion of the chemical from the living material (rE); the physical-chemical properties of the chemical (P), which really determine the activity of the chemical on living material; and then (S), the specific and peculiar characteristics of the living material concerned, including the organizational status (in terms of macromolecules or ecological milieus), its age, its metabolic state, its allergic sensitivity, its pathological status, and such integrating factors as enzyme systems, neuro-hormonal systems, and sex.

It is clear that there may be quite precise quantification of such factors as dosage, rates of absorption, distribution, detoxification and excretion, and physical-chemical properties. These factors are capable of precise scientific study, with results that may be expressed quantitatively. The product of dosage and the ratio of the rate of absorption and distribution of a drug to the rate of detoxification and excretion will give the concentration of the drug in the living material involved at any specific time after its administration. It is this concentration, with its so-called mass action effect, which is a predominant factor in drug action.

On the other hand, because of the peculiarities of the specific living material concerned, many judgment factors are involved. The application of pharmacology to medical affairs involves the judgment of the clinician and is a matter of long experience and wisdom. We are beginning to realize that similar judgment factors are involved in applying pharmacological knowledge to such aspects of living material as are involved in social organization or ecological milieus.

Route of Administration

The dose of a drug required to produce the effect the physician seeks will be determined by the manner in which it is introduced into the body. There are at least six ways of administering a drug. The simplest, least expensive, and most popular method is oral administration. Yet there are times when a doctor simply cannot prescribe a pill. Some pills, for example, cannot be absorbed by the gastrointestinal tract; certain types of antibiotics, and other orally-administered drugs cause nausea and vomiting. Other routes must then be employed.

A major route of administration is injection. The hypodermic needle is actually a very old instrument. As early as the 17th century Charles Boyle and Christopher Wren used quills to inject substances into the body. In 1853 Alexander Wood perfected the hypodermic needle, and this form of injection has been continually in use. Jet injection was introduced in 1947; by means of a high velocity "jet stream" the drug enters the body with great force through a microfine orifice, an orifice one thirtieth the size of a standard 18 gauge needle. There is virtually no pain with this very fast method. This form of injection has the additional advantage of rapidity—for mass inoculation and immunization programs.

Parenteral is a generic term applied to various forms of injection. Among these are the *intramuscular,* which is an injection made by penetrating through layers of the skin into layers of the skeletal muscle; *intravenous,* an injection made directly into a vein; *subcutaneous,* the insertion of a hypodermic needle through layers of the skin; *intrathecal,* insertion of the needle through the interspinous spaces into the spinal fluid within the backbone. Also, there is *bone marrow* injection, the insertion of a special type of needle directly into the bone; *intraperitoneal,* an injection made through the abdominal wall and into the abdominal cavity.

There are, of course, advantages and disadvantages to any one method. Subcutaneous injections produce a relatively quick response. Intravenous injections are rapidly effective; in fact, a drug injected intravenously can reach the brain in less than half a minute. Interspinal or intrathecal injections are used in spinal anesthesia.

The Vehicles of Drugs

Dosage, and in turn the response to a drug, can be affected by the form in which it is administered. Television advertising has made the public conscious of the fast-acting pill and the prolonged time-release capsule. Much can be accomplished in regulating drug effect by choice of an appropriate form and vehicle for administration.

First, there are the several solvents, used for making drugs more palatable. *Waters* are aqueous solutions of volatile substances. These make excellent solvent for certain drugs such as bromides and the salicylates (aspirin). Peppermint, spearmint, and cinnamon are among the more typical waters.

Hydro-alcoholic solutions of medical substances, sweetened and flavored, are called *elixirs*. There are aromatic, simple, or orange elixirs, each containing a high 22 percent of alcohol; elixirs are famous for masking that unpleasant taste. Other drugs can be in *syrups*. Some can be demulcent; these are soothing to the mucous membrane of the throat and are the common cough syrups, such as cherry, wild cherry, or cocoa. Also there are the *emulsions*, fixed oils in water, again to prevent a disagreeable taste. Milk of magnesia is usually referred to as a *mixture*. A number of precipitates and a supernatent fluid are combined in mixtures. *Tinctures* are made from vegetable drugs and are alcoholic or hydro-alcoholic. So much for the liquid forms.

Solid dosage forms have an even greater variety. First, there are the *powders*. Sometimes these powders effervesce in water. Capsules are nothing but tasteless gelatins into which powders are packed, tightly or loosely. A *tablet* is simply a powder that has been pressed mechanically into a small, discoid shape. Starch is usually a component of tablets and, upon contact with water, will usually swell. This, of course leads to immediate disintegration.

A *pill*, believe it or not, does have a specific scientific definition. Powdered drugs can be mixed with glucose or honey for adhesion. When cut into the desirable weights or sizes, they are called pills.

There are, of course, other forms of medication, and several are very common. *Liniments* are simply liquid preparations that one rubs onto the skin; for example, camphor and soap liniment. *Ointments* are greasy substances intended for local application to the skin. *Suppositories* are solid, for insertion into body orifices. They can be vaginal, urethral, or rectal. Coca butter, the oil of theobroma, and glycerated gelatin are the most familiar suppositories. A *lotion* is a liquid that is applied to the skin and quickly evaporates. The suspended ingredient remains as a film on the skin; calamine lotion is a typical example.

The Prolonged-Action Capsule

Medical scientists have performed experiments on the rate at which capsules dissolve. They have developed something called prolonged-action capsules—several capsules at once, one inside the other, like the stages of a space rocket. Thus, one will go off immediately after ingestion; another will go off four hours later; and perhaps a third eight hours later. This is highly valuable when a doctor must administer uniform medication which produces relatively uniform effects over a longer period of time.

The only thing about which a doctor can be certain when he prescribes a drug is that it will not be taken as directed. Any preparation that would simplify the taking of a drug by requiring fewer doses might improve this situation. This is another advantage of the oral prolonged-action preparations.

The first prolonged-action drug was introduced about 1950. By 1959 approximately 180 different products were available in oral prolonged-action form; about two thirds of the *anoretics* (appetite suppressants) and 40 percent of the antihistamines are of this type. Popularity of this kind of drug preparation is increasing.

The various types of preparations are also increasing. Some take the form of tablets within tablets—repeat action. Other tablets are made to disintegrate slowly in the gastrointestinal tract. And there are pellets within capsules, special slowly-dissolving salts of drugs, or drugs imbedded in inert plastic matrices. But almost without exception, prolonged-action dose forms are more expensive than the same doses in the usual capsule or tablet form.

Some situations do not, of course, require prolonged-action forms of drugs. If a drug is intrinsically long-acting, such as certain barbiturates, phenothiazines, reserpine, thyroid extract, digitalis, why try to improve upon nature's own pharmacology? If immediacy of effect and a short duration of action are desired, prolonged action would actually defeat the aim. If tolerance is likely to occur, as with nitrates or ephedrine, single doses as required are preferred, since sustained levels seem to facilitate the development of tolerance. Finally one would hesitate to use prolonged-action forms containing two to four times the usual single dosage, since this amount might be dangerous if by chance it were immediately absorbed.

Until recently, comparatively little investigative work has been done to verify claims made for oral prolonged-action medications. Quantitative studies by the Canadian Food and Drug Laboratories have established that for complete absorption of a drug tablets should dissolve under experimental conditions in less than 60 minutes, that physiologic availability is best measured by urinary output of drug over timed periods, and that by measuring rates of urinary excretion one can demonstrate the presence or absence of prolonged action. With so little time for effective absorption of a drug, any preparation that delays this process might very likely result in a smaller actual dose of the drug being absorbed than might be predicted from the total amount present in the capsule or tablet. It is generally agreed that, under experimental conditions, tests of prolonged release of drugs are completely inadequate.

Studies of trimeprazine used both chemical determinations and a study of blood and urine. These disproved that one triple dose in the prolonged-action form was equivalent to three single doses in tablet form given at 4-hour intervals. With most drugs, a larger dose acts over a longer period of time than a smaller dose. Thus, it has been shown that valid comparison of results requires that identical amounts of drug be administered in the same way.

Dr. Leo E. Hollister has compared equal single doses of drugs as prolonged-action preparations and as conventional tablets. In one of his studies the tranquilizer meprobamate, commonly known as Equanil or Miltown, was taken in 800 mg doses as compressed tablets and as two kinds of prolonged-action capsules by 16 volunteer subjects. Following both prolonged-action capsules, plasma levels of the drug were significantly higher 8 hours and 12 hours later. But the differences were of minor clinical importance.

A similar study of two phenothiazine derivatives failed to demonstrate prolonged action of either preparation: capsuled pellets in the case of chlorpromazine, tablets of thioridazine with retarding agents in the other case. Both of these phenothiazine derivatives have an intrinsically prolonged action regardless of their formulation. Further, judged by total urine recovery, evidence suggests that prolonged-action doses might be a less efficient form in which to administer these drugs.

The Human Variables

While the response of a biological system, e.g. the human organism, to a drug is dose-related, i.e., the magnitude of the response is directly related in some manner to the dose, the dose required to produce a given response is affected by several factors in the biological system. Some of these have been evaluated in detail. About others we have only a rather superficial understanding. Nonetheless, they have to be considered if an optimal effect is to be achieved.

Certainly age and weight play a role in determining the effects a given drug will produce. Generally speaking, infants are more sensitive than adults. Of particular importance here are drugs that affect the central nervous system, certain hormones that control growth, and agents that alter the water and acid-base composition of the body. Very young infants do not have the capacity to metabolize and detoxify certain drugs, e.g., the antibiotic chloramphenical. The physician has to be aware of these deficiencies and exercise appropriate care in administering certain drugs to the newborn. Formulas (based on age or weight) have been developed for calculating dosages of drugs for children and infants from known adult doses. While these generally provide fairly reliable values for children, they cannot be entirely relied on for infants. In the case of the latter, doses have been established empirically and must be memorized. Unfortunately such dosages are available for relatively few drugs. At the other end of the spectrum the picture is even less clear. Older individuals can respond to drugs in abnormal fashion. About all the physician has to go on in this situation is the knowledge that this portion of the population exhibits deviations from the normal, i.e., the response of the average member of the adult population.

Quite obviously body weight will have an influence on the ultimate concentration of a drug in the body and hence on the concentration it attains at its site of action. (The latter, of course, will determine the magnitude of the response.) Other factors being equal, a two hundred pound individual would be expected to exhibit less pronounced effects from a given dose of a drug than one weighing one hundred and thirty pounds. No absolute relationship has been established and the physician can only make adjustments of dosage based on experience for the excessively obese or lean individual. Although calculation of dosage on a weight basis in the research laboratory has been reasonably reliable for quantitative measurements, there is evidence to suggest that response may be related better to dose when the dose is expressed on some other basis, e.g. surface area of the animal.

Quite obviously sex hormones will result in different responses by the male and the female. Estrogens naturally cannot be expected to affect structures and functions in the male which only exist in the female. But there is evidence which suggests that sexual differences in drug effects extend beyond the more obvious. Women are stated to be more sensitive to the drug aminopyrine than men and may more frequently display an adverse reaction to such drugs as morphine.

The frequency with which a drug is given will depend on how fast it is inactivated and excreted. Giving it too often may result in its accumulation in the body, with possible toxicity. If administered too infrequently, the proper therapeutic effect will not be achieved; in some situations this can make the difference between life and death. For each drug an optimal dosage schedule has been established, based on the average individual. This works for the majority even though the true average is practically nonexistent, but there are certain individuals who deviate so much from the average because of a certain genetic make-up (see Chapter 23) that they require special attention. Only within the past few years has it been recognized that inherited differences may account for significant variation from the "normal" in rates of drug metabolism. On the basis of such knowledge an entirely new field of pharmacology, pharmacogenetics, has developed.

Repeated administration of a drug may create still another

problem—the development of tolerance or resistance on the part of the body to the effects of the drug. The mechanism underlying such tolerance is poorly understood, but it is nonetheless real. A notable example of drugs to which tolerance is rapidly developed are the narcotic analgesics—morphine being the prototype. Development of tolerance to the pain-relieving effects of morphine makes it necessary for the physician to progressively increase the dose to achieve the same degree of pain suppression when he is using it for treatment of chronic pain. Development of tolerance to certain sought-for effects of morphine on the brain makes it necessary for the addict to gradually increase the dose to achieve these. In either case addiction is the consequence (see Chapter 13). Not only may the body acquire tolerance, but an invading organism may develop resistance. This has been a particularly difficult problem with staphylococci (see Chapter 14).

When he is ill, an individual will often display a marked deviation from his normal response to drugs. Digitalis (see Chapter 5) in the patient with heart failure can increase blood flow to the tissues and hence improve the circulation. In the individual with normal heart function it can result in detrimental effects as a result of an increase in tone of peripheral vessels and a decrease in blood flow. Increased function of the thyroid gland markedly enhances the responsiveness to epinephrine (Adrenalin). Chronic diseases of the lungs may result in unusual sensitivity to agents, e.g. morphine, which depress respiration. Patients with the disease myasthenia gravis (see Chapter 8) are extremely responsive to the muscular paralyzing drug curare or the active material in curare, tubocuracine.

Certain foods or drugs may have a marked effect on another drug when it is administered. The consequences of eating certain types of cheese and other foods on the action of the monoamine oxidase inhibitors has been referred to in Chapter 11. In general, it is the unusual patient who receives no more than one drug. Most, when ill, receive four or five. A recent survey in one well-known hospital revealed that some patients were receiving as many as thirty different drugs. What variety of interactions might be encountered here? Multiple-drug therapy can result in anything from a rash to anaphylactic shock. Certain blood abnormalities from a combination of drug interactions may even be fatal. The liver, the most common center for detoxification of drugs, is a prominent danger zone. The old rule is that no drug is free of poisonous effects; two drugs merely serve to underscore this rule.

With the widespread use of drugs which affect behavior we naturally must take cognizance of the interaction between the environment and the response of the patient to these drugs. One only has to reflect on the influence of the surroundings in the individual's response to alcohol. Similarly, the subjective effects of LSD are determined to a great extent by the environmental input. In the laboratory one can find evidence of the importance of environment. The convulsions produced in a frog by injection of strychnine can be abolished by isolating him from the sensory input from his environment—by painting him with a solution of the local analgesic cocaine. Another convulsant, pentylenetetrazal (Metrazol) requires a significantly higher dose to produce convulsions in an isolated mouse than when he is grouped with other mice. We know relatively little about the influence of the environment on our responses to drugs, particularly those affecting behavior. Quite obviously this is a fruitful area to explore.

Chapter 23

Heredity and Drugs

O n 17 August 1961 an active 73-year-old man suffered a severe heart attack and was admitted to a hospital. Upon his recovery, which was slow and uneventful, his doctors decided to put him on a normal daily dose of warfarin. This common drug decreases the blood's capacity to clot, hopefully reducing the possibility of another attack. After a sample of the patient's blood was tested for clotting, no significant change was found. He was then referred to a research laboratory in hematology for observation. He continued to receive standard doses of warfarin for some time, but still showed no effects from the drug. The hematologist responded appropriately, however, and systematically increased the dosage. Now, in an average person, 7 milligrams per day will provide satisfactory protection against blood coagulation, but this patient required an astounding 145 milligrams daily before he obtained that protection. Only at a dose 21 times greater than normal did the patient finally respond to the drug. Moreover, the very high dosage of warfarin was in no way toxic to the patient; his body treated it like candy—the drug was absorbed and eliminated normally, but he seemed to be resistant to its effects. This might imply that the patient metabolized the drug much faster than normal (to account for his lack of response). The possibility was considered, but he was found to metabolize the drug no faster than normal individuals. Was there ever a similar reaction to warfarin? The doctors wondered. Then, in the same week, in another city, the patient's identical-twin brother also had a heart attack. Later, he was likewise given a standard amount of warfarin, and did not respond normally. He too needed what seemed to be an enormous overdose to show the expected drug effects.

The explanation of this problem lay in genetics, the study of hereditary factors. Strictly speaking, we do not inherit the color of

391

our eyes, the shape of our heads, or any other physical characteristic. Likewise, we do not inherit resistance to a disease or to a drug. What we do inherit determines these characteristics, the genes; half of them from one parent and half from the other. The large number and variety of genes possessed by each parent allows an astronomical number of gene combinations in the child, and this assures that each of us has a unique set of genes. The "selection" is random as far as the particular genes that are inherited, but once chosen, these genes direct the making—and shaping—of the human body and all the body tissues. Messages sent from the genes are continually decoded at the appropriate stages of human development, from the embryo to the adult. As these messages are decoded, the physical characteristics themselves appear. Genetic codes also indirectly control the day-to-day functioning of the body, as, for example, a response to a drug. Thus it can be said that each individual has a unique genetic constitution and a combination of physical and chemical characteristics no one else shares. There is an exception among identical twins, who inherit precisely the same set of genes. It should not then be so unusual that the identical twins who suffered heart attacks in 1961 reacted to warfarin in the same way.

Since unique genetic constitution can be assumed, a new science has recently begun to develop, called pharmacogenetics. The science deals with responses to drugs that are controlled or modified by hereditary factors. For a long time, individual variations from the expected response to a drug were considered only a bother. The exceptional individuals—and there were many—were more often dismissed as oddities, rather than studied with the scientific respect they deserved. Only in the last ten years have groups of geneticists and pharmacologists realized that study of variation to drug response might be valuable to both disciplines. Pharmacogenetics should continue to give us information about the potential toxic effects of many drugs now in common use.

Genetic factors can modify the response to a drug and influence the duration of drug action in several ways. Most of these variations can be attributed to genetically-determined differences in the structure or the amount of particular proteins present in the body. One of the basic components of the human body, proteins take part in many special functions related to the handling and disposal of drugs. For example, they may find a drug in the blood stream, pick it up and transport it to the body tissues where the drug exerts its effects. Proteins, as structural constituents of the tissues that receive the drug, may react with the drug at its site of action. Other proteins, as part of the body's system of enzymes, may bring about a chemical transformation in the structure of the drug, rendering it inactive and ready for removal by the kidney.

A drug is designed and developed to react with specified proteins in a specified way, like a key in a lock. When the key "fits" the drug produces the desired effect. If the proteins with which the drug is to react have been slightly altered by abnormal genetic information, the drug may react less effectively or not at all. Or worse, the reaction may result in poisoning because of an exaggerated response; or the drug may be toxic because it cannot be inactivated by the body in the usual way. Drug toxicities and other abnormal reactions to drugs may be the first indication of an unsuspected genetic alteration in one of these key proteins. Pharamacogeneticists want to determine the reason for the toxicity and how it can be predicted and prevented.

Non-genetic factors such as age, diet, or general nutritional state can also cause a variation in response to drugs. Hence, determining whether an unusual reaction stems from genetic or non-genetic factors is a task full of pitfalls. Pharmacogeneticists generally employ two methods to assess the probability that inherited factors are responsible for the abnormal response. One is the analysis of data after a large-scale population survey. This shows whether the person with an unusual drug response belongs to a distinct sub-group of the population. The other method is a detailed study of the individual patient affected, followed by an extensive investigation of his relatives. In this way, the trait can be carefully traced in the family tree. Both methods try to do the same thing to evaluate the influence of hereditary factors on an abnormal drug response, and to determine the patterns of its inheritance. Finally, pharmacogeneticists can sometimes be very precise in mapping out the biochemical basis for variation of the gene; they can estimate the frequency of the unusual gene in the population, and then introduce clinical and pharmacological reforms.

The following studies should illustrate the range and importance of pharmacogenetics.

A Drug Response Linked with the Sex Gene

Conditions for an epidemic of malaria are quite simple: steady heat and heavy rain. In the tropics and warmer temperate zones, the earth has vast tracts of land that satisfy these requirements. Long rainy seasons visit much of South America, Africa, and Asia, and also southern parts of the United States and Europe. For centuries, in fact, people thought that the fetid moist air rising from the marshlands caused this devastating plague; its name, *mala aria,* derives from the Italian, "bad air." In 1717, the Italian epidemiologist Giovanni Lancisi considered that mosquitoes might be the carriers of the disease, and he published his findings in *De Noxiis Paludum Effluvia.* It was not until 1880 that a French Army doctor, Charles Laveran, identified the malarial parasite in the blood. Twenty years later, Sir Ronald Rose proved that mosquitoes carry the disease which infects both man and animals. Now we know that between sixty and seventy species of female anopheles mosquitoes carry the malarial parasite.

Most of us are not likely to consider malaria a threat. But any disease that strikes about 300,000,000 people a year and leaves 3,000,000 of them dead is a problem for all of us. And we are more directly affected than we would like to think. Cases are still reported in the southern parts of the United States, and travel always brings us into contact with malarial areas in our own country and around the world. Millions of servicemen, moreover, who fought in the Pacific Islands or in Africa in World War II or in the Korean War, were exposed to the disease. Now, in tropical Viet Nam, malaria is once again a menace to United States and other servicemen.

Scientists and health officials take a many-sided approach to the problem of malaria. First they try to get rid of the mosquitoes that carry the disease. This is not as impractical as it may seem. As early as the 4th century B.C., the Romans drained their swamps as much to prevent disease as to salvage useful land. Neglect of these drainage installations later contributed to epidemics of malaria, one of the many causes of the decline of the Empire in the first centuries A.D. If only the swamps and stagnant pools lying near larger centers of population could be drained, an important start would be made to control the disease. Early in this century, pesticides and larvacides were put down in Cuba and Panama to fight both yellow fever and malaria. Most recently, the World Health Organization, an agency of the United Nations, has taken on the task of ridding the globe of malaria.

Still another method for controlling malaria lies in drugs; this disease has had for centuries a famous cure in quinine. Quinine is an extract of the South American cinchona tree, called by the natives the "fever tree." Jesuit missionaries brought quinine back to Europe in the 1630's; for a long time the drug was in fact known to Europe as "Jesuit's bark." (Oliver Cromwell's refusal to have anything to do with a Jesuitical drug led to his untimely death—from malaria.) But quinine is not strong enough to fight many types of malarial parasites. In the first half of the twentieth century, much experimentation went on to develop stronger drugs. When the Japanese cut off access to our supplies of quinine in the Pacific during World War II, pharmacologists finally substituted other drugs on a large scale.

Many soldiers who fought in the Second World War recall the use of anti-malarial drugs such as pamaquine and chloroquine. Compared to quinine, the advantages of pamaquine are exceptional. It is 60 to 140 times more effective against various forms of malaria. But certain parasites, such as *Plasmodium vivax* and *Plasmodium falciparum* were found to be extraordinarily resistant to the effects of pamaquine. A compound with a slightly different structure, primaquine, was introduced during the Korean War and proved to be very successful against the stubborn strains.

Primaquine was found to be poisonous to some people. The most deleterious effect is a reaction occurring in red blood cells known as hemolysis, an explosive break-up of the cells. The iron or *heme* centers of red blood cells are essential for respiration. In their passage through the tiny capillaries that line the air sacs of the lungs, the heme centers, with their high affinity for oxygen, absorb oxygen directly out of the "air." Then the onrushing blood stream carries away the red cells, now enriched by the oxygen to a brilliant red color. In this way the body tissues can "breathe."

Red cells that suffer an adverse hemolytic effect from the drug primaquine are called in medical terminology "primaquine sensitive," These cells disintegrate on contact with the drug. As waste matter in the blood stream, the infinitely tiny pieces are extracted from the blood by the kidney and darken the urine. In serious cases the urine becomes so dark that the fever associated with the cell disintegration is known as "black water fever." The destruction of red cells leads to a sometimes fatal anemia.

Primaquine causes hemolysis in patients whose red cells are deficient in a protein with the imposing name glucose-6-phosphate-dehydrogenase (G-6-PD). This is an enzymatic protein, a complex molecule that facilitates a chemical reaction in the body. There are hundreds of enzymes for the hundreds of chemical processes that take place within the body at every moment. Although there are about 500 scientific papers dealing with the deficiency of G-6-PD in red cells, no one knows as yet just why the deficiency causes hemolysis. In people who have a shortage of G-6-PD, the red cells adjust to this condition and they manage to carry on vital functions without too much difficulty under ordinary circumstances.

All would be well if the patient were not stricken with malaria and administered primaquine. For primaquine makes known the G-6-PD deficiency, perhaps by increasing the need for the enzyme to protect the store of another red cell substance, glutathione, which maintains the cell functions in proper balance.

If primaquine is given to a patient deficient in G-6-PD, nothing will happen for the first two days. Hemolysis begins on the third day, and continues with increasing severity for the next five days. As the kidney extracts the waste remnants of the dead cells from the blood stream, the urine blackens. The patient grows weak and feels back and abdominal pains. The level of red cells drops to half the normal level. This is the most serious period of the disease, the "crisis proper." But soon afterwards, strangely enough, the red cell count rises again. Pains decrease and the patient resumes a condition nearer to health.

Werner Kalow of the University of Toronto has described the changes in the number of red cells in the body at every period during therapy with primaquine:

On first administration the older half of the red cell population is destroyed during the acute hemolytic phase, i.e., during about a week. Thereafter, only a small number of cells per day age sufficiently to become susceptible. This is readily balanced by the formation of new cells . . . As long as these cells are young, i.e., 10 to 20 days old, they are not destroyed during a hemolytic reaction; at the age of about 70 days, the cells are preferentially destroyed during a hemolytic reaction induced by primaquine.

Thus, after the initial crisis is over, the red cells will die from primaquine only slightly earlier than they ordinarily would. If primaquine is not administered for a few weeks, however, the immunity is lost, and 50 percent of the red cells will again be old enough to die if treatment with primaquine were resumed.

Fortunately, trial-and-error experimentation is no longer needed to discover the individuals who are sensitive to primaquine. Blood tests have been developed that have proved capable of distinguishing between those who are sensitive to primaquine and those who are not. For example, a direct assay of the enzyme G-6-PD in the red cells can be made. A more convenient test is the glutathione (GSH) stability test; a substance threatens the life of the cells in a test tube in a manner similar to primaquine in the body. The advantage of the GSH test is that it is simple and quick, and can be performed on large populations susceptible to malaria. Individuals sensitive to primaquine seem to be sensitive to many other substances, such as the sulfa drugs, acetanilid, and chloroquine. Thus the GSH test is a very useful means of preventing toxic reactions from a wide variety of drugs.

The GSH stability test has given results of particular interest to geneticists. It has been proved that the gene which determines the hereditary trait for primaquine sensitivity is inherited along with the gene that determines the sex of an individual. Genes are like links in a long chain which is called a chromosome. There are on the average 3,000 genes linking together to form one chromosome. In every human being there are 46 chromosomes composed of genes of which half are inherited from one parent and half from the other. Each person has 23 pairs of chromosomes: 22 pairs of autosomes and one pair of sex chromosomes carrying the genes which determine the sex. Women have a pair of X chromosomes but men have one X and one Y chromosome as their sex-determining set. Obviously the Y chromosome is present only in males and is the key chromosome that determines male characteristics. A son's sex chromosomes are XY and his Y must have been inherited from his father and his X from his mother. A daughter would inherit an X from her father and an X from her mother, and so she is XX.

In the formation of sperm cells or ova, the chromosome pairs must split so that the total number of chromosomes in the sperm or egg cell will be reduced to twenty-three. In other words, each individual parent carries forty-six chromosomes, but *he* gives only half of his set of 46, just as *she* gives only half of hers. In this way, after the ova and sperm cells combine, the offspring will be insured of having only forty-six (23 pairs) and not ninety-two chromosomes. In the inheritance of sex, the father carries the sex pair XY, but each sperm cell can only carry an X or a Y. Depending on which sperm cell fertilizes the egg, the child will be of the sex determined by the sperm cell's sex chromosome. There is a fifty-fifty chance that the Y sperm cell (rather than the X sperm cell) will fertilize the egg, and so an equal or fifty-fifty chance that the baby will be male or female. All this should not seem so surprising, and a brief look around should assure us that the world is half man, half woman.

It so happens that sometimes an X-chromosome carries an undesirable gene on it which will be inherited by the child receiving that particular chromosome. However, since women have two X-chromosomes, the adverse effects of a bad gene on one may be counterbalanced or even suppressed completely by her having a good gene for the same trait on her other X-chromosome. In contrast, undesirable traits associated with the X-chromosome inherited by a man are not compensated for by his Y-chromosome and are likely to be expressed.

The genes affecting G-6-PD are located on the X-chromosome and a bad gene here can cause a deficiency of this enzyme and primaquine sensitivity. A woman can carry this gene, but its effects will be partially or completely stifled by the presence of a normal X-chromosome. Such women are said to be "carriers", since they do not suffer from the bad gene. Males, with only one X-chromosome, either do not inherit the dangerous gene at all or they have it and show its full effects. Obviously, such an X-chromosome linked trait cannot pass from father to son, but must have come from one of the mother's X-chromosomes.

The following chart shows the possible types of reactors to primaquine. A man may be either normal or a reactor. A woman, on the other hand, may be normal, intermediate, or (rarely) a very sensitive reactor.

TABLE 1

GENE CHART

MALE	FEMALE
XY normal male X'Y reactor male	XX normal female X'X intermediate female X'X' reactor female

Note: X' equals the chromosome with the gene that determines primaquine sensitivity.

A Population Study—Inactivation of INH

In the early 1950's, the drug isoniazid (INH) was introduced and found to be very effective against tuberculosis. Two years after it began to be used on a wide scale, the yearly rate of death from the tubercle bacillus dropped from 20 to 10 in 100,000 and by 1962 the rate was down to 8. INH has proven to be one of the strongest and most successful antitubercular drugs and it is currently used throughout the United States and abroad. Other features are in its favor, too; it can be given by mouth and can be quickly absorbed from the gastrointestinal tract.

In some individuals, however, the usual dose of INH was found to be toxic. An overdose in a sensitive patient caused severe convulsions. By experiment, the standard dose of the drug was established at 3–4 milligrams per kilogram of body weight. For the desired results with least danger to the patient, this dosage was considered the safest amount that could be inactivated daily for eventual excretion. Otherwise, the drug would accumulate in the blood stream and simulate the effect of an overdose. INH is inactivated by the liver and changed chemically to a derivative that can be easily excreted from the blood through the kidney. On its own, the kidney will extract some INH from the blood, but this organ is comparatively ineffective unless the liver is first able to perform a chemically-detoxifying process known as acetylation. If standard doses cannot be inactivated, the cumulative residue of INH in the blood stream causes numbness or weakness in the limbs, "tingling" sensations in the extremities, and even acute psychosis.

The *standard dose* cannot be reduced if the drug is to have a therapeutic effect. Fortunately by administering yet another drug, pyridoxine (vitamine B_6), daily elimination of the neurological toxic effects of INH is possible without destroying the drug's anti-tubercular activity. The entire process reveals a delicate chemical balance, and we should pause to appreciate it. INH must be maintained in the blood at a certain level. For some people on the standard dose, this level itself is excessive with serious side effects, and it becomes a matter of the cure being worse than the disease. Thus another drug must be brought in to preserve the therapeutic effect by stifling or at least by regulating the side effects.

Patients who would show the accumulation of the drug from prolonged treatment on standard doses of INH can be identified by a simple diagnostic test. Six hours after a standard dose is given to a patient, a specimen of his blood is obtained and the concentration of INH in the blood is measured. The concentration of the drug at this time gives us a way to distinguish between those who can inactivate INH rapidly and those who inactivate the drug slowly. Figure 1 shows the frequency of occurrence of different blood concentrations of INH six hours after a standard dose of the drug was given to a group of individuals.

The graph indicates that many patients had only one or two micrograms in one milliliter of blood after six hours, but many others had between four and five times as much. Ordinarily we would expect to find these results following a normal distribution curve with a mean value at the peak and variations around the mean sloping down along both sides, so that the curve is shaped like a bell. The INH distribution here, however, clearly revealed two definable peaks rather than one and we seem to have two distinct populations: rapid inactivators and slow inactivators. Sex, age, diet, and other environmental factors could not explain the two peaks. Scientists suspected that genetic differences were responsible.

Here the use of identical and fraternal twins provided a valuable aid in the investigation. If the rate of inactivation of INH is a trait primarily determined by genetic factors, we would expect

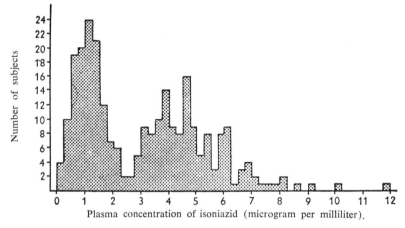

Plasma concentration of isoniazid (microgram per milliliter).

FIGURE 1. *Blood concentration of INH six hours after a test dose is administered.*

to find very close agreement between identical twins who have the same genetic make-up, but poorer agreement between non-identical twins. Such proved to be the case for INH inactivation. Although the comparison was made by measuring the percent of the dose of INH excreted in 24 hours rather than the blood plasma levels of the drug, the results are appropriate to evaluate the cause of variation in INH inactivation (Table 2).

The variation was found to be far less between identical twins than between fraternal twins, although marked differences are found in the values comparing one twin pair with another. Thus conclusive proof was obtained that the peaks in Fig. 1 are due to genetic differences. Statistical analysis of the data confirmed the

TABLE 2

EXCRETION OF ISONIAZID BY IDENTICAL AND FRATERNAL TWINS

Identical twins			Fraternal twins		
Twin pair number	Sex	Isoniazid excreted in 24 hours (%)*	Twin pair number	Sex	Isoniazid excreted in 24 hours (%)*
1	M	8.8	6	F	12.1
	M	8.3		F	13.7
2	F	26.0	7	F	10.9
	F	25.2		F	4.6
3	M	11.8	8	M	11.0
	M	12.4		M	8.5
4	F	12.2	9	F	3.9
	F	11.5		F	15.2
5	F	4.1	10	M	10.5
	F	4.4		M	15.6

* As percent of the dose.

results, giving the estimate of the relative contribution of hereditary factors as 97 percent. Essentially this means that nearly all of the variation in INH inactivation can be attributed to genetic rather than environmental factors.

For supporting evidence, family studies were made on the inheritance of the rapid and slow inactivation trait. Using a collection of pedigrees, one can predict how this trait is inherited. One can draw several conclusions from Figure 2. First, neither rapid nor slow inactivators are found to be exclusively males or females. Thus the peculiarity of rapid or slow inactivation is not, like primaquine sensitivity, a sex-linked trait. It shows up in equal numbers in males and females. Another conclusion from the study invalidates any use of the term "abnormal" to describe an unexpected reaction. In fact, about half of the population would be called abnormal on the basis of either slow or fast INH inactivation. Finally, if both parents are rapid, the offspring may be either rapid or slow. If both parents are slow, however, the offspring are all slow. And, if one parent is rapid and the other slow, offspring may be either rapid or slow. Large population surveys have shown that 47.8 percent are rapid inactivators and 52.2 percent are slow.

Other studies of slow and rapid inactivators have shown that the genes responsible occur unevenly among different ethnic groups. In the United States, about half are slow (55.1 percent), but in Latin America the percentage is much lower (32.8 percent). Although the number of subjects examined is small, values decrease to 21 percent in American Indians, to 4.6 percent in Eskimos. And no one knows why. The range of values found in these groups illustrates the striking variation in the frequency of the genes and the rates of inactivation of the drug in various ethnic groups. This variation of course must be

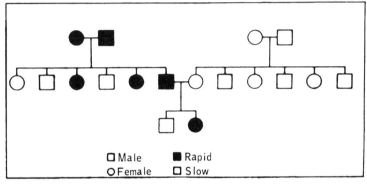

FIGURE 2. *Study of inheritance of rapid and slow inactivation trait.*

considered when a pharmacologist looks into the basis of a peculiar reaction or unexpected poisoning.

The contribution of genetic factors to the unusual response to drugs should make us recognize that the human being does not show uniformity in response to drugs or in his absorption, metabolism, and elimination of them. Pharmacological individuality, owing to our unique genetic codes, is really no different than our individual peculiarities in vitamin requirements and metabolism of food constituents such as amino acids and sugars.

While no drug is likely to be completely safe and free from all side effects and unusual reactions, it is important to understand the reasons for unexpected or unusual drug reactions and find how they can be predicted and prevented. Hereditary factors obviously account for some of these toxic or unusual drug effects. Further knowledge of these factors should be of practical importance and increase the usefulness and therapeutic value of many drugs used today. A better understanding of hereditary factors will also be helpful in the development of new drugs and reduce the chances that undesirable or toxic reactions will occur when they are introduced for general use.

REFERENCE CREDITS

The following are reprinted with permission:

Fig. 1 Price Evans, D. A., Manley, K. A., and McKusick, V. A., British Medical Journal, *2*, 485, 1960.

Fig. 2 Transactions of the 18th Conference on the Chemotherapy of Tuberculosis, Veterans Administration, Department of Medicine and Surgery, 1959.

Table 2 Böhnicke, R., and Lisboa, B. P., Die Naturwissenschaften, *44*, 314, 1957.

Chapter 24

Testing the Drug

Books must follow sciences, and not
sciences books.

Sir Francis Bacon
Proposition Touching Amendment of Law

R esearch with drugs evokes an image of a dedicated young scientist, clad in spotless laboratory coat, surrounded by a bewildering maze of equipment: a forest of glass tubing, beakers and Bunsen burners, distilling devices, Petri dishes, and dry crystals in dusty square jars. The scientist pursues his task relentlessly, and more like Sherlock Holmes than James Bond. He is continually inspired, knowing that his work contributes to the welfare of mankind. He is that romanticized genius drawn by Paul de Kruif in his memorable book, *The Microbe Hunters*.

Paul de Kruif could not write the same story today. The equipment is all there, including equipment that is never seen in high school, or even college, chemistry laboratories. There are vast financial resources available through grants from foundations and from the government—sometimes not vast enough for a given project, but the money does come in, for the value of the work being done is generally recognized. Networks of organization proliferate: research teams, entire laboratories, or even chains of laboratories across the country are devoted sometimes to a single project. There are researchers in clinics, in the great teaching hospitals, at the universities; scientists working for private foundations and institutes, or employed by private drug firms. The enterprise is not a lonely one, although the researcher, unlike a practicing physician, is primarily concerned with his project, rather than with people. Since he is probably part of a team, he must exchange ideas, data, and conclusions with his co-workers and with the director of his project. Now it is harder for the genius to be isolated.

The researcher's work, despite the support and resources available at his request, is not always full of glamorous discoveries. Much of his work may be routine, and routinely dull at that; major, headline-making findings do not occur every month, and in most of his labors, the welfare of mankind may seem far away. For every "discovery," every experiment that "works" to confirm an idea, perhaps twenty will fail, or prove inconclusive. From the failures, to be sure, there is often much to be learned, but such negative instruction can be frustrating. Even the clues that lead to success require patience and endurance, for it may take months or years for a full course of tests to be completed and all the idiosyncrasies to be worked out of a new discovery. When the medical researcher goes home at the end of his day (or night) he may find it difficult to answer the question, "What did you do at work today, dear?" in any way that is readily intelligible to someone without highly specialized training.

Many such workers feel, however, that it is highly essential and indeed their obligation to relate the significance of their work to the community, if only indirectly, through participation in educational programs in schools and colleges.

Skillful assistants are required to extend the capacities of the scientists, and all are unitary working parts in the huge machine of modern basic research. Although there is great need for the rare genius of a Pasteur or a Koch, a Walter Reed or a Paul Ehrlich, we do not have to rely solely upon the lonely achievements of rare giants of medicine. For without the mobilization of manpower, financial resources, equipment, and ideas made possible by modern research technology, we would not have more than a score of the hundreds of useful, even indispensable weapons we now possess for the war on disease and suffering. We owe much to all of these men —from the keeper of animals to the major figures in the national limelight of medical research.

By Thought or by Chance

All the basic research related to the discovery and development of new drugs can be classified under two headings: hit-or-miss and rational research. The hit-or-miss method, as indicated by the name, represents a haphazard approach ("try everything"), whereas the rational method starts with a clue or an idea.

This does not mean the hit-or-miss method of research should be scorned. In fact, this method has probably consumed a large portion of the research dollars spent in this country, and in return has produced quite respectable results. Several chemical compounds used in cancer chemotherapy have come from the application of this approach, and all the antibiotics presently in use are its products. This game of chance is technically called "random screening."

In random screening the disease or condition to be treated is induced in a laboratory animal. If the condition is contagious, several other such animals must be exposed and infected. In the case of cancer, which is not actually contagious, this is done by transplanting groups of the autonomous cancer cells from a single tumor into several other individuals of the same species. Once a sufficient number of test animals, say fifty, has been infected, various compounds can be tried. Compound A may be tested against the condition in the first ten test animals, compound B in the second ten, compound C in the third ten, compound D in the fourth ten, while the remaining ten animals are reserved as a control group to check the progress of the condition when left to take its natural course. The researcher is, as one scientist put it, "taking compounds off the shelf almost at random and putting them into groups of ten rats" to see if it causes the abatement or cure of the disease under study.

Meanwhile, careful check must be kept on the general health and condition of the animals so that any undesirable side effects of the drug being tested may be detected. If a drug has no apparent effect on the test animals, it is discarded. Since many drugs have been found that affect test animals but not humans, however, lingering doubt continues to trouble researchers concerning the rejected drugs. Is it possible to have a "false negative" reaction in an animal? That is, could certain drugs be ineffective in laboratory animals, but possibly be of use in treatment of humans? "False negative" reactions are the great risk in random screening.

The sheer drudgery and dullness of the job itself provides another practical drawback. There is little intellectual stimulation, no conscious choice or rational planning. Instead the researcher must confine himself to a scrupulously accurate check on mechanical matters—dosage, timing of treatments, progress of the disease, other factors in the condition of the animals. At the same time he must remain as alert as possible to unexpected and perhaps significant reactions to the drug by the test specimens. This last point is particularly important because many valuable drugs that have come from random screening are not at all useful against the disease for which they were being tested. In many cases the observation of an alert researcher has detected some unexpected and arresting characteristic of a drug under investigation, providing a clue for rational research in some hitherto unconsidered area.

Usually the earlier tests might be performed on mice or rats. But rodents are not human beings. Their diets, their structures, and, on the most elementary and basic level, their DNA codes and the details of their cellular chemistry differ from those of higher primates and the highest one, man. Consequently, a positive reaction to a drug in a mouse or a rat does not necessarily indicate that the drug will produce a similar reaction in man.

Actually many other species of animals are used: the rabbit, the guinea pig, cats and dogs. The more animals involved, the more chance there is of picking up possible untoward effects in humans, for no one can guess where danger—or success—will be encountered. The drug will probably be given to primates: rhesus monkeys are most commonly used. Alternatively, it may be tried directly on human volunteers, if there are no indications of hazardous side effects. Testing first in large numbers of animals, and then in people, is necessary over some period of time to ascertain accurately the probable effects of the drug and to ensure that no slow-developing harmful effects are associated with it. Carelessness or haste in this vital but entirely routine portion of experimentation with the drug can later produce disastrous results, as in the recent cases of thalidomide and an anti-cholesterol drug, triparanol.

Rational research demands a greater element of inspiration than random screening. It is also much more difficult to prosecute on the massive scale that characterizes the routine approach. Rational research proceeds along two lines: one originating in the laboratory or scientific library, and the other based upon physiological knowledge and clinical experience. A biochemist or pharmacologist may know, for example, that a certain complex molecule is necessary as a building block in one of the steps toward the synthesis of DNA in human cells. In combating cancer, it is desirable to prevent the growth and division of the malignant cells. One way to do this is to interfere with DNA synthesis, for DNA is a kind of programming center for the whole operation of the cell. A cell with its DNA fouled up is like a computer-controlled weapons system being fed the wrong program—or no program at all. The scientist may reason that substitution for the necessary complex molecule will inhibit the formation of DNA. The cell, asking for bread, is in effect given a stone. Of course, the scientist also knows that the substituted molecule must resemble the molecule it replaces in certain essential respects no less than it differs in at least one other essential way. If the substituted stone cannot fool the cell by looking enough like a loaf (in some chemical sense) to pass for one, it will not be accepted by the cell and will be prevented from playing its subversive role.

From here, if the scientist is dealing with aspects of the cellular chemistry that are fairly well understood, he may proceed to construct his desired molecule-analogue by further theorizing. He may be forced to experimentation in his effort to find something that *works*. In this latter case, his experiments will at least be purposeful, not random, for he has already limited the scope of his search and discarded alternatives purely on the basis of prior knowledge and careful, logical thought.

Clinical experience, on the other hand, may provide the first clue for the researcher's tracking down a new drug. Physicians may observe in the victims of a specific type of poisoning that the poison is concentrated in certain organs. Over the years observation of many cases of some disease or chronic condition may convince a physician that the sufferers are peculiarly immune to some other, perhaps unrelated disease. Edward Jenner, in the eighteenth century, observed the apparent validity of an old Gloucestershire belief that milkmaids who had had cowpox could not contract smallpox. He acted upon his observation to produce the first smallpox vaccine. From such an observation research can take off with a specific end in view. As biochemistry advances and we learn more and more about the activities and chemical relationships of the complex molecules and enzymes within the cell, we can expect increasingly valuable discoveries and insights from rational research.

Some Problems in Drug Testing

The drug researcher does not work with machines and identical mass-produced parts, but with a random variation of living organisms, each an ongoing system. Even the simple task of killing a given type of bacterium in a laboratory culture presents unforeseen difficulties. Certain chance mutants within the population may be resistant to the drug used to exterminate the whole colony. If these mutants are genetically stable, they will become the basis for a whole new population of resistant bacteria. A drug that initially looked highly promising will, in the long run, turn out to be totally ineffective.

Now complicate matters by placing the bacteria to be destroyed, not in laboratory bottles, but in a living host organism, which has all sorts of processes going on at once. The trick is to find something that poisons the bacteria but does not affect the host—or at least affects the host much more slowly and to a lesser extent than it does the specific bacteria. The researcher attempts to establish that *qualitative difference,* which is esteemed so highly and has proved so elusive for scientists, for example, in the province of cancer chemotherapy. If an essential difference between the cells of the host organism and the cell or cells of the invading organism can be found, chances seem very good that the game is up for the invader, for some way will certainly be found to exploit chemically that essential difference. Perhaps the target organism has some vital structure lacking in the cells of its host; or the host may possess some structural or chemical attribute that would shield its cells from the effects of a drug. This would be lethal to an invading organism lacking that structural or chemical peculiarity. The success of some modern antibiotics, for example, is based upon the discovery and exploitation of the fact that bacteria have a cell wall not possessed by cells in the higher forms of life, such as man, and that this structure is necessary for their continued existence.

Even if a qualitative difference cannot be found, it is sometimes possible to treat an infection due to an invading virus or bacterium by isolated dosage of the affected area, leaving the toxic effects of the drug limited to that particular tissue or organ. Such a method of treatment capitalizes on the advantages enjoyed by the multicelled host organism. However, the more complex multi-celled organism also presents disadvantages, as far as the drug tester is concerned. There is always the possibility that a drug designed to attack a target in a given tissue will perform perfectly there, destroying the target organism and causing no apparent toxic reactions in the target area, but it will be found to have unexpected and highly undesirable effects elsewhere in the host's body. A drug, for instance, designed to eliminate an invading foreign organism in the blood may not affect the blood or circulatory system adversely in man, but may on the other hand have deleterious effects on the liver or kidneys. An apparently harmless example of unexpected and remote side effects emerged during the testing of oral contraceptives. One such agent, which in preliminary trials appeared to do what was expected of it without undesirable complications, showed one unusual quirk: if the person taking the contraceptive agent drank even a minute amount of alcohol within several hours after taking the drug, an unsightly case of highly blood-shot eyes resulted.

Testing over a long period of time and with large numbers of cases is necessary to discover other possible pitfalls of a drug. A drug may, like modern advertising, create a demand in the organism where none existed before—a demand that can be satisfied only by larger and larger increments of the drug. Or the body may be unable either to break down the drug, metabolize it, or eliminate it from its system, allowing concentrations of the drug to build up through protracted treatments, sometimes reaching fatal levels. Some drugs may react unfavorably with unusual dietary items or other kinds of medication—facts that would not have become immediately apparent in a routine course of testing. In the case of some types of therapeutic substances, genetic effects that may show up in the next generation must be taken into account.

The possibility always lurks that one individual in thousands may be seriously allergic to the drug—a circumstance once again traceable to the infinite genetic variation within a species. But, of course, the existence of a few allergic individuals in a population of hundreds of thousands or even millions is not sufficient cause to discontinue such vital public health measures as mass vaccination for smallpox, innoculation against typhoid and diphtheria, and immunization against poliomyelitis. Widespread and controlled use of any new drug by selected physicians gives some assurance against all but these few allergic reactions. This must be done even after all the procedures of laboratory testing and trials with human volunteers have been successfully concluded. Otherwise the new drug cannot be declared safe for marketing and general availability. As for the rare allergic individual, satisfactory protection for him can be assured only by the continued vigilance and alertness of his personal physician, even when he prescribes tried and familiar drugs. At the first sign of an allergic reaction, an alert doctor will discontinue the prescribed drug for that individual no matter how unusual such a reaction may be in the population as a whole.

These generalizations about "rational research" take on an added dimension when specific histories of the discovery and testing of actual drugs are examined. Antibiotics are treated elsewhere in this book, and some of the stories of certain drugs used in cancer chemotherapy are given in other chapters. Here we shall deal with other drugs of various kinds, selected primarily because of interesting or illustrative features in their development and use. Many of these compounds did, indeed, originate in cancer research work, and some are still used in that field today, while others have turned out to have totally unexpected uses in seemingly unrelated areas. Although we shall be concerned primarily with products of laboratories and clinics in this country, our first case takes us half way around the world, beginning with a lowly plant long used in home remedies in India.

Flowers for Cancer

For centuries in India the common periwinkle, *Vinca rosea,* was thought to have therapeutic value. Extracts of the blue-flowered, trailing evergreen plant were used in folk medicine as a remedy for many different diseases, among them diabetes mellitus. In diabetes, the ability of the human body to use sugar is impaired, so that abnormal amounts of sugar appear in the blood and urine. Popular belief held that extracts of periwinkle could lower the levels of blood sugar.

Modern scientists in this country have decided to examine and evaluate critically some approaches to healing that have long been either neglected or disavowed. Consequently, teams of American drug company agents and physicians from university research establishments today comb underdeveloped areas of the world searching for folk cures that might be useful and adaptable for modern medical practice. One such hunt turned up the vinca plant in India, with its supposed value in the treatment of diabetes.

Initial testing took place in Canada. Vinca alkaloids, extracts from the periwinkle, were tested on experimental animals and the effects on blood sugar levels observed. The substance was found to be relatively inactive; in terms of its original intent, the experiment was disappointing. Scientists noted, however, that every time the laboratory animals were given the vinca alkaloids the number of white cells in the animals' blood would drop. This observation aroused considerable interest. If normal white blood cells were reduced in number by the drug, it might be possible that the abnormal high white cell count found in leukemia would also be reduced by similar treatment. Accordingly vinca alkaloids were tested in cases of leukemia, and the drug was found to be partially effective against some forms of the disease. The results were not outstanding, but good enough to encourage further testing. When tried in other kinds of neoplastic disease, the drug was found to be very effective.

Today, the marketed alkaloids of the vinca plant, vincristine and vinblastine, rank high among drugs used in the therapy of certain types of leukemia and of Hodgkin's disease, a form of lymphoma related to leukemia. In addition, these vinca alkaloids have been found to be second only to methotrexate among drugs effective in the treatment of choriocarcinoma, a cancer associated with the tissues that contribute to the placenta in humans. The researchers looking for a drug purported to be effective in the treatment of diabetes were able, through astute observation, to detect a previously unknown property in the drug under examination. They applied this knowledge to produce useful therapeutic agents for a disease totally unrelated to the area of their first concern.

Making the Most of Disaster

During the Second World War, American government and military authorities feared that the Germans would use gas warfare on the western front. Consequently it was decided that the United

States should manufacture and stockpile quantities of war gases for use as a retaliatory measure. Some of our stockpiled gases were to be shipped abroad and stored in the British Isles. One ship loaded with nitrogen mustard gas was convoyed to a Scottish harbor. While it was waiting to be unloaded, the Germans launched an air raid against the town. Considerable damage was done to the town and the shipping in the harbor, including the gas-laden ship. The word on shore was that the Italian navy had landed, for the odor of garlic, the characteristic smell of mustard gas, was everywhere. But there was no humor in the situation for those unfortunates who were exposed to quantities of the gas. Those not killed immediately suffered terrible burns on the skin and in the lungs, the typical effects of mustard gas. Some persons exposed to heavy doses of the gas survived these burns, only to have it discovered that their bone marrow had been destroyed, leaving their bodies unable to manufacture either red or white blood cells. This circumstance, horrible enough in itself, was duly noted by an attending physician, who thought that some good should come from the discovery.

Superficially, such a discovery does not sound at all useful, except, perhaps, for making more and better poison gases. After further study at the Army Chemical Center in Maryland, however, reports were sent to scientists at Yale University. There mustard gases were tested as bone marrow depressants in the treatment of certain human neoplasms. Hodgkin's disease and leukemia appeared to be good possibilities for the application of this powerful drug. As it has turned out, nitrogen mustards are a very important type of therapy today in a number of types of neoplastic disease, notably Hodgkin's disease. Palliative treatment and symptomatic relief have also been obtained in a number of other types of tumors. Initially, the source of the observation which led to this valuable discovery was hushed up because U.S. authorities did not want the public to learn that we were prepared to wage gas warfare and actually had ships loaded with mustard gases in the war area.

In the development of the nitrogen mustards as anti-neoplastic agents, these clinical experiences provided a crucial suggestion leading to an important application of drugs to allay human misery. A physician in Scotland, attending the victims of a terrible accident, offered the invaluable insight. The research and testing facilities of

American academic medicine used that insight to develop another major drug.

Insecticides and Adrenal Tumors

Substances not intended for human consumption but which humans come into contact with must also be tested for toxicity. When DDT and its companion insecticide DDD were first being developed, it became apparent that humans would handle the spray or powder, and that human food sources would be treated with the new chemicals. Accordingly, studies were made in which dogs were treated with high concentrations of the insecticides to test their effects on mammals. It was observed that considerable necrosis (death of a circumscribed tissue or organ) of the adrenal glands resulted in the tested dogs. This initially caused the researchers to fear that DDD and DDT would be too dangerous for general use as insecticides. However, when many samples of the purified and mass-produced chemicals were used in further tests, no further cases of adrenal damage could be observed in test animals. It appeared that an impurity in the samples originally tested was solely responsible for the gland damage. Considerable amounts of pure DDD or DDT could be given to dogs in the laboratory without such toxic effects. This impurity was identified as a contamination of DDD by the "ortho-primed" isomer. The mechanism of its action against the adrenal cortex is so far unknown, but the fact of such action is thoroughly documented by experimentation and observation.

The adrenal cortex produces the adrenal cortical steroids responsible for certain stress reactions. It also produces other steroids, including androgens, male sex hormones, and hormones governing protein, fat, and carbohydrate metabolism and regulating salt and water balance. In some neoplasms of the adrenal gland, the malignant cells, which are growing and dividing without normal controls, continue to produce these hormones. This over-production results in considerable discomfort for the stricken person: characteristic effects include accumulation of excess fat, especially in the face and back; diabetes; salt retention; and osteoporosis (absorption of the bones by the system, resulting in extreme fragility and porosity). In women, the increased androgen production can cause particularly unwelcome symptoms including baldness, interference with normal menstrual cycles, and development of male secondary sex characteristics, such as growth of the beard.

Because of the selectivity of ortho-primed DDD for the adrenal glands, therapy with the drug arrests the development of the tumor, controls the disease, and makes the patient much more comfortable. Some regression of the metastases (spreading of the cancer to new sites) has been secured in cases of adrenocortical carcinoma treated with orthoprimed DDD, but there is no evidence at this point of its being at all effective as a cure, or even as a means to longer life in patients suffering from the disease. Nevertheless, its proved ability to offer symptomatic relief is of obvious value for the comfort and morale of the patient. In this case, researchers were able to capitalize on an accidental, unwanted impurity in a new drug that at first sight appeared merely destructive.

Space Age Diets, The Leaf Vitamin, and Leukemia

In the late 1940's some scientists were attempting to devise a purely synthetic diet which would support life. In this diet there were to be no ordinary meats, vegetables, or nutrients found in the normal diets of man and animals. On the surface, such an attempt may appear to be ridiculous, one more contribution to useless knowledge, but the research proved useful in at least two ways. It was appropriate space-age science, for the problem of food supply will be one of the great difficulties to be faced by space voyagers and colonists on lifeless bodies in space and in environments radically different from that of earth. Synthetic non-perishable nutrients would have obvious advantages over normal foods that usually present problems of storage and preservation of one kind or another. Furthermore, this "space-age research" could make valuable contributions to our everyday dietary and medical knowledge, since the experiments would inevitably show what substances, in what quantities, were necessary to support life.

The scientists found that one of the essential ingredients in their experimental diets was a vitamin derived from leaves, called folic acid (from the Latin, *folium,* 'leaf'). Folic acid, it has now been learned, is necessary for all cell growth. At the time, however, the researchers were most impressed with the effects of a folic acid deficiency in the diets of laboratory monkeys. The undeveloped red blood cells still in the bone marrow, where red cells are manufactured, looked very unhealthy in folic-deficient animals. These cells took on what is known as blastic appearance (from the Greek, *blastos* 'germination'), indicating arrested development. The chemists and biologists conducting the experiment were struck by this condition—the characteristic appearance of the leukemia blood cell. The experimenters reasoned that if absence of folic acid prevented the cells from maturing, then reintroduction of the absent vitamin would cause the blastic cells to mature. And, indeed, this is precisely what happened. It seemed only logical that leukemia therapy with folic acid could result in maturation of the blastic white blood cells.

Unfortunately, it did not work this way in human patients. Persons suffering from advanced leukemia who were treated with folic acid developed much higher counts of leukemic cells in their blood; the disease and all its symptoms were much aggravated.

Such unexpected consequences of a perfectly logical, apparently sound step in testing were, quite naturally, something more than upsetting for the researchers. But at least a new inference was strongly suggested. If the rate of proliferation of leukemia cells can be speeded up by giving folic acid, it stands to reason that something which, by removal or interception, attacks folic acid should have the opposite effect, and slow the course of the disease. Numerous folic acid antagonists were accordingly synthesized, and in 1948 and 1949, only a few years after the significance of folic acid was realized, one of the most important chemotherapeutic drugs, methotrexate, emerged from the laboratory. The approach used by the chemists in synthesizing methotrexate can readily be grasped by a person with no training in chemistry, if he will make a moment's examination of the following diagram (Fig. 1). The lines indicate chemical bonds between the elements designated by the letters: a double line indicates a double bond between atoms.

Methotrexate is now one of the drugs chosen for treatment of acute leukemia in children. It is also the drug of choice in treatment of choriocarcinoma in women, where it has perhaps the best record of cures attained by any type of chemotherapy directed against any kind of cancer. Its development was a milestone in the progress

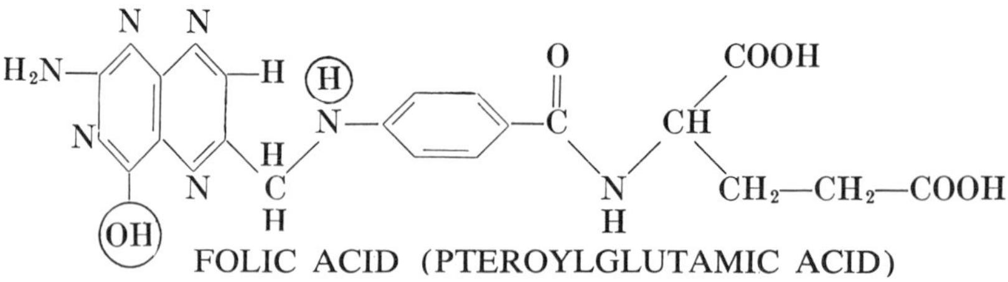

FOLIC ACID (PTEROYLGLUTAMIC ACID)

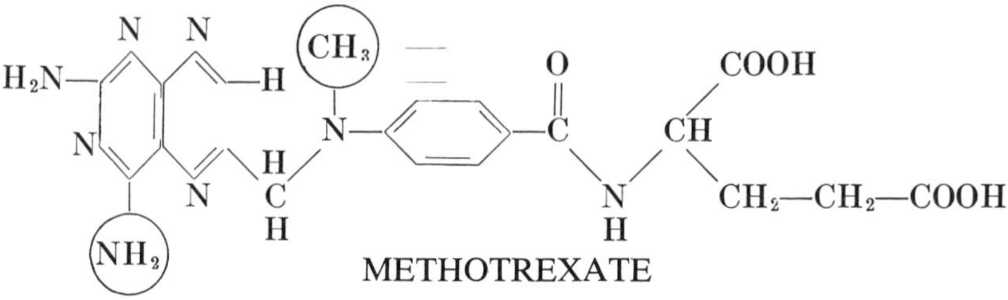

METHOTREXATE

Key to the symbols: 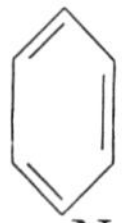 = benzene ring

N = nitrogen   H = hydrogen
O = oxygen   C = carbon

FIGURE 1. *The substitutions that differentiate methotrexate from folic acid are circled on the diagram. It is easy to see why methotrexate, a folic acid antagonist in most technical classifications, has also been called a folic acid analogue.*

of chemotherapy, comparable to Ehrlich's discovery of salvarsan, the "magic bullet" used against syphilis, or the discovery of the sulfa drugs and penicillin. The family of folic acid antagonists comprised the first antimetabolites to produce proved, often long-term, benefits in cancer therapy.

Substitution

Lest our diagrams should make the chemists' job appear too simple, further consideration should be given to the problems of substitution in the creation of these camouflaged chemical booby-traps. Many of the most interesting of the chemotherapeutic drugs operate in this fashion. Perhaps they are more like secret agents operating under assumed identities, but they must fool not only the functionaries in the local cell that is their destination, but also the transportation authorities and the border guards. Moving the "agent" into position to do his work is a complicated problem, since some of these check-points in the system will be likely to discover one portion of a disguise, while others will destroy the agent because of some other slip-up.

The complex molecules are not really *very* like either secret agents or the tinker toys they resemble so much when diagrammed on a page or simulated in a plastic model. The task of creating effective analogues or antagonists for proteins, enzymes, and other substances naturally occurring in the body, is a trial of both mind and patience. One cannot simply substitute a red ball for a green one some place in the structure, even if they are of similar size, for the molecule is three-dimensional in its energy relationships and chemical bonds, as well as in actual structure.

The substitution of one atom may affect electron distribution throughout the molecule, altering in turn many of the normal chemical reactions and binding capacities all along the structure. One cannot blithely knock off an atom here and put another there, any more than one could expect to build a hi-fi amplifier from a kit, using tubes and resistors different from those called for in the directions. The antimetabolite must perform differently from the metabolite at one site only—the "receptor site" at which the chemical reaction to be inhibited takes place. Elsewhere, the substitute is expected, indeed *required,* to behave identically with its original. Nine times out of ten, however, modifications of the original molecule will result in changes in its behavior on the way to its receptor site; its solubility, catabolic break-down rate, chemical reactivity, and other factors important in its behavior in the human body, all come into play. Substitution is not a game played at random, in spare moments with a pencil and a scratch pad.

Risk

Risk has a painful simplicity about it. In any rational approach to drugs, irrational factors must be heavily weighed. Sometimes they can even be calculated. The risk of administering a drug, in testing or in therapy, is carefully balanced against the reasons for using it. If a drug has a rare but nonetheless serious side effect, it should not be used for any trivial disease. If the infection is potentially fatal, then risk is justified. But to what extent?

Consider chloramphenicol, sometimes referred to as Chloromycetin. This drug is now the best available to fight *Salmonella typhosa,* the bacterium which induces typhoid fever. Several years after the drug was introduced, cases of serious—sometimes fatal—aplastic anemia were attributed to its effects. About one in a hundred thousand seemed to be so affected. Yet some typhoid patients would respond successfully to no drug other than chloramphenicol. Doctors finally decided that chloramphenicol could only be used when death itself threatened a patient. A person stood a far greater chance of death from typhoid fever than from chloramphenicol. And so the drug was kept, with precautions.

Overall, the results of drug testing more than make up for dangers, setbacks and frustrations. Since World War II the contribution of researchers in the field has been immense. In the quest for cures, the scientists ransack nature for plants and organisms, they follow suspicious clues from folklore, and at times they synthesize something completely "new" in the laboratory. By their discourse and method they keep finding remedies for some of the worst diseases. More so than workers in any other branch of modern science, they might subscribe to an eighteenth century premise: that the world is not chaotic, it is only "harmoniously confused." With a steady application of intelligence, scientists know that they can see farther than the eye has seen. In spite of all the frustrations encountered in the laboratory, they must be optimists, believing as Alexander Pope expressed in his *Essay on Man*:

> All Nature is but Art, unknown to thee;
> All Chance, Direction, which thou canst not see;
> All Discord, Harmony, not understood;
> All partial Evil, universal Good:
> And, spite of Pride, in erring Reason's spite,
> One truth is clear, 'Whatever is, is right.'

Chapter 25

Past and Future

Then Prometheus in his perplexity as to
what preservation he could devise for man,
stole from Hephaestus and Athena wisdom
in the arts together with fire—since by
no means without fire could it be acquired
or helpfully used by any—and he handed
it there and then as a gift to man.

—Plato *Protagoras* 321 d-e

$\mathbf{W}$hoever first administered drugs simply had to recognize the connection between the plant or potion and the cure. The event happened so long ago that the individuals might not have had names, but one hopes that in some way they were honored for stealing fire, the fire of mind by which they understood the connection. It was purely empirical observation, but no less important for that reason, and even today many of the mechanisms by which a drug acts remain unknown, although the drugs are given anyway. It is, one supposes, part of our pragmatic way of dealing with much of life: if it works, it is kept, until something better is found. Perhaps at some future time, the reasons why the drug works will be forthcoming.

Like most sciences, pharmacology has had a long time to tread the road from magic to theoretical and experimental analysis. But, pharmacology had to wait for the ground to be cleared in biology, in physics, and above all, in chemistry. The first chair in pharmacology, in a medical school, was only established some seventy-five years ago. Pharmacologists need not wait for other basic sciences to prepare the way any more, and every year are making important contributions that have far-reaching implications in other fields.

Lore and Logic

Asclepius, the Greek god of medicine, is supposed to have brought "golden health" to all who sought his services. It is said that he even raised a man from the dead with the help of the soothing potions of Chiron the centaur. Needless to say, such accomplishments have never been matched in the mundane realms of nonfiction. Practical medical research has never produced life-restoring drugs and many illnesses remain unsolved mysteries. Still, myths are made by men and the story of Asclepius underlines

425

two important constants in man's social behavior. First, the noble art of healing is as old and universal as human suffering; and, second, man has always dreamed of the day when the fruits of this art would make the fact of his suffering unnecessary. In the myth, Zeus slew Aesculapius for thinking thoughts too great for man. Are we placing ourselves in the same predicament?

Even the most primitive cultures studied the interaction of chemical agents and living materials, in their struggles against sickness and injury. In this manner, a considerable drug lore accumulated in almost every social structure known to modern man. Medical knowledge became so extensive in some instances that elaborate codifications were made. Much of our own information of early Egypt stems from those remarkable medical papyri surviving from around 2000 B.C. One such document—the Ebers papyrus—contains some 900 prescriptions of various kinds of crude animal, plant, and mineral materials for the relief of different diseases and injuries. These prescriptions include plant purgatives and natural products for everything from expelling worms to covering unsightly sores. Many are carefully measured, indicating a recognition of dose-effect relationships.

Elaborate compilations of a similar sort were made in Ancient India, China, and Latin America. A surprising number of the plant remedies listed still figure prominently in modern times. Long before Europeans came to the new world, the Indians were familiar with the use of leaves of wintergreen for rheumatism. Wintergreen contains methyl salicylate and is currently well established as an antipyretic—capable of reducing fever—and as an analgesic, particularly for application to the skin. North American Indians also discovered the purgative action of cascara bark. The drug's true value was not recognized by modern medicine until the latter half of the 19th century when it was finally introduced as a standard preparation. On the other side of the globe, the ancient Egyptians had already recommended moldy bread for application to skin abrasions, even though penicillin was not technically derived from mold for another few millennia.

Expertise in certain areas was far more general. People everywhere in the world soon learned that fruit juices and grain mashes tend to change their characteristic effects when exposed to warmth and sunlight. The fermented remains produce alcohol—the oldest and most universal medication known to man. Elaborate techniques in the brewing of beers are at least 6000 years old and wine-making was commonplace throughout the Mediterranean area in the Early Stone Age. Our purpose here is to trace the development of such early medical remedies and to mark the evolution of drugs from an ancient subject wrapped in superstition into the modern science of pharmacology.

Pharmacology, today, is the study of the interaction of chemicals with living material, whether the action is good or bad, and whether the living material is plant or animal. If the action is harmful to living material, the inquiry becomes toxicology and the action of the chemical is said to be toxic. The field in general is closely related to all aspects of physiology, pathology, microbiology, biochemistry, and even such matters as psychology and sociology. This is true because "living material" involves everything from macromolecules to ecological milieus, forcing the pharmacologist to cope with a variety of different frameworks. Individuals and societies as well as cells and organ systems are within his proper scope. Moreover, pharmacology, as such, may concentrate on any one of a number of factors in the management of disease. One analysis may concentrate on diagnosis; another may deal with prevention, cure, treatment, or simply the relief from unpleasant symptoms.

Within each category, pharmacologists face a whole host of problems that distinguish their field from other scientific disciplines. Some of the more important difficulties are: 1. dose-effect relations; 2. localization of the site of biological activity of chemicals; 3. factors involved in the absorption, metabolism, and fate of chemicals introduced into living material; 4. mechanisms of chemical action with biological material; and 5. the relation between chemical structure and biological activity.

Clearly, a pharmacologist's talents must be many and varied if he is to deal competently with all of these factors. Mathematics and especially statistics are always necessary for a controlled investigation of the probabilities involved. More often than not, a physician's personal judgment is also required. Any one of a number of variables—such as the age, sex, allergic state, or pathological condition of a patient—can greatly modify the intensity of drug action. Finally, a pharmacologist must have a detailed knowledge of the physicochemical properties of any drug he handles. There is no other way to understand a chemical's pattern of absorption, distribution, action, and removal. Awareness of solubilities, reaction potential, and spatial configurations are especially important in this context.

Chemists synthesize thousands of new chemical compounds each year on the basis of such knowledge and techniques. The scores of useful discoveries that eventually emerge from the laboratories may affect anything from agricultural procedures and chemical warfare to contraception and pest control.

More than time and knowledge separates this complicated and often tangled web of twentieth century study from the drug lore of antiquity. The crucial difference is one of attitude and approach. The drug collection of the Roman naturalist Pliny, in the first century A.D., contains a vast series of remedies built supposedly on the author's own experiences. But the collection itself is based on no theory. It is supported by no doctrine; and there is no meaningful experimentation. Verifiability—the crucial feature that distinguishes science from empirical observation—is totally lacking. Indeed, the characteristic methodology that we call science does not *begin* to appear until the Renaissance, and Lavoisier in the late 18th century is history's first real chemist. Not until he introduced the concepts of chemical combination by means of precision measurements do we find any genuine analysis of drugs and medicines.

Before the 16th century there is no inclination to even separate the studies of chemistry and medicine from philosophy, theology, and learning in general. Hence, we find Quintus Serenus Sammonicus, a Latin physician of the third century, suggesting that certain forms of malaria might be cured by placing the fourth book of Homer's *Iliad* under the sufferer's head. In this light, should we be surprised that the same Greeks who listened to Aristotle and Plato also believed in the doctrine that connected the "medical practice" of bleeding with tides and the moon?

The history of pharmacology abounds with civilizations that saw ecclesiastical overtones in illness and suffering. Under primitive conditions and in early cultures, the causes of disease were mysterious and feared. Superstitious appeals to beneficent deities and appeasement of malevolent powers were the rule and not the exception. Our own vocabulary has not escaped this influence. The word "blister" derives from a Teutonic variation meaning breath or spirit and the very term pharmacology comes from a Greek reference to something "evil" that should be "expelled."

Many cultures, including the Babylonian-Assyrian and the early Christian, subscribed to the theory that disease was due to the entry of a demon into the patient's body. Prescriptions for exorcism were prevalent in these societies. Nauseous drugs were also popular, presumably because their administration made the patient so sick that his possessing demon would pack up and leave in disgust, seeking healthier surroundings.

The New Testament is literally saturated with examples of demonic medicine. In the Gospel of Luke, Jesus rebukes the fever in Simon Peter's mother-in-law, and the illness of Mary Magdalene is in the form of seven evil spirits. In all four gospels, Christ encounters devils of blindness, dumbness, madness, and epilepsy. Again, it is Luke, the first century physician, who tells us of the miracle where Jesus casts "legions" of demons out of a single sufferer into a large herd of swine feeding on a convenient hillside.

Significantly, those whom Jesus and the earlier Jewish prophets heal are "oppressed by the Devil." Who would believe that Job's boils might result from lack of the right food? Disease, accordingly, is usually the work of demons guided by a conscious malevolent force. Unfortunately, it is but a short step from this theory to the moral belief of the Middle Ages that illness generally falls upon the sinful. The monkish medicine of the Dark Ages placed a stigma on the diseased that has not been completely erased to this day. Vague notions of shame and sin still obscure the true nature of certain infirmities in our own age. Too often we fail to realize that mental illness, drug addiction, and alcoholism are diseases requiring treatment, not moral weaknesses to be condemned.

Much of the superstition surrounding drugs in the Middle Ages and early Renaissance can be traced to the same failure to distinguish between scientific, ethical, theological, and philosophical norms that limited the studies of the ancients and early Christendom. Concepts of illness and nature, physical experience and the moral world, were completely interdependent in the medieval mind.

To illustrate, a preparation of sarsaparilla, smilax, and sassafras was widely regarded as a treatment for syphilis in 17th-century Europe simply because it had been introduced from the New World. The remedy was based on the dubious principle that when God has created a disease, He has also created the means for treating it. Since syphilis was presumed to come from the New World, physicians frequently limited their search for cures to the same geographical area. In the belief of the times, there was also a close relation between the external and internal world, the macrocosm and the microcosm. Medical astrologers drew parallels between the four "humours" of the body (blood, phlegm, choler, and melancholy) and the solstices and equinoxes.

In many cases, a medieval physician's diagnosis amounted to little more than a elaborate numerical formula that assigned the patient's fate, regardless of treatment. The day of the moon on which the patient fell sick and the numerical value given his name by astrological tables were far more crucial factors than the crude drugs used to eliminate symptoms of disease. Beginning in the early 18th century, we find a genuine disposition to base medical opinion upon observation and a corresponding willingness to categorize different fields of study. And not until the early 19th century do these scientific methods finally lead to important developments in the field of pharmacology. By that time it had become possible to obtain pure compounds of unvarying physical-chemical properties. Some could even be synthesized in the laboratory.

Modern Pharmacology

F. W. Serturner is credited for first isolating a chemically-pure active agent from a crude drug. This discovery, made in 1803, stimulated the development of an entirely new scientific approach to pharmacology. Chemicals of constant physical properties became available for the first time. Dosage could now be measured accurately in terms of mass of chemical per mass of living tissue, and the concept of a quantitative relationship between drug dosage and biological effect could be developed. Francois Magendie, the great Parisian teacher, quickly built upon this initial success. He and his students isolated such chemicals as strychnine from the *nux vomica* bean, quinine from cinchona bark, and emetine from ipecacuanha. By 1821, he was able to publish a medical formulary that included only pure chemical compounds, for use in the treatment of disease.

These same methods of analysis and subsequent critical study were followed with respect to all sorts of crude drugs. At first, most of the new drugs prepared in this way were alkaloids. Later, steroids were isolated from many natural products and then attempts were made to improve on these natural products. More recently, various vitamins in chemically-pure form were obtained and most of the active principles in hormones were also isolated and identified. The intricate complexity of initial preparations of enzymes, coenzymes, and even viruses and genes are currently yielding to similar techniques. This probably will go on to include vaccines and other immunological preparations.

There are two factors that can cloud a modern physician's judgment regarding drugs and that lie at the basis of all quackery. They were known and recognized as long ago as 500 B.C. by the Hippocratic School of Cos. The first is the realization that people tend to get well regardless of what may be done for them. The Romans called it "the healing power of nature" (*vix medicatrix naturae*). The second is the common fallacy of confusing sequence of events with the principle of cause and effect. The mere fact that the patient gets well after a doctor has administered his drug is no reason for believing that the drug has really helped the patient. The patient might well have recovered anyway. This fallacy is embodied in the Latin phrase, *post hoc ergo propter hoc,* "after this and therefore on account of it."

Moreover, we have learned that the attitude of physicians toward their patients may profoundly influence the effect of the drugs they use. Patients tend to get well with hope and gentle treatment, regardless of the drugs administered to them. The "double-blind technique" is designed to eliminate all of these variables, by screening out unpredictable personal aspects.

Many of the rudimentary aspects of contemporary pharmacology were not seriously considered until our own century. This is especially true of dose-effect relationships. It is remarkable that it took so long for a firm scientific basis to be provided for such an ancient concept. Nineteenth-century physicians, like the ancient

Egyptians 4000 years before them, gave drugs on the general basis of an average dose for the average effect desired in an average person. This involves three intangible abstractions making the whole concept of dosage meaningless from a scientific point of view.

J. W. Trevan, an English mathematician, made the first real advances in this area in 1927. He was a consultant for Burroughs-Wellcome in London and had much to do with the establishment of sound standardization methods for biological assay. His quantitation of the dose-effect relationship was improved upon by A. J. Clark at the University of Edinburgh. Clark expanded the problem to include the consideration of time-concentration relationships. Frequently, such relationships are the fundamental factors in examining the relative merits of similar chemical agents that may be recommended for the same purpose. Modern pharmaceutical industry is providing hundreds of closely related chemicals annually. It is important that physicians and pharmacologists understand what is involved in getting as wide a spread as possible between the dose that will produce the effect desired and the dose which may cause some unwanted or lethal effect.

Notable advances have been made in precision measurement of dose-effect relationships even in the last decade. This aids in many aspects of the study of the action of chemicals on living material. Interaction can now be studied at a micro level, with the use of individual cells or in tissue culture. Precision measurements have also been instrumental in aiding recent studies of chemicals on macromolecules which constitute the anatomical architecture of cells. The most exciting problems here revolve about the action of chemicals on genes and viruses. We are just beginning to understand that the ribonucleic acid complexes, which constitute the basis for genes and viruses, may be altered by chemical activity or by radiant energy. This is how mutations occur.

Genes and viruses are macromolecules, consisting of single or paired molecules of deoxyribonucleic acid, coated with protein complexes. When the protein is stripped off, the macromolecules remaining may be acted upon by molecules of other chemicals. This is a matter that is becoming extremely important in chemical efforts to control overgrowth and cancer.

The history of other aspects of pharmacology also illustrates how young the science is. The Frenchman Magendie died only 110 years ago and he was one of the first pioneers in experimental pharmacology. He was the first to explore the vast area encompassing the localization of the site of action of chemicals in living material. He organized studies into the mechanisms of absorption and distribution of chemicals in the human body and initiated the analysis of ways to remove chemicals from the body. Magendie's Parisian laboratory also cleared the way for the study of the mechanisms of drug action. Until the beginning of the 20th century, almost every pharmacologist of importance had been his pupil. In the mid third of the 19th century many alert American physicians made that pilgrimage to Paris without complaint. They rarely returned without important ideas and new principles which were reflected in greatly improved medical practice.

This state of affairs does more than demonstrate the size of the debt modern medicine owes to Magendie. It also shows that knowledge of drugs was so scarce and limited until the 20th century that a single man could master and dominate the entire field. Such a feat would be an impossibility today. Pharmacology is the most rapidly expanding scientific discipline associated with the health professions. During 1959 alone, some 57 new chemical compounds were introduced as useful drugs, not to mention several hundred new combinations of drugs recommended for related fields. Not surprisingly, single discoveries are often found to be of use in totally unconnected areas. Recent variations of nitrogen mustard gases, for example, could be horribly effective if used in chemical warfare. They are odorless, colorless, and undetectable until the desired symptoms begin to develop. On the other hand, these same gases appear to be helpful in the treatment of leukemia. They may well lead to a whole series of useful drugs in this area of medicine.

Certain pharmacological discoveries are also leading to new fields of study. Recent experimentation with brain activity has literally created the new field of neuro- and psychopharmacology. Other breakthroughs have changed the entire make-up of older established fields of study. New chemicals in functional tests have added to the area of diagnosis. Antiseptics and vitamins have improved disease prevention. Chemotherapy with antibiotics has brought whole new strata of sophistication to the "cure" of previously fatal illnesses.

Pharmacological trends of cultural interest include an increasing understanding of mechanisms and effects of the interactions of drugs and living material from the basic molecular level of biological organization, through cells, tissues, organs, individuals, and societies, to ecological milieus. For example, on the molecular level, more appreciation of the significance of the factors that determine the intensity of action of any drug should lead to more precise quantifications. On the other hand, a better coordination of knowledge on drug modification of biological activity could lead to a suppression of viruses, or other diseases that plague large-scale populations.

We should expect more and more technical achievements in pharmacology. Since drugs are becoming more and more specific, the burden of diagnosis will be all the greater on the physician. It will become immediately obvious whether a given drug is effective against the diagnosed condition. Allergic preventives, effective antiallergens, currently in the laboratories, will be of immense relief to those, say, who suffer hay fever intensely from May to September. Also under development are potent and nontoxic inhibitors of immune reactions, and agents that may enhance immunity and promote tissue regeneration. Drugs will probably play a great role in 'transplant' operations.

Nontoxic compounds for pest control have been in use for a long time. Recently, their abuse stirred a controversy. Newer and more specific insecticides should make man's control over nature more rational and selective. Chemicals used in food production and preservation are already on the market. Drugs that can act against poisonings—food or other types—are becoming more and more refined.

There is no real limit to pharmacology's growing impact. Advances in knowledge, particularly in the area of fertility control, are likely to change the entire foundation of human societies. Several steroid compounds have now been devised which can control ovulation in women and we are on the verge of discovering other compounds which can control spermatogenesis in men. The former drugs will be used for the purpose of promoting satisfactory ovulation and for the purpose of suppressing it entirely. Many other drugs have created an alarming population explosion by virtually eliminating many of the diseases that have dogged civilizations for centuries.

Eventually fertility control through drugs will be necessary to restore the balance. Clearly, pharmacological discoveries are often mixed blessings and can create new problems to replace the old.

Overpopulation is not the only problem that has resulted from the rash of miracle drugs discovered in the last century. Measures must be taken to allow for the ever-increasing number of old people in our society who are unprepared psychologically, economically, or socially to take care of themselves. Chemicals and drugs may help in providing comfort, relaxation, and some degree of physical contentment even into advanced old age. But medical wonders alone will do little to solve the subsequent economic and social problems of those whose lives have been prolonged by the advance of science.

Increased pharmacological knowledge brings increased responsibility. Already we are learning more and more about the highly-complex chemical integration within certain cells of the brain. Activity here is apparently closely linked to such basic drives as self-preservation and sexual gratification. Altered activity of the cells in question is dependent upon the metabolic change by a considerable complex of many types of chemical agents within them. Even now, we have discovered agents such as the tranquilizer reserpine— from the snakeroot of ancient India—and LSD, which profoundly affect behavior, presumably because they disturb the normal metabolic balance in certain brain cells.

How soon will it be before our knowledge allows far greater control over our own actions and thoughts? How far should we go, given the knowledge? What inevitable problems will come with pharmacological success? These are questions that elude the scientist's slide rule. Answers, if any, lie within the realm of philosophy, ethics, and esthetics. The complexities involved become all the more difficult and dangerous when we realize that they will only arise in the face of unmitigated success.

INDEX

Antimetabolites, 23, 278, 285, 420
5-fluorouracil, 278
6-mercaptopurine, 278
methotexate, 278
Antineoplastic agents, 416
nitrogen mustards, 416
Antipyretic, 426
Antirickets vitamin (D), 50
Antiscorbutic (scurvy-preventing)
factor, 39
Antisympathetic drugs, 124
see sympathetic blocking drugs
Aorta, 60, 87
Aplasia, 248
Aplastic anemia, 422
Aqueous humor, 126
Aqueous penicillin G, 240
Aramine (metaraminol), 124
Aristotle, 4, 14
Arrhythmia, 86, 181, 182
Arterial acidity, 185
Arteries,
coronary, 60, 62
pulmonary, 87
Arteriosclerosis, 60
Asclepius, 425
Ascorbic acid, 40, 42
Aspirin, 208
Ataxia, 186
Atherosclerosis, 60, 62, 67, 68, 69,
71, 72, 73, 74, 76, 79
Atopy, 369
asthma, 369
hives, 369
other rashes, 369
running nose, 369
Atrium,
left, 87, 88, 89
right, 86, 87, 88
Atropa belladonna, 121, 122, 128
Atrophy of the gonads, 320
Atropine, 121, 122, 123, 127, 128,
129, 133, 371
Atropos, 121
Aureomycin (chlortetracycline), 245,
246, 253
Auricles, 86, 90
Auricular fibrillation, 90
Auto-immune diseases, 301, 342
auto-immune thyroiditis, 301

Auto-immune diseases, encephalitis,
301
lupus erythematosus, 301
rheumatoid arthritis, 301
Autonomic nervous system (ANS),
105, 112, 202, 211
parasympathetic, 106, 113, 317
sympathetic, 106, 113, 317
Autonomous cells, 261
Autosomes, 397
6-Azauracil, 297
6-Azauridine, 285, 298, 299

Bacillus anthracis, 238
Bacillus brevis, 227
Bacitracin, 249
Bacteria, 227, 229, 235, 236
Gram-negative, 229, 238
Gram-positive, 229, 238, 239
Bacterial resistance, 236, 253
Bacteriophages, 236
Barbiturates, 28, 167, 175, 180, 182,
186, 188, 204, 216, 222, 369,
370, 372, 382
amytal, 167
thiopental, 180
Basal body temperature, 11
Basal metabolic rate (BMR), 333
Basophil cells, 333
Belladonna, 121
Benactyzine, 182
"Bennies" (Benzedrine), 218
Benzedrine (amphetamine), 218
Benzene ring, 141
Benzylpenicillin, 239
Beriberi, 37, 38, 43, 45
dry, 45
wet, 45
Beta blocking drugs, 125, 135
propranolol, 126, 135
Beta-cell exhaustion, 356
Beta rays, 267
Beta receptors, 111, 125, 131, 132,
133, 135
Betel leaf, 3
Bethanecol (Urecholine), 120
Bhang, 214

Laveran, Charles, 394
Lavoisier, 428
LD₁, 378
LD₅₀ (lethal dose 50), 378
Leake, Chauncey D., 302
Leucocytes (white cells), 267
Leukemia, 267, 415, 416, 419, 433
  acute, 278, 279
  blood cells, 419
  chronic granulocytic, 278
  chronic lymphocytic, 278
Levanil (ectylurea), 182
Libido, 321
Librium (chlordiazepoxide), 191
Lidocaine (Xylocaine), 141, 144, 146
Lincomycin, 250
Lind, James, 40
Lingual nerves, 144
Liniments, 381
  camphor, 382
  soap, 382
Link, Karl P., 78
Lipoproteins, 68, 69, 71
  high-density, 68
  low-density, 68, 69
  β-lipoprotein cholesterol, 74
Lipoprotein lipase, 75
Lipoprotein measurements, 68
Listeria, 238
Lithium ion, 177
Load test, ascorbic acid deficiency, 42
  thiamine deficiency, 44
Local analgesics, 140–143, 146
  cocaine, 139, 140, 141, 387
  chloroprocaine (Nesacaine), 141
  dibucaine (Nupercaine), 141, 147
  lidocaine (Xylocaine), 141, 144, 146
  procaine (Novocain), 141, 145, 147
  tetracaine (Pontocaine), 141, 147
Local anesthetics, 140, 143, 144, 147, 219
  cocaine, 219
  lidocaine (Xylocaine), 142, 144
  mepivacaine (Carbocaine), 144
  procaine (Novocain), 145, 147, 219

LSD (lysergic acid diethylamide), 191, 192, 193, 194, 195, 196, 197, 207, 222, 387, 435
Lumbar region, 106, 113, 146
Lumbar vertebrae, 147
Lumen, 233
Lung cancer, 262
Lupus erythematosua, 301
Lymphatic systems, 259
Lymph nodes, 265
  swelling, 369
Lymphocyte, 231
Lymphocytic leukemia (chronic), 278
Lymphosarcomas, 278
Lysergic acid diethylamide (LSD), 195, 207

Macrocosm, 430
Macrolides, 248
  erythromycin, 248
  oleandomycin, 248
Macromolecules, 432
Macropsia, 194
Magendie, François, 430, 433
Magnesium pemoline, 303
Malaria, 394–396
Male sex hormones (androgens), 347, 353
Malthus, Thomas Robert (1766–1834), 5
Mammary carcinoma, 340
Mandibular nerve, 144
Mandragora, 168
MAO inhibitors, 112, 165, 173–176
  iproniazid, 174
  isocarboxazid, 174, 175
  nialamide, 174, 175
  pargyline, 175
  phenelzine, 174, 175
  tranylcypromine, 174, 175
Margolin (methylparafynol), 182
Marijuana, 191, 204, 214
Marplan (isocarboxazid), 175
Master gland, 309, 320
Mautner, Henry G., 301
Maxillary nerve, 144
Mecamylamine, 123, 130

452 INDEX